THE HEALTHY JEW

The Healthy Jew traces the culturally revealing story of how Moses, the rabbis, and other Jewish thinkers came to be understood as medical authorities in the nineteenth and twentieth centuries. Such a radically different interpretation, by scholars and popular writers alike, resulted in new, widespread views on the salubrious effects of, for example, circumcision, Jewish sexual purity laws, and kosher foods. *The Healthy Jew* explores this interpretative tradition in the light of a number of broader debates over "civilization" and "culture," Orientalism, religion and science (in the wake of Darwin), anti-Semitism and Jewish apologetics, and the scientific and medical discoveries and debates that revolutionized the fields of bacteriology, preventive medicine, and genetics/eugenics.

Mitchell B. Hart is Associate Professor of History at the University of Florida. His first book, *Social Science and the Politics of Modern Jewish Identity* (2000), won the Salo Baron Award for Best First Book in Jewish Studies, presented by the American Academy of Jewish Research.

The Healthy Jew

THE SYMBIOSIS OF JUDAISM AND MODERN MEDICINE

Mitchell B. Hart

University of Florida

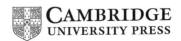

CAMBRIDGE
UNIVERSITY PRESS

CAMBRIDGE UNIVERSITY PRESS
Cambridge, New York, Melbourne, Madrid, Cape Town, Singapore, São Paulo, Delhi

Cambridge University Press
32 Avenue of the Americas, New York, NY 10013-2473, USA

www.cambridge.org
Information on this title: www.cambridge.org/9780521877183

First published 2007

Printed in the United States of America

A catalog record for this publication is available from the British Library.

Library of Congress Cataloging in Publication Data

Hart, Mitchell Bryan, 1959–
The Healthy Jew : the symbiosis of Judaism and modern medicine / Mitchell B. Hart.
    p.   cm.
Includes bibliographical references and index.
ISBN-13: 978-0-521-87718-3 (hardback)
 1. Medicine – Religious aspects – Judaism.   2. Health – Religious aspects – Judaism.
 3. Jews – Health and hygiene – History.   4. Medicine – History.   5. Medicine in the
Bible.   6. Jews – Dietary laws.   7. Tuberculosis – Treatment.   8. Medicine – Religious
aspects – Christianity.   I. Title.
BM538.H43H37   2007
296.3′76–dc22   2006102788

ISBN   978-0-521-87718-3 hardback

To Nina

Do not suppose that the sufficiency of the Chaldaic magic derived from the Kabbalah of the Jews; for the Jews are without doubt the excrement of Egypt, and no one could ever pretend with any degree of probability that the Egyptians borrowed any principle, good or bad, from the Hebrews. Whence we Greeks [by which he seems to mean Gentiles] own Egypt, the grand monarchy of letters and nobility, to be the parent of our fables, metaphors and doctrines.

Giordano Bruno, *Dialeghi italiani*[1]

Moses . . . was a product of Egyptian civilization, and he offers us a sense or reflection of the sanitary system established among Pharaoh's people by the priests of Isis and Osiris.

E. Bertin-Sans, in *Dictionnaire encyclopédie des sciences médicales*[2]

The Hebrew physician feels it in his bones, has an acute intuition that it [Hebrew medicine] is the foundation of medical knowledge.

Dr. Yosef Tennovim, in *Ha-Rophe ha-Ivri*[3]

[1] Giordano Bruno, *Dialeghi italiani*, cited and translated in Martin Bernal, *Black Athena: The Afroasiatic Roots of Classical Civilization*, vol. 1 (New Brunswick, N.J.: Rutgers University Press, 1987), 159.

[2] "Moïse . . . issu de la civilisation égyptienne, nous offre comme un reflet de l'organisation sanitaire établie chez les peuples des Pharaons par les prêtres d'Isis et d'Osiris." E. Bertin-Sans, "Hygiene," in *Dictionnaire encyclopédie des sciences médicales* (Paris, 1888).

[3] Yosef Tennovim, review of A. Goldenstein, *Torat ha-Hygienia* in *Ha-Rophe ha-Ivri* 1 (1927): 58–60. All translations in this book are my own unless otherwise indicated.

Contents

Preface and Acknowledgments

This book began when I was researching my dissertation in the early 1990s. I came across a work on the history of social medicine in the ancient world by Alfred Nossig, a Polish Jewish intellectual who played a key role in founding the Jewish statistical movement in Berlin in the first years of the twentieth century. Nossig's book was fascinating, in large part because it contained ideas and arguments about Judaism and the Jews that were very different from anything I'd encountered before. I set aside the dissertation research for a while, worked through Nossig, and wrote an article on it. I imagined that I could then integrate that research into my dissertation; that, however, did not happen. Yet, having encountered Nossig's work, and then having examined some of the literature that he relied on, I was aware that there existed an entire counter-tradition in Europe that represented Jews and Judaism as vital and healthy, and that linked Jewry in numerous ways to civilization and progress rather than to barbarism and decline (the focus of my first book). *The Healthy Jew* grew out of this extended fascination with Nossig's book and the larger interpretive tradition he'd built upon.

Any book that takes a decade and a half to research and write owes its existence to a large number of people who make the research and writing possible. It's a great pleasure for me to thank those individuals and institutions for their assistance and support. First of all, my gratitude to Alexander Grass, whose generosity and interest in Jewish studies have made it possible for me to focus on research and devote time to writing. Thanks as well to my colleagues in the Department of History and the Center for Jewish Studies at the University of Florida for the vibrant intellectual and social environment. My thanks especially to Robert Singerman, recently retired as Judaica bibliographer at the University of Florida, who was extremely generous with his time and knowledge. I thank him for his invaluable help. My enormous gratitude as well to the research librarians in the Jewish Division of the New York Public Library, and especially Eleanor Yadin for her knowledge and humor. Thank you as well to Andy Beck at Cambridge University Press for shepherding the book through, and to Sally Nicholls for her editorial expertise. I would also like to acknowledge and thank Indiana University Press for allowing me to reprint an expanded version of "Moses the Microbiologist."

Gil Anidjar, Peter Eli Gordon, David Rechter, Alan Steinweis, and Steve Zipperstein all read the manuscript and offered helpful comments and criticisms. I'm deeply grateful for their input, and even more so for their friendship.

Thanks as well to other friends and colleagues who have made the past few years in Gainesville and New York so pleasurable (or at least tolerable). A special thanks to Taal and Todd Hasak-Lowy for all the time I've spent in the chair, and especially for Monday nights; to Tony Michels for the many discussions about Jewish history and culture; and to Kyle Todd for the time in New York and Massachusetts, and the continuing conversation.

Finally, to Nina Caputo, who for two decades has done her very best with a rather unhealthy Jew. There is nothing I could possibly write here that could convey my appreciation.

THE HEALTHY JEW

"Links in a Long Chain"

Jews, Judaism, Health, and Hygiene

In December 1883, James E. Reeves, the Secretary of the State Board of Health of West Virginia, delivered a speech to the annual meeting of the American Public Health Association. The speech was later printed in the *Journal of the American Medical Association* (*JAMA*), the nation's most prestigious medical journal. Reeves spoke about the "usefulness of state boards of health in guarding the public welfare" and the intimate link between laws of health, the fitness of the individual citizen, and the "prosperity, freedom, and glory of the State." He began by noting that

> the principles of sanitary science are not of modern origin. Indeed, they are as old as the Mosaic code, and their unerring rewards and penalties have marked the life-history of all the nations that have covered the earth. In their scope, they are wide enough to embrace all humanity, and just as applicable to communities of to-day as they were to the Jewish race thousands of years ago.[1]

Forty-five years later, in the Hebrew language journal *The Hebrew Physician* (*Ha-Ropheh ha-Ivri*), Dr. Yosef Tennovim gave voice to the same basic idea, though more forcefully and with greater specificity: "Almost all contemporary medical issues or questions found expression already in ancient Hebrew medicine. Concerning the modern understanding of the circulation of the blood, there are already hints of this understanding in the Talmud, testifying to a specific professional erudition [*b'kiyut*] long before [William] Harvey...." For almost all the modern insights into psychology and medicine, including hygiene, "one can find support, a trace, evidence in our ancient medical writings."[2]

Both Reeves and Tennovim were participating in and contributing to a particular interpretive tradition about Moses, medicine, and the history of Judaism and the Jews. *The Healthy Jew* explores this interpretive tradition.[3] In continental Europe, Great Britain, and the United States of America, physicians, medical researchers, and popular writers rendered Moses and the rabbis of the Talmud as medical authorities, equal or superior in their knowledge to both ancient and modern scientific figures. Jewish law and ritual, in turn, were translated into codes of health and hygiene, and presented as equal or superior to ancient and especially to modern systems of medical knowledge. Thus, Moses was the ancient equivalent of Joseph Lister, Louis Pasteur, and Robert Koch. The Jewish dietary laws, sexual hygiene laws, the practice of circumcision, and the myriad rules dealing with purity and impurity found in the Hebrew Bible and the Talmud were ultimately not religious but medical in nature. And this abiding concern with purity and health had its effects, largely positive, on the Jews themselves, ensuring their survival and vitality. This interpretive tradition found expression in texts produced in German, French, Italian, English, and Hebrew (at the least),[4] which appeared in mainstream medical journals, academic monographs, newspapers, and popular magazines and journals, both general and Jewish. This book explores these texts in the light of a number of broader trends in the nineteenth and twentieth centuries, debates over civilization and culture, orientalism, religion and science (in the wake of Darwin), anti-Semitism and Jewish apologetics, and the scientific and medical discoveries and debates that revolutionized the fields of bacteriology, preventive medicine, and genetics/eugenics.

The role played by physicians, anthropologists, and racial hygienists in the identification of the Jews with disease has occupied a prominent place in recent studies of modern Jewish history, the history of anti-Semitism, and Nazism. Such works have, furthermore, emphasized the fundamental importance of medicine and biology in preparing the ground for the Nazi extermination.[5] Moreover, as Sander Gilman and others have pointed out, many Jews themselves came to accept this image of the diseased Jewish body and soul, and set about seeking to reform or regenerate Jewry.[6] The large body of scholarship that explores the nexus of Jews, disease, the natural and social sciences, and the politics of "the Jewish body" is, of course, extremely important. But a substantial literature that linked Judaism and Jewry with health and hygiene was also produced in the nineteenth and twentieth centuries. This scientific and popular work was published throughout Europe and the United States, the labor of non-Jews as well as Jews. Thus, the "disease" or "health" of Jewry remained an open question, for both Jews and Christians (as did the even larger question about the very identity of "the Jews"), and a variety of opinions competed for intellectual hegemony in the decades prior to the 1930s (and, indeed, beyond).

Most of the recent scholarship on this question has been concerned with the "diseased Jewish body" as constructed by both Gentile and Jewish elites. My focus in this book is the flip-side, the medicalization of Jews and Judaism that rendered a hygienic Judaism and a healthy Jew. I don't question the medicalization of Jews and Judaism as an important development over the past two centuries, though we may be in danger of overemphasizing the extent of its import. Rather, my interest is in redressing what I see as an imbalance in the scholarship that has produced a one-sided notion of this medicalization. This study recovers the healthy Jew and the interpretive tradition that situated Judaism at the center or forefront of Western medicine and civilization.

JUDAISM AND HEALTH

The debate that began in the eighteenth century over the emancipation and integration of the Jews into the modern nation-state was infused with the language of medicine and science. The historical reconstruction of "the Jewish Question," as the debate over Jewish integration came to be called, tends to focus on the negative representation of Jews and Judaism. For even the most sympathetic advocates of Jewish legal and civic equality, individuals such as Christian Wilhelm von Dohm in Germany and the Abbé Grégoire in France, conceded that the Jews were degenerate and diseased – even if such terms were used as much in the moral as in the physical sense.[7] Judaism was inferior, the cause, together with Christian oppression and persecution, of the contemporary degeneracy of the Jews. Emancipation and integration would, so it was argued, free the Jews of the negative influences of both rabbinism and Christian oppression. The transcendence of both traditional religion and historical experience would produce a healthy Jew. This was a view held by Gentile advocates of Jewish emancipation and also by a significant proportion of Jewish elites who entered into these debates.

The interpretive tradition I analyze in this book is different in significant ways from the emancipatory discourse that emerged in the late eighteenth century around the question of Jewish civic rights and the place of the Jews in the newly emerging nation-state. The story of Moses and hygiene that grows in the nineteenth and twentieth centuries is, I argue, a repudiation, at least implicitly, of the idea that the Jews and Judaism are degenerate and that they require Europe to civilize *them*. As we shall see, the thrust of the discourse explored here is that the Jews were civilized thousands of years ago; *they* helped to civilize Europe; and they could be of assistance again if Christians would only follow the Jewish model of preventive medicine. While the anti-Semitic image of "the dirty Jew" is well known, it is not so well known that an alternative set of images circulated of a clean and healthy Jewry, living amidst the dirt and disease of European Christendom.

Moreover, the interpretive tradition of Moses and hygiene was a response to, and a transcendence of, the Enlightenment's thinking about Egypt and Israel, Europe and the Jews, "civilization" and Judaism. The Enlightenment repudiated what Jan Assmann has called the "Mosaic distinction," the notion that "Israel embodies truth, Egypt symbolizes darkness and error. Egypt loses its historical reality and is turned into an inverted image of Israel. Israel is the negation of Egypt, and Egypt stands for all that Israel has overcome." One of the central components of the Enlightenment's arsenal, Assmann argues, was the "deconstructive memory" that challenged this Mosaic distinction.[8]

If, as is well known, the primary target for Voltaire and others was the Church, Jews and Judaism were nonetheless objects of ridicule and hostility. But "the Enlightenment," of course, was hardly a monolithic movement, and the ideas and opinions generated by philosophers and publicists about Jewry were varied and complex. Enlightenment thinkers were profoundly ambivalent about Judaism and Jews.[9] Though Jewish history and religion could not be tolerated, a philosophy rooted in notions of universal tolerance could not articulate a principled intolerance of Jews. *Philosophes* used Judaism to articulate key ideas, but they could never either fully repudiate Jews and Judaism, or integrate them into their own visions of an ideal society. What is relevant here is the emergence within Enlightenment thought of an "originary" Judaism,[10] a Judaism believed to be equivalent to natural religion that had not been corrupted by priests and useless ceremonies. This originary Judaism was contrasted with papal Christianity, and also with rabbinic and contemporary Judaism. As Adam Sutcliffe has persuasively demonstrated, thinkers such as John Toland and Voltaire, among others, posited an ancient purified "Judaism" that was later negated by degenerate Jews and Judaism. Moses, in this view, was an Egyptian, and all true wisdom derived from Egypt and Chaldea. The purity laws and other barbaric superstitions (like circumcision) associated with Moses were in fact introduced by the cultic priests, and were the surest sign of Jewish degeneracy.[11] This held true as well for many *Maskilim* or Jewish enlighteners, who believed that Jewish religious rituals and customs were in large measure responsible for whatever physical and mental ills plagued their co-religionists. As John Efron has argued with regard to the eighteenth-century Jewish physician, "there existed a certain strain in *Haskalah* thinking that held that Jews had ceded control of their bodies to nothing less than Judaism itself."[12]

The narrative of "the healthy Jew" challenged this older Enlightenment view of Moses, Jewish ritual and law, and the status of the Jews. It repudiated the notion of an originary Judaism distant and distinct from the Mosaic laws and the later rabbinic tradition. In the texts I explore here, rabbinic and medieval Judaism are natural extensions of the healthy, positive laws and ceremonies that originate with Moses. If in the eighteenth century and beyond a chasm was posited by some between an idealized and purified Judaism that had existed before the priests and rabbis, and contemporary Jews and their institutions, others sought to close that gap in the nineteenth century. And that gap was closed, as we shall see, by Christians as well as by Jews. These physicians and medical writers did not seem to accept the Enlightenment (and *Maskilik*) rendering of Judaism and the Jews. Religion, in the guise of Jewish law, was not something that needed to be transcended if Jews – or Christians for that matter – were to be healthy, either individually or as a collective. Yet "religion" did require translation, a reinterpretion in terms of public hygiene and preventive medicine. Nor did the historical experience of the

Jews under Christian rule necessarily result in debility and degeneration: rendered through the prism of Darwinism, the historical experience of isolation and oppression, suffering, violence and death could be seen to act as a natural selection process, removing the weak and leaving a stronger, more vital Jewish people. What I hope to bring into stronger focus here is a discursive tradition that developed among Christians and Jews that shared important components of other discursive traditions (i.e., Enlightenment and *Maskilik*, anti-Semitic and anti-modern) but was nonetheless distinct and, in important ways, oppositional.

To be sure, texts dealing with Jews and health can be highly ambiguous as to the messages they convey. To take at the outset one of the major textual or narrative traditions explored in this book: when hundreds of writers celebrate Moses and his law code as the foundation of hygienic knowledge and practice, do they mean to suggest that Jews as a collective are indeed a healthy people? Or are they pointing up just the opposite, the degree to which Jews "today" (whenever that might be) have fallen away to a significant degree from their ancient health and purity? It is possible to find both of these judgments in the medical literature of the past two centuries. Yet overall, I argue that for most of those who participate in this interpretive tradition, Judaism and the Jews are indeed healthy. And since far more attention has been paid in the scholarly literature to the nexus of Jews and disease, this book will dwell almost completely on the alternative, positive image of the Jews and Judaism.

Anti-Semitic literature oftentimes represented modern Jewry as degenerate while allowing that ancient Hebrews, or even premodern Jews, were or at least could be healthy, as long as they followed their own laws and lived lives separate from their Christian neighbors. Degeneration of the Jewish body and soul occurred because of modernity, that is, emancipation and assimilation, and the freedoms from traditional observance that had characterized pre-emancipatory communal life. On the other hand, the equation, in anti-Jewish literature, of ancient and modern Jews was also quite common. In particular, racialized texts collapsed both time and space in the depiction of "Jews" as physically and spiritually distinct, and in one way or another inferior and corrupt.

However, this collapsing of time and space did not necessarily have to work to the disadvantage of Jews; that is, positive depictions of Jews and Judaism also relied on this technique. The healthy Hebrews of the past could also be the healthy Jews of the present. Both Jewish and Christian medical writers who participated in the interpretive tradition of the healthy Jew sought, in the first place, to demonstrate the positive effects of ancient Jewish law on the Jews themselves; moreover, and at some level more significantly, these authorities suggested that these laws remain valid and practical, and not only for the Jews. A number of writers believed that the world would be a healthier place if all governments instituted – and all citizens followed – at least some of the hygienic practices laid out by Moses; and these authors explicitly urged their governments to undertake appropriate measures.

Over the course of the nineteenth century, medicine and race coalesced around nationalism to produce a coherent anti-Semitic ideology that cast the Jew as essentially different from and dangerous to civilization and culture. The medical images utilized by modern anti-Semitic writers are familiar: parasites, germs, plague, cancer, pathology, abnormality. Judaism and Jews were often, though certainly not universally, represented as pathological and pathogenic, as diseased and as the cause of disease. The diseases of the Jew and the diseased Jew were racialized over the course of the nineteenth century; the pathology and abnormality of the Jew was heritable and immutable.

The effort to represent Judaism and Jewry as healthy, as linked in multiple ways to the history of western medicine and science, was one clear and forceful response to a medicalized and racialized anti-Semitism. And, without doubt, this anti-Semitism and the response to it reached their apogee in Central Europe. However, it was not the case that the only extensive or systematic engagement of Jewish thinkers and writers with the issues of race and medicine occurred in Central Europe, as a response to German-speaking anti-Semitism. If we link causally the emergence of a discourse on Jews and health, or Jews and disease, with the political struggles over emancipation or civic rights – and the anti-Semitism that accompanied this – then we are bound to focus on the German-speaking countries of Central Europe, for it was there, as is well known, that this struggle was most protracted and uneven, and ultimately fraught. However, such a focus on the political or emancipatory drama cannot explain why a medicalized discourse about the Jews also emerged in such countries as Great Britain and the United States, and to a lesser extent France, in which the 'path to emancipation' was either notably different

(Great Britain and France) or nonexistent (the United States). Rather than focusing on the narrower political struggle over emancipation, I would argue that we need to understand the medicalization of the Jews and Judaism as linked to multiple intellectual, political, and cultural forces, and ultimately as part of an ongoing ordeal of civilization and civility, to borrow John Murray Cuddihy's felicitous phrase.[13]

Thus, I draw on scholarly and popular work produced in Europe, Great Britain, and the United States. This book is in part an attempt to demonstrate just how international, or transnational, the tradition of the healthy Jew and hygienic Judaism was; there was a vigorous borrowing and exchange of ideas across national and linguistic boundaries. It was not only Jews who produced this literature, nor was it produced for an exclusively Jewish audience. Much of it certainly was intended for Jewish readers. Surely this was so for the abundant popular medical literature written in Yiddish and published in Poland and the United States (and, to a lesser extent, Great Britain). These books, pamphlets, and articles were meant to educate the Jewish masses about all manner of things related to health and hygiene. The texts produced by Jews and non-Jews in English, German, and French were written with a different audience in mind, and with a different purpose. The articles published in general journals such as the *Lancet*, *Journal of the American Medical Association* (*JAMA*), *Hygienische Rundschau*, and *Soziale Hygiene* were intended for a religiously and ethnically heterogeneous audience.[14] Once we go looking, we encounter in journals, books, and newspapers produced around the world a significant number of studies concerned with aspects of the Jewish body and mind, and infused with the same images, concepts and questions that impelled those in Central Europe. This engagement, moreover, was overdetermined. It was a result in part of anti-Semitism. But it also emerged because of dramatic developments in medicine and science, particularly in the realms of bacteriology and microbiology; intellectual and cultural tensions between the realms of religion and science; and the instability of the social status of doctors. The interpretive tradition of the healthy Jew was thus a product in part of anti-Semitism and apologia; but it also testifies to the truth that discourses emerge through an engagement with multiple forces, including the challenge of new discoveries and technologies, new ideas and methods, as well as developments in the political and social realms. In addition, the discursive tradition of Moses and hygiene was built upon and directly engaged with older intellectual traditions that only indirectly or tangentially had anything to do with contemporary Judaism and Jewry.

The medical narratives produced in the nineteenth and twentieth centuries were linked intellectually with earlier narratives, even if later authors did not explicitly mention these earlier works. All these texts constitute a particular delimited discourse because they are working over and coming to terms with a common set of themes, ideas, and images. They share a language, even if written in many different languages, and a set of questions. What is the ultimate nature and purpose of the Mosaic laws? What is the relationship between these laws and the nature and condition of the Jews? What was the relationship between Moses and Egypt, between the Jews, Judaism, and Western civilization: Greece, Rome, Europe, America?

EGYPTIANS, GREEKS, AND JEWS/ARABS, CHRISTIANS, AND JEWS

The texts I deal with here are in one way or another counter-narratives, challenges to the dominant history of medicine (and, by extension, the dominant history of "civilization" defined in philhellenic terms), a history that began with the Greeks (with a nod to the ancient Egyptians) and culminated in the research laboratories and universities of Europe, Britain, and North America. If or when the Jews appeared in the dominant narratives, it was first and foremost as middlemen, as transmitters or "carriers" of medical texts and knowledge from one major civilization, the Arab, to another, the European. This notion of the Jews as "carriers" or mediators of medical knowledge echoed or perhaps derived from a more general and widespread notion of the Jews as carriers of civilization in general, and carriers of capitalism more particularly.[15] As we shall see in Chapter 1, Jewish apologia appropriated and advanced this notion of the Jews as transmitters of Eastern wisdom and science to the West; yet, at the same time this apologetic narrative reconfigured the story, adding an interpretive component that made the Jews not merely the transmitters but also the originators of medical knowledge.

One of the themes that threads through this book is the discursive relationship between Jews and civilization, and the way in which narratives about Jews and medicine address the larger notion of what J. Hoberman has called the Jews' purported "imperfect adaptation to Western civilization."[16] It is most explicit in the sort of apologetic literature I examine in the first chapter, the sizable group of texts that celebrated the "Jewish contribution to civilization." But it constitutes a recurrent theme throughout the book.

While Egypt, ancient Israel, Greece, and Rome surely stand for themselves in these narratives, at some level they also serve as codes for other constructed or imagined entities. Greece, and to a lesser extent Rome, stand for the West as originators and bearers over the centuries of all that is defined as wise, healthy, civilized, cultured.[17] Central and Western Europe, and then the United States, are the natural inheritors and guarantors of this wisdom and civilization. What was at stake, even if only at the level of discourse and imagination, in being a people or group defined as civilized, of being credited with having contributed to the course of civilization and progress in the West (which, in the period we are discussing, was of course the only place that Civilization and Progress could and would occur)? Sven Lindqvist, in his work on colonialism and genocide, has argued that at the heart of the European relationship with non-European "primitive" peoples (what German writers called *Naturvölker*) was the notion that nature and history determined whether individual nations or peoples survived, or were enslaved, or exterminated.[18] It is hard to argue with him; the course of the twentieth century, including the fate of the Jews of Europe, bears this out.

What better way, then, to demonstrate the civilized and cultured status of the Jews than to make the Jews the saviors of this civilization, a salvation effected through the invention and transmission of the principles of health and hygiene. In this way, "civilization" for the Jews is an act of recovery; the Jews are not, like *Naturvölker*, in an original state of barbarity, deprived of civilization until they acquire it through contact with the civilized nations of Europe. Rather, the Jews are the very source of civilization. It is civilization itself that has, willfully or not, forgotten this.[19] And thus, the task of the texts on Judaism and hygiene was to remind an only recently civilized Europe and America that the Jews had been healthy and civilized since long ago, and that the West owed more to the Jews in this regard than mainstream scholarship seemed willing to acknowledge.

The contribution that Jews made to (Christian) civilization, and to science and medicine in particular, was often juxtaposed with the persecution and oppression inflicted upon Jews by that very civilization. It was an irony that some authors felt obliged to point out. Indeed, in much of the work about Jews and hygiene there is a deep underlying connection between persecution and health, oppression and vitality. We will see it, for example, in the discussion of the ghetto and social Darwinism (Chapter 4). This, again, constituted a counter-discourse to that produced by Enlightenment and *Haskalah* thinkers, who had insisted that persecution and oppression were the causes of Jewish disease and degeneracy.

Images of oppression also shaped the narratives constructed about the Jewish contribution to medicine and, by extension, to Western civilization as a whole. In the first place, it was the destruction of Jewish sovereignty and the Temple by the Romans, and the subsequent dispersion that placed Jews in the position of translators or mediators of knowledge between the ancient pagan world and that of medieval Christendom. But the fact of persecution also adds further glory and pathos to the narrative of Jewish contribution. The Jews survive despite all that has been done to them. More than this, they repay their persecutors by giving the gift of knowledge, by caring for the health of their kings, queens, princes, and popes; by translating ancient medical texts; and, in the modern period, by contributing to medical research and practice to a degree far beyond what might be expected from such a numerically insignificant minority group.[20]

The sense of an unjustified marginality or invisibility in the historical record, coupled with accusations of savagery and incivility were spurs to the production of texts that demonstrated the civilized status of Jews and Judaism. Yet, as I have already pointed out, such texts cannot or should not be reduced to this motivation. The image of a civilized Jewry and Judaism, rooted in a reinterpretation of religion as science, and the image of the Jews as both a religious and racial entity were not merely reactionary. To make such a reduction is to elide the degree to which Jews – not all Jews, but many more than is usually imagined or acknowledged – embraced a set of images and ideas about "Jews" and Judaism that, while unfamiliar and even bizarre to us, were normative for the period. Chief

among these was the notion that the Jews are a race, and that this racial
identity was not something imposed upon them by anti-Semitic opponents, but resided in very real physical and mental attributes. The relative
status of the health or disease of the Jews, therefore, constituted a significant component of the broader debate over the Jews as, simultaneously,
a religion and a race (for, as Gil Anidjar has argued, we must "recognize
that religion and race are contemporary, indeed, co-extensive and, moreover, co-concealing categories"), and as a civilized or barbaric people.[21]

In an important sense the formulation of "the healthy Jew" I explore in
this book is continuous with earlier interpretations of Jews and Judaism,
most notably the idea of an ancient Mosaic Republic, an idea that circulated widely in the seventeenth and eighteenth centuries, and the figure
of "the noble Jew" that became popular in the 1700s. The practice of
reading back into the Bible contemporary political and social ideals, such
as republicanism or monarchy, or an economy rooted in agricultural production, is evident in the works of Italian, Dutch, and English thinkers
by the seventeenth century at the latest. Debates about the ancient Jewish
polity concerned both the nature of good and workable government, and
the nature of the Jews; that is, the relationship between ancient Israelites
and contemporary Jews, and the grounds on which the latter could realis-
tically be expected to integrate into Christian society.[22] The "noble Jew"
was one element in a much broader discourse of orientalism and the
Jews that will also concern us here. The "noble Jew" allowed Christians
and Jews to forge a link with ancient Israelites and construct Jewishness
as "a patent of nobility."[23] This, in turn, allowed contemporary Jews,
as descendents of these ancient Israelites, to participate in this nobility (Lessing's Nathan, in the eighteenth-century tolerance-drama *Nathan
der Weise*, serves as a famous example). The "noble Jew," according to
Ivan Kalmar and Derek Penslar, "was part of a pro-Jewish movement
among the Gentiles, who wished to demonstrate the nobility of the Jewish
spiritual heritage. On the Jewish side, it was seized upon by a desire to
proclaim the Jews as a 'race' or 'nation' of great antiquity, ennobled by
its association with the Bible, but also more generally with the Orient
as the source of spiritual inspiration for the West."[24] The "healthy Jew"
was also a product of both the (Christian) Gentile and Jewish imaginations, and its proponents also sought to identify the Jews as a race or
nation whose origins reached back to antiquity and who continued to

be ennobled through association with the Bible (and, as will be discussed, post-biblical Jewish literature).

Thus, "the healthy Jew" has its precedents in ideas and images that circulated among Jewish and Christian thinkers in the period between the Renaissance and the nineteenth century. However, there are also certain discontinuities that I will identify, chief among them the turn from spirit to body, from religion to science and medicine – even if religion is of course still present as a powerful force – and the reintegration of Mosaic and rabbinic law into an organic whole. The discontinuities are significant enough, and developments over the course of the nineteenth century transformed the context enough that the image of "the healthy Jew" merits its own analysis.

One of the major discontinuities is the disruption of the normative orientalist narrative about the Jew, a disruption that is evident in texts produced by both Christians and Jews, and advanced through discussions of health and hygiene. The normative orientalist discourse is familiar enough, although until quite recently "the Jew" was less likely to be understood as one of its objects than was "the Arab" or "the Muslim." But, of course, Jews and Judaism were historically and racially linked with Arabs and Islam; this discursive link existed at every level, including the physical and the pathological.[25] Orientalism is not only about the Muslim, but also about the Jew in Europe and America – the Jew as essentially Eastern or Oriental, and not Western and European. Thus, at first glance at least, the interpretive tradition I explore in this book represents a discontinuity with orientalism as it has been defined since the work of Edward Said. The narratives by Jews and Christians that configured Moses as Pasteur or Koch, that represented the Mosaic and rabbinical codes as ancient versions of modern sanitation science and preventive medicine, and that sought to move Judaism and the Jews from the margins to the center of Western civilization, such narratives repudiated the idea of all things Jewish as essentially other than the West. Indeed, the West owed more to the Jews than was generally acknowledged. When the medical texts considered here represented Mosaic and Rabbinic law as the ancient equivalent of modern Western medicine, they posited an essential sort of identity between the Jews and the West.

At the same time, such narratives were ultimately framed by a powerful orientalism. The normative status of the West remained unchallenged. *It* was the site of health, culture, and civilization. The interpretive strategy employed by Jews and non-Jews, the translation of Jewish tradition and history into central components of the larger Western story of science, medicine, and civilization, was an assimilationist strategy. But it was an assimilationist strategy with a twist. If the Jews and Judaism were to be reinterpreted as central to civilization (and not just until Jesus arrives to make Judaism, at best, dispensable), if health and hygiene were integral to Jewish law and tradition from the outset (and again, Christianity's advent did not affect the status of the law in this regard), then the Jews did not require Europe to make them healthy and civilized. Who, in the end, was civilizing whom? Thus, the narratives I analyze in this book challenge, consciously or not, the orientalist discursive tradition even if, in the end, they participate in and reinforce it.[26]

SCIENCE AND RELIGION

As these comments should make clear, the relationship between religion, science, and medicine in the texts under discussion here was anything but straightforward.[27] Scholars have shown that the popular idea that science and religion were fundamentally at odds during the nineteenth and twentieth centuries, that they represented irreconcilable worldviews, is misleading. The historical relationship between science and religion was far more complex and ambivalent than often believed. As one historian of the controversy has put it, "Serious scholarship in the history of science has revealed so extraordinarily rich and complex a relationship between science and religion in the past that general theses are difficult to sustain. The real lesson turns out to be the complexity."[28] Indeed, there now exists a substantial amount of scholarly work on this complex relationship between religion and science.

Yet when we look at the literature produced by historians of religion and modern science, it quickly becomes evident that "religion" usually means Christianity.[29] A vast scholarly literature has addressed the response of Christian clergy and theologians to Darwinism, to evolutionism, geology, anthropology, physics, and, more recently, to debates over genetic engineering. Yet, this historically complex relationship existed not only between science and Christianity, but also between science (including medicine) and Judaism (and Islam and other faiths as well).

What is the relationship between religion and science in the medical texts analyzed in this book? When Moses is made into a social hygienist, the ancient equivalent of Pasteur or Koch, who and what is raised up in the process? Is the ancient Hebrew law code redeemed through its association, its equivalence, to modern science? Or is modern science elevated and enhanced by its association with Moses (and by implication, of course, God)? One historian of science has written, in the context of a discussion of science and Romanticism, that "mid-nineteenth century science and medicine assiduously cultivated the idea of the single creative scientific mind, of the doctor or scientist as hero."[30] Few other figures (Jesus, Newton) rose to the level of Moses in the Western cultural imagination. So, when Moses is transformed into a scientist and doctor, does such a translation process elevate Moses, or does it somehow further celebrate the individual genius of doctors and scientists by linking them with a mythical hero? It seems clear, in any case, that the translation of Judaism, as a set of practices, into hygienic terms was intended to "raise" Judaism to the level of modern medicine and science, to provide it with relevance and an ongoing significance that could not be taken for granted.

Where do these texts and their authors fall along the spectrum of secularization? When medical authorities touted the laws of *kashrut* (the Jewish dietary laws) as a tested means of preventing infection from tuberculosis, when they celebrated the practice of circumcision for its health benefits, invoking statistics on the extremely low incidence of penile cancer among Jewish men and cervical cancer among Jewish women, were they obviating the religious significance of these rituals or encouraging it? The interpretive tradition dealt with here testifies to a complex interaction of religion and science, religion and medicine that cannot be explained simply by reference to "traditionalism" or "secularization."[31] When we look at the numerous texts produced about the Bible and Talmud as codes of hygiene and health, we see a negotiation that belies any notion of a simplistic dichotomy between science and religion.

Was the point of these texts to shore up religion or science, biblical authority or medical authority? In fact, such narratives reinforced the one and the other, and it is untenable to interpret the interconnections in a unidirectional way. Reading the Bible literally, as the medical writers I am concerned with did, meant historicizing Moses, reading him in realistic and historical rather than mythological or metaphorical terms. Indeed, one of the most startling aspects of this translation process, of what we might call a medical midrashic reading of classical Jewish sources, is the literalness with which scientific authors approached these texts, the Bible in particular. Ironically, at a time when the metaphorical or symbolic exegesis of scriptures had become the norm for scholars working in what becomes known as religious studies, physicians and other scientists approached Scripture in a naïve, positivist and literalist way.

Moreover, there was a strong, if at times only implicit, "religious" impulse to the intense concern about germs, cleanliness, dirt, and disease that preoccupied many in the nineteenth and twentieth centuries. The language and images that framed "the gospel of germs," to employ Nancy Tomes's phrase, testifies to this.[32] But rather than cast this in the mode of secularization, the material I deal with in this study speaks to the continuing import of religion at a level that goes to the content as well as the form. In other words, for the medical authorities concerned with these issues, religion was still a living thing, still had something to teach science and scientists. More particularly, it was the Hebrew Bible, the Old Testament, and especially the law, that was the content and the object of interest. One of the central themes explored and delineated in *The Healthy Jew* is the continued relevance, for Christian and Jewish medical writers alike, of the Mosaic, and to a lesser extent rabbinic, laws and rituals. Granted, "religion" had to be translated into scientific medicine. But this translation process, which will occupy us throughout, means that physicians and writers on medicine did not simply and disdainfully disregard religious tradition. Again, this makes more complex the story we tell, or ought to tell, about the historical relationship between religion and science, between tradition and secular trajectories over the past two and a half centuries.

TRANSLATING MOSES, JUDAISM, AND THE JEWS

The context for the medicalization of Jewish tradition was, first and foremost, the profound shift in the relationship between professional medicine and society: the development of public hygiene and preventive medicine that began in the early to middle decades of the nineteenth century; then later, the revolutionary impact of evolution and eugenics, germ theory and bacteriology; and the concomitant shift in the image of the physician, the sanitarian, and the public health official into noble, even heroic figures. The intellectual and cultural strategy employed in the medicalization of Judaism and the Jewish past was translation, a strategy focused first and foremost on the figure of Moses. The notion of translation here is not linguistic but cultural. A code of beliefs and behaviors that had been fixed or categorized as "religious" was translated into the realms of science and medicine. This does not mean that its traditionally understood use and value were lost or dismissed; this was a broadening out or multiplication of meaning. Aleida Assmann has called this process transcodification:

> In its narrow sense, the problem of translation is the preservation of meaning; in a wider sense, the potential of translation is the generation of meaning. It is precisely in these constant shifts of transferal and displacement that meaning is generated. To look at translation in these terms, then, is not so much to consider it as establishing semantic equivalents in different codes (which of course it also is) but as generating new meanings in the process of transforming a given information.[33]

In some sense it can be argued that the "translators" of Moses were bringing back together something that had artificially been rent asunder by "modern" sensibilities, capturing more fully the world of the ancients in which "religion" as a separate sphere and cultural category did not exist.

The nineteenth and twentieth century texts with which I deal here constitute in some way part of a much longer intellectual tradition of interpreting or translating Moses and his law code. More specifically, there existed a tradition reaching back to the ancient world that understood Moses as a man (or in some cases also as a demi-god) possessed of extraordinary wisdom, a founder of culture and civilization, whose code offered a key to health and longevity. This was countered, we should remember, by an alternate intellectual tradition that identified Moses as a leper, as a criminal who commanded a band of diseased and criminal outcasts, and whose code was the negative inversion of Egyptian wisdom.[34] At the same time, the medical works examined here constitute something new insofar as they inscribe Moses, the Mosaic code, and subsequent Jewish authorities within contemporary medical and scientific discoveries and practices.

The Western discourse on Moses saw the construction of numerous Moseses: Moses the lawgiver, Moses the creator of the Jewish nation, Moses the Egyptian priest, Moses the magician, Moses the prophet, and, for Freud, "the slain Moses." The Moses I am interested in is Moses the physician, Moses the microbiologist, Moses the lawgiver – with the law translated into a prescription for health and hygiene. This Moses is both an extension of and a departure from those that came before. I am not claiming that Moses the microbiologist becomes at any point the dominant Moses, that this image replaces the older or alternative ones of Moses. Freud's Moses, for instance, comes later and has obviously had a far more wide-reaching impact on subsequent discussions. Nonetheless, this medicalized Moses was a distinct and identifiable version of Moses, one that gained in popularity in the nineteenth and twentieth centuries.[35] In turn, this Moses constituted one element of a much broader discourse that sought to translate other figures in Jewish history into physicians or medical experts; that translated both the Bible and Talmud into codes of hygiene and health; and that reinterpreted the history of the Jews and their relation to the West in terms of medical and scientific knowledge and practice.

The Moses of modern medicine is another Moses, a projection of the needs of physicians and medical authorities, both Jewish and non-Jewish. Taken as a whole, as an interpretive tradition developed over decades, the narratives about Moses and medicine were, *inter alia*, legitimations of male authority and patriarchal knowledge in a modern culture that was deeply divided about the complex and intertwined issues of gender, race, and religion. The Moses of modern medicine is Jewish, yet also transcends Jewishness. As the ancient equivalent of Koch and Pasteur, the "founder of preventive medicine" as numerous writers put it, Moses was universalized into a scientist, a physician, and a public health official. He served as a projection of the ideals of modern medicine, as well as the primordial "healthy Jew." Thus, what we encounter here was a Moses who retained a particular "Jewish" identity while simultaneously undergoing a process of universalization, a process that was the intended or unintended effect of translation. Moses' code clearly originated as a means to create a new people, a distinct and separate nation, or *am*, by means of concepts and modes of behavior organized around notions of purity and impurity, holiness and its opposite. This was a holy people, a nation of priests, who would be free of disease as a sign of and a reward for obedience to God's law.

Normative Christianity, of course, repudiated this notion of salvation through obedience to law. The modern narratives I explore in this book seem to me to be a sort of universalization of this ancient particularism, extending salvation (i.e., a greater freedom from the ravages of disease) through obedience to God's laws, interpreted as medical ordinances. In 1940, the physician and medical researcher Charles Weiss, writing in *Scientific Monthly* about "Medicine in the Bible," repeated a formulation about the innovation of Mosaic law in the ancient world that had been a staple of medical literature for at least a century:

> One of the most remarkable achievements in the field of preventive medicine and hygiene is the introduction by Moses of a compulsory weekly day of rest (the Sabbath) for *all* the people. It is true that the ancient Babylonian calendar included certain days when the king could not perform certain functions; such as riding in a chariot, using fire or wearing the robes of his kingdom. A weekly day of rest for *all the people*, however, is indeed a step forward in democracy, as well as in physical and mental hygiene. The Jewish and Christian peoples were the first to benefit from this Mosaic law.[36]

The universalization here is obvious (even if it takes place through what in this case at least is an implicit "Americanization" of Mosaic law). A practice previously reserved for the king, for those in power, is extended to the masses, to all the people. The invocation of democracy, the echoes of America's sacred documents, and the anachronistic bringing together of Jews and Christians allows Weiss to celebrate a practice for both its particularistic and universalist benefits. And again, it bears noting that this appeared not in a publication of Jewish provenance, but in a monthly journal aimed at the broadest possible audience.

The translation of Moses into a physician or sanitarian was central to the discourse on the healthy Jew. But the translation process went beyond the figure of Moses, extending to Judaism and the Jews themselves. Judaism itself was translated into a system of laws whose purpose was, first and foremost, the preservation of the nation or race through

specific hygienic principles and measures. Thus, the law codes of the rabbis and the medieval Jewish commentators (many of whom were, in fact,
trained in medicine) were reinterpreted as health codes. Moreover, the
Jews themselves were represented as translators of medical wisdom. And
this image constituted a central component of Jewish apologetics as it
developed in the nineteenth and twentieth centuries. "As a physician,"
the English writer Israel Zangwill told the Universal Races Congress in
1911, "the Jew's fame from the Middle Ages, when he was the bearer
of Arabian science, and the tradition that Kings shall always have Jewish physicians, is still unbroken. Dr. Ehrlich's recent discovery of '606,'
the cure for syphilis, and Dr. Haffkine's inoculation against the plague in
India, are but links in a long chain of Jewish contributions to medicine."[37]

Translating Moses, then, meant situating the Jews and Judaism at the
beginning of the history of medicine, making them founders or initia-
tors of a regime of scientific knowledge and practice that Europeans
and Americans only recently had had the good fortune to understand
and experience. Placing the task of translation at the heart of the Jewish
experience in Europe, as Zangwill and so many others did, meant situating the Jews at the center of a centuries-long historical process, one
that began in the early Middle Ages and continues today. Both Judaism
and Jewish history were recast as essential to Western civilization, a fact
more often ignored or denied than acknowledged.

APOLOGETICS AND PHILOSEMITISM

It need hardly be said that Jewish historiography has given over enormous
time and space to the issue of anti-Semitism. Much of that has consisted
of the collection, organization, and analysis of anti-Semitic texts – ideas,
arguments, and images generated about Jews by non-Jews. My study is
no less or more than another collection and analysis of texts – narratives,
discourses, representations, and strategies of interpretation. In part this
is so because I remain convinced that that is really all we have; even
our contexts are constructed out of texts. We privilege some and leave
most others aside; we use texts to explain other texts, even if we call the
explanation by a variety of other names. Of course this does not mean
that historical reality is a chimera, only that history in its fullness is gone
and what is left to us are its remains and ruins: texts, broadly defined.[38] I

also focus on texts, and mainly published ones at that, because so much of the analysis of anti-Semitism focuses on them. Certainly, historians of the Jews pay great attention to the translation of hostility and hatred into actions: attacks on synagogues, businesses, and Jews themselves. But the often unquestioned assumption governing much of the historiography is that there exists a clear causal relationship between this actual violence and negative images and ideas about Jews. Histories of anti-Semitism are written largely in this vein: anti-Semitic discourse and anti-Jewish violence are deeply intertwined. I am not arguing that such a relation does not exist. But too often the history of anti-Semitism gets written as the history of narratives about Jews, a series of negative representations produced over the centuries and brought together by the historian. And when we do encounter physical violence, whether isolated attacks or coordinated pogroms or expulsions, the implicit assumption seems to be that some causal connection exists between the narrative representation and the action; that negative images produce negative consequences.[39] Again, I am not equipped to demonstrate that this is either so or not so; that is another project entirely. My interest here is in introducing an alternative set of narratives and images that circulated at the same time as the negative ones. And I want to raise the question: on what grounds do historians identify one period as more or less "anti-Semitic" than another when evidence for a variety of ideas and images about Jews can be found to be circulating at the same time?

The Healthy Jew, therefore, is also about anti-Semitism, philosemitism, and the relation between them. It is a collection of counter-narratives to the anti-Semitic ones and to the dominant Jewish narratives that have largely been constructed from the anti-Semitic. Alan Levenson has recently defined philosemitism as "*any* pro-Jewish or pro-Judaic utterance or act." Levenson minimizes or rejects qualifiers such as motive or primacy of place or even overall sympathy. Thus, philosemitism might emerge as an ancillary byproduct of another cause, as when a defender of liberalism or universal rights offers up the Jews as an example of a group that must be included. Nor does the defender of the Jews necessarily have to love or even like Jews; this, according to Levenson, does not diminish the value of the act or utterance.[40]

In this book I draw on material produced by both Jews and non-Jews, and I make the philosemitism and Gentileness of many of these authors an explicit theme. In the first place, it is important to note, as I do throughout, that Christian authorities participated and contributed in significant ways to the discourse of the "healthy Jew." At certain junctures I suggest some reasons that this might have been so, mainly along utilitarian or functional lines. Their real motives may, ultimately, prove unknowable. However, following Levenson, I would argue that this is less important than the dissemination of the ideas and images themselves, and the fact that non-Jews – Christians – were indeed responsible for these positive representations of Jews and Judaism. What was the standing of the non-Jewish contribution? Exploring more closely the role of non-Jewish narratives about Jewish health allows us to identify a double standard of sorts, and one that speaks to larger themes of apologia and anti-Semitism. At certain times, in certain contexts, non-Jewish narratives become privileged because they are non-Jewish. When Christian authors write and speak in positive ways about Jewish health and hygiene, the power of such narratives to convince may very well be greater than narratives produced by explicitly identified or identifiable Jews. Non-Jews are given an authority precisely because they are non-Jews. This is the positive corollary of the Jewish authority who is dismissed by opponents precisely because he (and all the medical authorities examined in this book were male) is Jewish, because this fact is taken as evidence of excessive bias and subjectivity. In this case, Jewishness diminishes one's capacity for objective analysis; non-Jewishness is assumed to be neutral, the natural and unproblematic ground on which the real scientist stands. Jewish authorities might be assumed to possess this naturalness or neutrality when they come to speak on Jewish matters. And it might be the non-Jew whose subject position is in question. Yet, in the interpretive tradition explored here, the non-Jewish voice is often granted a privileged status. And the non-Jewish voice becomes a crucial instrument in Jewish apologia as well as in non-Jewish polemics.

THE JEWISH BODY, HEALTHY AND DISEASED

This study is concerned, as I have explained, almost entirely with published texts that constitute a discrete narrative tradition or discourse. This stems in part from my belief that historians are really only left with texts; this is what we have once "the present" becomes the past. Just as important though is the difficulty posed by getting at "the body," – the healthy body, the diseased body, the body in pain – through texts. There exists a not insignificant gap between the body and its representation. Thus, the focus is on textual representation, absent any claim to hereby be able to arrive at some closer or better approximation of "the truth" about Jewish health and disease as it was experienced by millions of Jews.

If we cannot bridge the epistemological gap between the representation of the Jewish body and the reality of how Jews lived in their bodies, how they experienced health and disease, we can at least attempt to answer the question of why a particular discourse about the Jewish body took hold among historians and cultural theorists at a particular time. To paraphrase Caroline Walker Bynum, why all the fuss about the Jewish body?[41] More specifically, why all the fuss about the diseased Jewish body?

One interpretive strain of recent Jewish body studies reproduces, in one way or another, the image of the healthy Jew. Scholars such as Daniel Boyarin and Howard Eilberg-Schwartz seem intent on recovering a healthy Judaism (and by implication, Jew), even if in Boyarin's case this means radically reinterpreting ideas of "healthy" or "normal."[42] Another influential interpretive tradition has focused on the discourse produced about the purported "diseased" Jewish body. This is a Jewish body that seems to be both real and imaginary, the product of genuine social, political and economic forces, but also the product of the overactive anti-Semitic imagination (and, then in a psychopathological process of internalization, a Jewish imagination that absorbs anti-Semitic imagery and becomes self-hatred). Medicalization, from this perspective, translates into pathologization.

"It is impossible," Sander Gilman writes in his study of Franz Kafka and tuberculosis, "to invoke the concept 'Jew' without immediately invoking concepts of masculinity and pathology."[43] No single scholar has done more to disseminate "the Jew's body" than Gilman; and for Gilman, the Jew's body is a diseased body.[44] Certainly, as Naomi Seidman has pointed out, he is not interested in the "corporeal experience of Jews but rather how their bodies looked to the doctors and journalists of the late nineteenth century." Seidman has identified certain themes in Gilman's writings, and chief among these is an interest in how the Jewish body was constructed as different, pathological, inferior, and feminine. Exploring the European fascination with the diseased Jewish body, of course, is a way to explore the issue of anti-Semitism, understood in part as the collection of anxieties called up by the encounter with the "deformed Jew."[45] Many Jews also evinced such anxieties about the deformed Jew, internalizing anti-Semitic images and reidentifying themselves and other Jews as pathological. Gilman's twinned phenomena of Jew hatred and Jewish self-hatred rest on the purported normative status of the abnormal.

Gilman seems intent on universalizing the diseased and the pathological. "The difference of the Jewish body is absolute within the Western tradition," as he put it in *The Jew's Body.*[46] And different for Gilman means inferior and pathological. He does not ignore "the healthy Jew" in his work. Indeed, he is interested in the stereotype of the Jew as both healthy and diseased, and the way in which "the sterotype's peculiar power to accommodate antithese comes into play." Thus, the Jews as capitalists and communists, as "arch-bankers and arch-revolutionaries," finds its counterpart in the image of the healthy and diseased Jews.[47] Nonetheless, ultimately for Gilman it is the diseased Jew who wins out, and this not only for anti-Semties but for Jews as well: "Western Jews were constrained by the power of science to accept the argument for Jewish physical insufficiency."[48] It is this generalization, which Gilman has advanced in almost everything he has written on Jews (and which I, among others, have adopted and used to great advantage), that I want to challenge.

"Modernity," Gilman writes at one point in his book *Franz Kafka, Jewish Patient*, "is either the cause of or the result of Jewish illness, depending on whom one reads at the turn of the century."[49] Yes, but not entirely. "Depending on whom one reads" is the key phrase here. This is the nodal point, I would argue, at which we can see the importance of Gilman's own choice of the texts to be interpreted, and the way in which such choices shape the overall argument.[50] If you are only reading anti-Semites, or Jews who share in the discourse of Jewish illness, then the image of the Jews and their relationship to modernity can be framed in these terms. And, again, I in no way wish to deny the reality and power of such sets of images. But there was a counter-discourse (at least one) that constructed an image of the healthy Jew, a discourse produced by Gentiles and Jews. If we look at other texts (or even at the same texts with different eyes), then we arrive at a very different image of the Jews and Judaism. As I argue throughout *The Healthy Jew*, there did exist a significant body of literature that represented Jews and Judaism as healthy and vital, that did not feminize the male Jew, or associate him with the sorts of social and political pathologies so common in the anti-Semitic imagination. There might very well have been real Jewish men out there who did not internalize anti-Semitic imagery, who did not come to understand their own minds and bodies through the prism of the negative stereotypes of Jews. This does not obviate the importance that the diseased Jewish body had for anti-Semites, for the history of Western medicine (including Freud and psychoanalysis), and for the construction of a modern Jewish identity. Yet it necessarily complicates the narratives produced about all of these.

Gilman's representation of the Jewish body has become to a large extent the paradigmatic (modern) Jewish body, and his work has been extremely important and influential within Jewish studies and perhaps even more so among those working in literary studies, German studies, and the history of medicine. And if, as is generally acknowledged, Gilman's work was seminal in creating a subdiscipline of Jewish body studies, with its focus on disease and abnormality, then this focus can be understood in part at least as a product of a particular moment in American intellectual and cultural history. The fascination with the diseased Jewish body certainly cannot be understood without reference to the Holocaust and the ongoing need to understand the role that anti-Semitic representations played in preparing the ground for Nazism. Is it possible, at the same time, to see the fascination with the abnormal or diseased Jew as, in part, a product of a shift in American culture, and concomitantly as further evidence of a continuing development within American Jewish self-consciousness? By the latter I mean a cementing of both the faith in security for Jews in the United States, and the willingness thereby to confront themes in the Jewish past that do not lend themselves easily to apologia and that have of course traditionally been associated with anti-Semitism. Disease and the malformations of the Jewish body and mind surely fit into this category. Paradoxically, then, it is precisely "Jewish health" among American Jews today – defined, if you will, broadly enough in this case to include not merely physical health, but a general sense of well-being and security – that allows for the dissemination of images and ideas about Jewish disease in the past.

If, as discussed in Chapter 1, the need for a "healthy Jew" emerged in the late nineteenth century in part because of a sense of insecurity, a need to respond through apologetics to a widely disseminated image of a diseased Jew, then the embrace of "the diseased Jew" today may very well speak to a heightened sense of security.

The disrepute in scholarly circles of apologia also helps us understand the attraction of the pathological rather than the healthy Jew. The interpretive tradition of the healthy Jew was fundamentally apologetic in its thrust, even if its objects of analysis – bodies, sexuality, blood, and so on – could be seen as linking the Jews with the disreputable and the dangerous. The overall thrust of this literature, as I show in this book, is to translate Jews and Judaism into contemporary terms of the healthy, the respectable, and the civilized. Yet, at a certain point such overt apologetic impulses were deemed unacceptable, irretrievably at odds with the ideals of a critical scholarship. Moreover, the healthy and respectable ceased to be as interesting or illuminating as the diseased and abnormal.[51]

The recent preoccupation of Jewish historians or cultural studies scholars with the Jewish body, and more particularly with a diseased Jewish body, must be situated, then, within larger trends within academia and scholarship, and beyond this within a larger cultural arc. For the emerging field of body studies, influenced above all by Michel Foucault's framework of abnormality and illness (physical and mental) as normative for the discourse of knowledge and power, "health" is far less interesting than disease, the rational and respectable less illuminating than the irrational and disreputable (Foucault was, of course, the self-proclaimed heir to Nietzsche and Freud). If reason, respectability, and health are less engaging because quintessentially bourgeois, then this too might help to explain the interest in the diseased Jewish body. This turn to the diseased and abnormal within academic circles reflects a broader shift in the culture, one that is now inundated and saturated with images of illness, threats from within and without one's own body to the individual and the collective self.[52]

The Healthy Jew is about the desire for the bourgeois, the respectable, and the civilized. It is not intended as a challenge to the power and significance of the diseased Jewish body. The representation of Judaism and Jews during the past two centuries on the part of both Jews and Christians has been multifarious and complex. The Jews were both diseased and healthy, different and similar (though perhaps never identical), barbaric, civilized, yet never quite civilized enough. Judaism, for both Jews and Christians, could be seen as decadent and desiccated, the cause of Jewish incivility, or it could be represented as the very foundation of civilization and the reason for Jewish survival and vitality. The intellectual strategies for dealing with such a range of images have also been diverse.[53] This book explores one such set of strategies.

I

"'Tis a Little People, But It Has Done Great Things"

The Role of Health and Medicine
in Modern Jewish Apologetics

The notion of a particular and particularly profound connection between Jews and medicine has a long narrative history. We know that medicine was for centuries one of the few respectable professions that Jews in Europe were allowed to pursue; they could study in Italian universities and practice in the courts and palaces of Christian and Muslim rulers. Even the popes had their Jewish physicians. Histories of the Jews in Europe, especially those written in the mode of "great men" narratives, are replete with the names of eminent intellectual and political figures who counted the practice of medicine as one of their achievements: Hasdai ibn Shaprut in Andalusia, Jehuda Halevi in Christian Toledo and then in Moslem Cordova, Nachmanides in Aragon, and, of course, Maimonides in Fostat, near Cairo. The notion of a unique Jewish contribution to medicine, framed in apologetic terms, reaches back at least to the end of the sixteenth century, and David de Pomis's *De medico hebraeo. Enarratio apologetica* (Venice, 1588). I will not aim in this chapter, however, to attempt a comprehensive survey of this apologetic literature.[1] Rather, I want to engage with examples from the nineteenth and twentieth centuries in an attempt to draw out some of the formal elements of Jewish apologia related to medicine and science – in particular, the nexus of Moses, Judaism, and hygiene – and to explore the mechanisms of this genre.

The sentiment, "'Tis a little people..." is taken from Joseph Jacobs, *Jewish Contributions to Civilization: An Estimate*. Jacobs died in 1916, and the Jewish Publication Society of America published the book posthumously in 1919.

28

I.

One cannot speak of a "Jewish medicine," either of the Middle Ages or modernity, because "Jewish physicians belonged to those lands and languages in which they lived and wrote. . . ." So argued the eminent Jewish historian Moritz Steinschneider in 1896, in a leading German-language medical journal.[2] Steinschneider felt it necessary to object vociferously to the attempt to reinterpret the Torah as a hygienic system, to make Moses and the rabbis into ancient versions of Louis Pasteur and Robert Koch. "Whoever intends to glorify Moses by reference to his knowledge of trichinosis," he wrote sarcastically, "transgresses the fundamental prohibition of historical criticism: the introduction of modern science into ancient records."[3]

Yet such "transgression" occurred quite often, both before and after Steinschneider issued his censure. Ever the exemplary bibliographer, Steinschneider appended to his article a list of over one hundred books and articles, a few reaching back to the seventeenth century, that violated the fundamental prohibition of historical study: Thou shalt not commit an anachronism. His admonition had little or no impact. In the decades that followed his article, a large number of works continued to develop the ideas of Moses as sanitarian and scientist, Jewish sacred writings as keys to health, and the Jews as a healthy nation and race. Thus, Hans Goslar began his introduction to a 1930 volume, *Hygiene und Judentum*, by noting the abundant literature produced in German by Jews and non-Jews that explored the "wise foresight" of the Jewish religious laws, their hygienic and eugenic efficacy (*"die volkserhaltenden, hygienisch und eugenisch wirksamen Bestimmungen des jüdischen Religionsgesetzes"*).[4] While the claims about Jews, Judaism and hygiene made by physicians and rabbis in that 1930 volume certainly had a particular resonance in that particular context, such apologetics were by no means limited to the German-speaking world. The literature was international, and there was, as we shall see, a high level of intertextuality, with ideas and images moving over time and across national and linguistic boundaries.

Surely, one of the main reasons for the production of Jewish apologia, by both Jews and non-Jews, was as a response to anti-Semitism, and particularly to the widespread notion that Jewish difference resided not only in particular traits and proclivities, but also in an absence of certain attributes. Gathering Jews and Arabs together under the rubric "Semites," the eminent French thinker Ernest Renan granted that this nomadic race had had the "primitive intuition" to arrive at the idea of monotheism. But he denied to them any of the attributes or talents usually associated with culture and civilization. The Semites, he wrote, possess "neither plastic arts, nor rational science, neither philosophy nor political life, nor even military organization." "La race sémitique n'a jamais compris la civilization dans le sens que nous attachons à ce mot."[5]

Almost as quickly as scholars and others brought the Jews and Arabs together as "Semites," the two were disentangled. While at certain moments Jewish thinkers (a few Zionists in particular) identified a historical and racial connection between Jews and Arabs, as Semites, by the end of the nineteenth century the case for the Jewish contribution to Western Civilization (meaning Europe) was being made on behalf of the Jews alone. "Semites" were now Jews, and the case for the Jews rested in part on the assertion of a fundamental difference between Jews and Muslims, between Arabs and the West, and the desire and ability of the Jews to embody the highest values and accomplishments of European civilization. Anti-Semitism, then, was for Jewish apologists the product first and foremost of ignorance, as well as a cynical political posturing. Anti-Semites and their supporters needed to become aware of all that the Jews had given to the West, of the central role Jews played in the making of European civilization. The Anglo-American scholar Joseph Jacobs, for example, framed his posthumously published *Jewish Contributions to Civilization* explicitly in these terms. Anti-Semitism, in Jacobs' view, is an elite phenomenon, a set of ideas about the Jews produced by literate elites to serve their own particular purposes. It was not and is not a "natural outcome of the clash of racial tendencies or temperaments."[6] Rather, anti-Semitism was "artificial," as opposed, for example, to the natural "realities of commercial envy and rivalry" that also help to explain antagonism at certain junctures between Jews and Christians.

After providing a sketch of the various forms or reasons for anti-Semitism, Jacobs identified the one that "swells out above the rest and becomes dominant": the "Counter-Revolution," anti-Liberal version, whose most representative and recent example was Houston Stewart Chamberlain's *Foundations of the Nineteenth Century*. Chamberlain's book had gained such popularity because it offered up to the vanity of the Germans (and the English) the notion that they were the Chosen Race, "from whom alone real genius and real progress can be anticipated. As part of his argument he has been compelled to show that the other claimants for the title of Chosen Race, the Jews, have no claim to creative genius, even in religion...".[7]

Jacobs's work was conceived, then, out of the conviction that "it is time to come to an understanding with these anti-Semites; to speak, as it were, with the enemy in the gate."[8] Believing, as he did, that anti-Semitism "has always come from above downwards," it made perfect sense for Jacobs to believe that a counter-history, one conceived along the lines of Jewish contributions to civilization, would have a real impact.

Interestingly, Jacobs was one of the few writers in this period that downplayed the Jewish contribution to medicine. Still, he certainly included it as a category. He noted that Jewish works on health were translated into Latin, and "in adapting the works of the Arabic medical writers into Latin the Jews were exceptionally active."[9] On the other hand, Jews, according to Jacobs, played little or no mediating role in the realm of Greek medicine. In addition to the production and translation of medical texts, the Jews' contribution to medicine in the West lay in their capacity as carriers or mediators of drugs or medicines originating in Arabic lands: "In medicine, the Arabs introduced syrups and julep, nitre and soda, senna and camphor, alum and borax, tamarinds and laudanum, and mercury as a drug."[10] The Jews moved these medicinals, in addition to much else, from East to West.

As noted already, the themes of mediation and translation were central to the debates over Jews and medicine, and over the contribution of Jews to Western civilization and culture. The advocates of Jewry in this regard had to insist that the normative narrative of medical history was either incomplete or incorrect. Most were far more vigorous than Jacobs in their arguments. If the normative narrative traced the origins of medicine back to Greece (or, less often, Egypt), and minimized or eliminated the Jewish contribution, then the counter-narrative insisted that ancient Hebrew society had already possessed much of the medical wisdom of modern practitioners. If certain medical historians told the history of the medical renaissance in the West in the early Middle Ages without including the

Jews (or in some cases even the Arabs), or collapsing the Jews and Arabs into one "Oriental" influence, then those historians responding to this would need to distinguish clearly between Arabs and Jews, and make the case for a distinct Jewish contribution.

In order to comprehend the significance of medicine and health for modern Jewish apologia, therefore, it is not sufficient merely to invoke anti-Semitism and its racialized or medicalized nature. Without doubt, this context is important. But Jewish apologia is overdetermined, and the power of science and medicine in this context derived from the general power – discursive and social – that public medicine, physicians, and hospitals acquired over the course of the nineteenth century. More specifically, the attempt on the part of numerous authors to link Jewish law and ritual with modern scientific medicine, to medicalize Moses and the Torah, depended on more specific developments within European and American medicine, even as it participated in a discourse (or an inter-related set of discourses) that extended back centuries and circulated among scholars of numerous countries. Both a medicalized anti-Semitism and a medicalized Jewish apologia are to be understood within the larger context of societies or cultures that were obsessed not only with Jews and their enemies, with metaphorical parasites and diseases, but also with actual germs, bacteria, parasites; with the infectious illnesses produced by germs; and then with the scientists and physicians who discovered the causes and cures and treated the sick and dying.

Jews, of course, were not alone in calling attention to and celebrating their own group's purported achievements and contributions to civilization. Other minorities or groups seeking greater political and social or occupational inclusion made contributory literature one of the intellectual strategies for addressing more immediate needs. In the United States, for instance, both black and women's emancipation movements sought to convince others and themselves of their own worthiness through the articulation of contribution; health and medicine, as in the Jewish case, were crucial categories. For those groups – Jews, blacks, women, and others – who historically, in the dominant scientific literature and in the popular culture, had been identified as not only different, but also diseased and dangerous, the discursive link with health, fitness, and hygiene held a great deal of power.[11] Certainly, when Jewish writers delineated the medical contributions of Jewish physicians and researchers, when they celebrated the health and hygienic genius of Moses and the rabbis, and when they insisted on the contribution that components of the Jewish law – *kashrut*, circumcision, family or sexual purity rules – could make to the present and future health of general society, they were participating in an intellectual (and political) exercise that paralleled strategies produced about and by other minorities.[12]

At the same time, the apologetics of Jews and medicine depended upon and participated in a much older and broader debate than that of a modern racialized anti-Semitism. As the earlier reference to Greece and Egypt suggests, histories of Jews and medicine were also interventions in the ongoing debate about Athens and Jerusalem (as well as Alexandria and Rome – both pagan and Christian), a debate that was in large measure about the origins of culture and civilization and that had already begun in the ancient world. As Yaakov Shavit, among others, has shown, the claim that the Egyptians and Greeks actually owed their wisdom and culture to the Jews was common among Jewish Hellenists. There was a systematic attempt to draw correspondences between Greek and Jewish myths, and to demonstrate that the Greeks imitated the Hebrews. Ignaz Goldziher, the Jewish Hungarian Islamicist, wrote mockingly of this attempt that, over the course of centuries, numerous works had sought to show that "Greek literature and Greek theologies are nothing but inferior translations or facile versions of the Hebrew."[13]

These apologetics carried on into the Middle Ages and beyond. According to Shavit, medieval Arab philosophers and commentators were capable of recognizing and admitting that the Arabs borrowed their science and philosophy from the Greeks. They wrote proudly of the fact that Islam "internalized" alien science and made it their own. "Not so the Jews," Shavit writes. "They were writing out of a sense of inferiority, and that is why they had to resort to apologetics and were not satisfied merely to act as intermediaries between ancient antiquity and Europe. From the Jewish standpoint, the role of a people who preserved the Greek treasures of wisdom and passed them on to the West was not a sufficiently meaningful one."[14] Thus, Jehuda Halevi could claim that the Greeks received all wisdom, philosophical and scientific, from the Jews. Halevi's "apologia appears again and again in medieval, Renaissance, and post-Renaissance works as a true historical account; already in the fourteenth century Meir ben Solomon Alguadez from Castile declared in the preface to his Hebrew translation of the *Nicomachean Ethics* that Aristotle was explaining the precepts of the Torah." Other Jewish writers disseminated the notion that Aristotle ended up converting to Judaism after having encountered the wisdom of the Torah.[15]

That wisdom and science originate with the Jews is, then, a very old and well-established trope, appearing in ancient, medieval, and early modern Jewish literature: that the Greeks derived their wisdom from the Jews, that ancient Greek philosophers and scientists went and studied in Jerusalem, and/or that through the Jewish dispersion the wisdom of Jerusalem made its way to other nations, who then appropriated it as their own. This is the "tradition of the theft of wisdom." And underlying and impelling this tradition is the anxiety of "civilization."

As I argue throughout this book, narratives of medicine, of health, and of hygiene were always also about civilization. Where did it originate? Who contributed to it? Who is capable of shaping and being shaped by it? Who, today, upholds its standards, embodies its ideals? These were the questions asked by the French Jewish medical writer Marc Brochard in his 1865 work on Jews and public hygiene. *"Qu'est-ce que la civilization? Qu-est-ce que le progress?"* These consist of creating the conditions by which the physical, intellectual, and moral faculties of each human being can be developed to their fullest extent. Public hygiene has an essential role to play in these developments, and, as Brochard sought to demonstrate, Moses' sanitary code was intimately linked with universal civilization and progress.[16]

Thus, situated behind the discourses on Jews and health, medicine, and race are the theories and assertions about civilization and progress.[17] As scholars of philhellenism such as Suzanne Marchand and Frank Turner have made abundantly clear, for the vast majority of educated Europeans and Americans, "civilization" by the nineteenth century was equated with the ancient Greeks.[18] Philhellenism, as Turner has written, "involved an international community of scholars and writers," but assumed different shapes and took on a different significance within particular national contexts.[19] For our purposes what matters is the more general point that, beginning in the late eighteenth century, "in the learned imagination of Europe the ancient Hellenic achievement assumed a vitality and sense of relevance previously entertained in the minds of only a fewscore Renaissance humanists."[20]

The story of philhellenism is about many things in addition to a genuine and profound affection for the ancient Greek world: the emergence of neo-humanism and neoclassicism; the birth of art history, ancient history, and archeology as scholarly disciplines; the celebration of democracy, and the celebration of freedom (whether political, cultural, or spiritual); the enthusiasm surrounding the Greek War of Independence (1821–1827); and the development of modern national identities through an engagement with ancient classical culture. The Jews, certainly, were not always and not necessarily a component of the story. Nonetheless, one might argue that the celebration and elevation of one group necessarily comes at the expense, if only implicitly, of others. In the case of the ancient Greeks, their elevation was often enough accompanied by the explicit derogation of the Jews, among other ancient groups. F. A. Wolf, for instance, the founder of the academic discipline of *Altertumswissenschaft* (the scholarly study of antiquity),

> explicitly excluded from its domains many of the cultures we now believe constitutive of the ancient world. His *Darstellung* [representation] separated Greeks and Romans from Egyptians, Jews, Persians, and other "Orientals," describing only the first two in the list as possessing "a higher *Geistescultur* (intellectual culture) of their own." The latter, he argued, had only reached the level of *"bürgerliche Policirung oder Civilisation* [policied civility or civilization].²¹

Turner has noted a similar development in Great Britain, exemplified in the writings of William Gladstone. The Greeks, according to the Prime Minister of England, had "nurtured certain fundamental potentialities in human nature that the messianic mission of the Hebrews prevented the chosen people from realizing. These included the capacity for art, science, philosophy, commerce, government, and all those other human activities that provided for the quality of life on earth."²²

Marchand notes that already in the late eighteenth century some of the leading figures in German philhellenism racialized the subject of antiquity, insisting on a link between aesthetic sensibilities and racial qualities. This racialization of the subject of civilization and culture only strengthened over the course of the nineteenth century, so that for philhellenists "the definition of the greatness of the Greeks increasingly set up racial and cultural models that neither past nor present Jews could imitate."²³ The way in which political opponents of Benjamin Disraeli made him into a "Turk" as well as a Jew, and thus sought to challenge his identity as a proper Englishman by "de-civilizing" him, points to the same sort of development in Great Britain.[24]

Even many of those thinkers who situated the Jews within the larger white or Caucasian race nonetheless seemed compelled to then relegate them, together with Arabs and other non-European peoples, to a lower level. The French naturalist Georges Cuvier, for example, divided the world into three main races – Caucasian, Mongolian, and Ethiopian. He placed the Jews in the first category; but like the Arabs, Phoenicians, Egyptians, and others, the Jews too were given over to mysticism, and to an exaggerated imagination. It is, unsurprisingly, to the Gothic and Teutonic nations that we must look for genuine civilization and culture: "It is by this great and venerable branch of the Caucasian stock, that philosophy, the arts, and the sciences have been carried to the greatest perfection, and remained in the keeping of the nations which compose it for more than three thousand years."[25] For normative racial theory, beginning with the Enlightenment, the line from the ancient Greeks to the modern Anglo-Saxons or Teutons was direct. Or, as Martin Bernal has summarized it with regard to the nineteenth century, the predominant "view of world history was one of a dialogue between Aryan and Semite. The Semite had created religion and poetry; the Aryan conquest, science, philosophy, freedom and everything else worth having."[26] Bernal identifies and charts the centuries-long development among European scholars of the ancient world of what he calls *Besserwissen*, the notion that history is about progress and that "we" know better than those who came before.[27] When this combines with more insidious assumptions of racism, anti-Semitism, and ultra-nationalism, it produces a framework within which ancient Egyptian, African, or Semitic peoples by definition must have been incapable of producing anything that contributed fundamentally to the construction of Classical Greece and Western Civilization. My point here is not to endorse or condemn Bernal's reconstruction of what he casts as the dominant scholarly model of understanding and analysis; that would require an expertise far beyond mine.[28] I argue only that when we examine the literature produced about Moses and the rabbis in connection with health and disease, we can identify a counter-narrative that, at least implicitly, repudiates this notion of *Besserwissen*, and that complicates the historiographical tradition of progress and civilization.

2.

In an 1882 pamphlet, *Christentum und jüdische Presse*, the eminent Protestant scholar Franz Delitzsch set forth his view of the Jews' relationship to Christianity and Western civilization:

> If the Jew cannot be convinced that Jesus is the fulfillment of the Law and the Prophets, so he must recognize, that from him [Jesus] a new era commenced, whose blessings have brought benefits even to himself [the Jew]. Are not the Christian people the bearers of culture and civilization? And what were these people before Christianity began to exert its transforming influence? That we know quite well! It is then [with the advent] of Christianity that a new, enduring, spiritually revolutionary, sanctifying principle enters into the world.[29]

As Alan Levenson notes, Delitzsch was hardly an anti-Semite. Over the course of his long career he wrote numerous works celebrating Judaism, and in the world of nineteenth-century Protestant scholarship, Delitzsch falls into the camp of the philosemitic, with all the ambivalence to Jews and Judaism that this entailed. Delitzsch's insistence, then, on the fact that ultimately culture and civilization rest with Christians and Christianity, and that Jews benefited as well from this and would do well to acknowledge it, is revealing precisely because it came from a Christian with deep sympathies towards *Judentum*. Thus, when apologists for Jews and Judaism wrote about the healthy Jews and a hygienic Judaism, they were addressing not only the "diseased Jew" of the anti-Semites, but the assumptions about Jews, Judaism, and civilization articulated at times even by those with a certain sympathy for Jewry.

Thus, the literature on the Jewish contribution to medicine must be read within the broader intellectual and polemical context of the debate over the Jews and their place within Western civilization. In general, writers on Jews and medicine believed that Jews made their greatest contribution to Europe as intellectual and material intermediaries or translators. In the formulation of one authority, writing in 1955, the biblical and talmudic literature contains evidence of a deep, if unsystematic, empirical engagement on the part of Jewish authorities with matters of health and disease: "But the unique contribution of the Jews to medicine was less in discovery than in transmission."[30] Close to a half-century earlier, Joseph Jacobs advanced the same argument. Although we can discern original contributions made by Jewish thinkers and scientists, "it is in their inter-mediation as translators between Islam and Christendom that we have to find the chief valuable function of Jewish intellectual activity in the Middle Ages."[31]

The clearest strategy utilized by proponents of a Jewish contribution to medicine hinged on the notion of translation, both literal and figurative. At the literal level, Jewish scholars translated medical texts. Ancient Greek medicine, like ancient knowledge as a whole, was lost to European Christendom with the fall of the Roman Empire. Only the Jews, or the Jews and the Arabs, managed to preserve this wisdom, thus allowing European knowledge to undergo a renaissance after the demise of the "dark ages." The twelfth century witnessed the revival of medical learning in the West, according to Max Neuburger, the eminent professor of the history of medicine at the University of Vienna. This revival hinged on the dissemination of texts originally written in Greek, translated into Arabic, and then translated into Latin so that they could be studied in the universities of Europe. "The revival of scientific medicine, therefore, chiefly depended upon the work of translators, in which the Jews, the natural mediators between East and West, participated to a large degree."[32] In *Die jüdischen Aerzte im Mittelalter* (*Jewish Physicians in the Middle Ages*), Isak Munz celebrated the role of Jews as original researchers and physicians. Nonetheless, it was as translators that Jews made their signal contribution: "Jewish scholars translated scientific works of the Arabs, and were the conduits of culture between the Orient and Occident. . . . On no other realm of science did the Jews have such an impact and influence during the Middle Ages as on the realm of medicine."[33] The fact that they understood Hebrew, Arabic, Greek, Latin, and Spanish meant that Jews were perfectly suited to translate and comment on medical and scientific works. "It was the Jews who through their translation of ancient Arabic works of medicine facilitated the transmission of this knowledge to the West."[34] In the words of L. Wallerstein, writing over thirty years later, "the bulk of the translation of the Greek [medical] classics into Arabic was accomplished by Jews," thus facilitating the rebirth of scientific medicine in the West.[35] The American Jewish physician Max Thorek celebrated "the zeal of the Jew for the science of medicine," which he traced back to Moses and his "distinct contribution to what is termed 'preventive medicine.'" And Thorek noted the crucial role Jews had played in the translation and transmission of this knowledge during the "dark ages" of Christian Europe:

> During the early Christian era and in the Middle Ages medical science made very little progress. However, some light did filter through to Europe from the Orient, and the Jews were in great measure responsible for this also. For, apart from their own contributions, they served as translators and interpreters of such scientific learning as developed in Persia and Egypt. Indeed, some of the contributions made in these countries, notably on dietary subjects and in ophthalmology, were also made by Jewish physicians who dwelt there.

The Jew, Thorek concluded, had been so prominent in medicine not for any utilitarian reasons but because "it is in his blood." The Jews were poised to make their signal contribution to civilization in the Middle Ages because two thousand years before Jewish tradition and law had formed the Jews in a unique way. The Jew is "not merely a doctor who happens to be a Jew. He is a doctor because he is a Jew."[36]

By the 1930s and 1940s, of course, the argument about the Jewish contribution to civilization was particularly pointed, a direct (and almost wholly ineffectual) response to Nazi propaganda.[37] Nonetheless, the insistence on a specific Jewish contribution to medicine, focused on the translation of texts, reached back much further. In 1830, an American Christian physician, J. K. Walker, argued that contrary to common opinion much of medicine in fact derived from the ancient near East, and the Jews in particular. Walker's strategy was to celebrate the Jewish mediation of knowledge by downplaying or dismissing the historical role of the Arabs. While it was not often acknowledged, he claimed, the Arabs derived their knowledge from the Jews, as had the Greeks: "The works of the Greek physicians have had the good fortune to reach our age, and we know how prone that nation was to extol their own merits at the expense of others. Had any of the works of Jewish physicians been preserved to our day, the respective pretensions of the two might have been on a different basis."[38] Walker's intention in his article, as he made clear, was to demonstrate to his mainly Christian audience "the advanced state of our art [i.e., medicine] among the [ancient] Jews."[39]

In his celebration of the hygienic genius of Moses and the Jews, Marc Brochard offered a detailed rebuttal of the argument put forth by Ernest

Renan and others that Jewish culture was but a "reflection" of that of
the Muslims, revealing an even greater dependence on and similarity to
Islamic than to Christian civilization. "The terms of such a judgment,"
Brochard insisted, "simply must be reversed." It was the Jews who had
reached a level of culture and civilization long before either of the other
two faiths.[40] Seventy years later, writing on the Talmud and medicine, the
physician Lawrence Irwell could assert that "[T]hroughout the middle
ages in Europe and in the East the science of what we now call medicine
was in the hands of the Jews."[41] For Irwell, the Arabs were the destroyers
of medical knowledge; their religion was hostile to scientific learning: "An
immense destruction of medical books, as well as of others, took place
when the Arabs conquered Persia in 639 A.D." According to Irwell, when
the Caliph Omar received a message, asking what was to be done with
all the books that the Arab forces now controlled, the Caliph answered
"Throw them into the river. If they are good for anything, Allah can
and will direct us without them; if good for naught, the sooner we are
rid of them, the better."[42] The Arab engagement with medicine is mentioned but, in Irwell's opinion, it is the Jews who are the prime source of
knowledge and production of science: "It was through the Jews that the
knowledge of medicine penetrated among the Arabs," and through the
Saracens in Spain that medical knowledge was disseminated throughout
Christian Europe.[43] Thus, ultimately it was the Jews who were responsible for medicine in the West. Irwell quotes the French authority P. J. G.
Cabanis, who, in his work *Coup d'oeil sur les revolutions et sur la réforme
de la médecine* (1804), made it clear that it was the Jews alone who "knew
how to treat the sick with some sort of method, and to make a practical
use of the labors of antiquity."[44]

   In 1930, Max Danzis, a prominent American Jewish surgeon and medical writer, insisted that the Arabs, described as "bent on destroying everything of the mind," were themselves less important than the Jews in the
history of Western medicine. The Arabs inherited some medical knowledge from the Nestorians (an Eastern Christian sect), but it was the Jews
whose contribution to the survival of science and medicine was crucial.[45]
The Jews wrote medical works in both Hebrew and Arabic that were
later translated into Latin; they translated ancient works into Latin for
use in the West. What came to be called "Arabic medicine" was introduced into the Western world around the middle of the eleventh century,

largely a product of Jewish efforts: "Jewish scholars, acting under the patronage of Christian bishops, were again active in translating from Arabic the medical works of that day."[46]

This sort of diminution of the Arab contribution to medical history was not limited to Jewish authorities or to Anglo-Americans. One of the most influential general medical histories of the second half of the nineteenth century, Heinrich Haeser's *Lehrbuch der Geschichte der Medicin*, is illustrative of a number of the major themes I am tracing here. Haeser racialized the history of medicine and civilization, and he fully orientalized or semiticized the Jews. But his was not an unambiguous representation of Jews. Haeser traced the origins of medicine to "the ancient Aryans" ("the Asian *Urvolk*") and through them to the Greeks and Germans. When he discussed the origins and development of healing in the ancient world, he began with the Indians, then moved through the Chaldaens, Chinese, and Egyptians.

Haeser devoted very little space to medicine among the ancient Israelites, and presented their knowledge as wholly derivative: "The Jewish people owe the origins of their elevated culture (*höheren Cultur*) directly to the Egyptians. With the exception of monotheism, Moses derived everything from his own masters, the Egyptian priests."[47] As we shall see in Chapter 2, the Polish Jewish scholar Alfred Nossig took up Haeser's model, though he offered a very different representation of the role of Moses and the Jews in the history of hygiene and health. Nonetheless, Nossig agreed with Haeser on this point about Moses, citing the German scholar as the main source for this judgment: "In every major way, Moses constructed his system of social hygiene on the model of the Egyptians [*Im grossen und ganzen hat sich Moses bei dem Ausbau seiner Sozialhygiene an das Vorbild Aegyptens gehalten*]," as well as the Chaldaens.[48] Indeed, Nossig began his extended discussion of the social hygiene of the Jews with the quote from the Book of Acts (7:22): "And Moses was learned in all the wisdom of the Egyptians." But Nossig departed from Haeser in insisting that while Moses may have learned a great deal about medicine from the Egyptian priests, the knowledge and wisdom he set down in his own code far surpassed them. Moreover, the Egyptians and Chaldeans had limited their knowledge to the priestly caste; Moses put his wisdom to the service "of his entire nation" (*auf sein ganzes Volk*).[49]

Haeser, in contrast, represented whatever medical knowledge was to be found in the Mosaic code as wholly derivative. While, of course, Mosaic regulations dealt with diet and prophylactic measures of purity, he claimed, there was no medicine per se in ancient Israelite culture. Later, Jews adopted certain practices, above all from the Phoenicians and Babylonians. Still, "one cannot speak of a scientific approach to healing [*wissenschaftliche Gestaltung der Heilkunde*]" among the ancient Jews.[50]

Haeser granted that one could locate a far more advanced set of health and medical practices in the Talmud, but here, too, he said, the Jews demonstrated no innovation or originality: "The medicine in the Talmud is essentially borrowed from late Greek medicine...." A page later he repeated this: "Without doubt, Talmudic medicine is borrowed from the Greeks."[51] Haeser devoted the next two hundred pages of Volume 1 to the Greeks, and then one hundred and thirty pages to the Romans.

It was in the second book and his analysis of Arabic medicine that Haeser made his argument about the primary role of Jews and Christians, rather than Arabs, in the renaissance of knowledge that occurred in the early Middle Ages. The Jews are fully semiticized here, but they are at the same time distinguished from the Arabs and raised above them. In his discussion of the pre-Islamic period in Arabic lands, Haeser followed those who had argued that Jews and Christians were the primary progenitors of culture and science, citing three works written in French from the first half of the nineteenth century.[52] This intellectual primacy of Jews and Christians continued and strengthened after Islam's conquest. It was in the Spanish lands of the eighth century, as a result of contact with Greek and Roman influences, as well as German elements, "that the Arabic essence or nature [*arabische Wesen*] flowered to its most beautiful and richest level. And the Jews played the greatest role in this."[53] By the second century, the Jews had already settled in the Spanish lands oppressed by Gothic conquerors. The Arabs "appeared as liberators to the Jews" because the Arabs were "of the same racial stock [*Abstammung*] and instilled with the same hatred of the Christians...." When it came to libraries, schools, and first-rate physicians, Moorish Spain far exceeded "the West" of that time. This was due, according to Haeser, to the fact that Spain attracted not only Muslims and Christians but, above all, Jews.[54]

When Haeser came to speak of the general nature of Arabic society, he insisted that ultimately Arabs were incapable of producing an original scientific culture:

> All of this beneficence provided by science notwithstanding, the Arabs in no way reached the heights of intellectual development which might have been expected from so gifted and receptive a people. Their efforts and their creations, apart from poetry, lack the primary requirement of genuine living and productive achievements: independence of spirit [*Selbstständigkeit*]. The scientific achievements and legacy of the Arabic people derives almost exclusively from Greek sources [*Das wissenschaftliche Besitsthum des arabischen Volkes entspringt fast ausschliesslich aus greichischen Quellen*].[55]

In everything, the Arabs have only passively taken over Hellenic knowledge, though they then transformed it in substantive ways. But the Arabs never managed to internalize the Greek manner of feeling and thinking. In tones echoing the most fervent German Graecophilia, Haeser contrasted the Arabs unfavorably with the Greeks:

> The simple naturalness, the bright clarity, the beauty of Greek life, these they [the Arabs] never managed to absorb. These are in conflict with their racial particularity [*Stammes-Eigentümlichkeit*]. In terms of intelligence, receptivity, and business [of culture], the Semite takes a back seat to no other *Volk*; however, they at no time reconciled themselves to the pure and chaste sense of the ideal, the emblem of the Graeco-German.[56]

Haeser seems to have conflated Jews and Arabs into Semites, and denigrated both. But then he proceeded to link the Arab character with the Islamic religion. The greatest impediment to free and productive thought, he argued, was the Koran. It powerfully expressed the idea that anything outside of what it taught was worthless knowledge. But one tends to forget, Haeser concluded, that the Koran was not the root cause but the fruit or expression of the Arab essential nature; in this regard, the Arabs were like all other Oriental peoples who live their entire lives under a patriarchal system of authority. Arab society was characterized by enslavement and blind obedience to authority; so Arabs were closed off to everything beautiful and enlightening in Greek culture. The Jews and Judaism, then, seemed to fall somewhere in-between the Greeks and the Arabs. Racially, Jews were Semites; but they did not share the Arab "essential nature." They were not Greeks, and thus were incapable of appreciating "the pure and chaste ideal" of Hellene; but the Jews were in large measure responsible for the medical and scientific advancements in Arabic lands and thus worthy of being celebrated.

Most scholars did not go this far in their disparagement of the Arab influence on the West. They recognized the primary importance of Arabic contributions to medicine and science, even as they called attention to the mediating role of the Jews. At times, the Jews and Arabs were simply conflated, brought together as a single entity whose difference from and contribution to Europe were duly noted. Thus, the eminent German medical authority Rudolf Virchow, speaking at the International Medical Congress in Rome in 1894, told his audience: "In the early middle ages it was the Jews and Arabs who were largely responsible for the progress of medical science. In our own time Hebrew manuscripts have been brought to light which reveal the keenness and learning of Jewish physicians in the early Middle Ages for the maintenance and progress of medicine."[57]

The British Christian writer Percival Wood reproduced Virchow's argument in a work entitled *Moses: The Founder of Preventive Medicine*. While Wood is a perfect example of the Christian writer who celebrated the health and hygiene of the ancient Israelites while disparaging post-biblical Jewry, nonetheless even he granted that "in justice to the Jews, it should be added that in the dark ages, even in post-biblical times, they were the pioneers in the art of medicine."[58] Almost three decades after Wood, Virchow's words, in a slightly altered translation, were cited by the renowned Italian-Jewish historian of medicine, Arturo Castiglione, in the article he wrote on Jewish contributions to medicine for Louis Finkelstein's well-known multi-volume work, *The Jews: Their History, Culture, and Religion*.[59] Castiglione, too, celebrated Jews as mediators, as translators literal and figurative. The Jews, according to Castiglione, are the "great seekers after truth"; they were uniquely qualified and positioned to mediate between the Arabic and Christian European cultures. Castiglione invoked Moritz Steinschneider's authoritative work on the Jews as translators of Arabic culture in the service of the West. In the Jews' "hands was the light of ancient scientific knowledge and by adding it to Arabic culture they saved Greek science for the Occident."[60]

At times, the Jewish contribution to the West through this act of translation and transplantation was articulated in more specific, nationalist terms. Thus, Heinrich Rosin's *Die Juden in der Medizin* was explicitly apologetic. The real purpose of his book, Rosin wrote, was to prove that, more than any other *Volk*, the Jews have always been "true citizens of their country," have always worked and wished for the best for their *Vaterland*, have always felt the deepest *Vaterlandsliebe* (love of fatherland).[61] Rosin, who posited that the Jews possessed a "hereditary [*erblich*] predisposition for the *Geisteswissenschaften*," would build his apologia on two main themes: first, the Torah contains sanitary and medical proscriptions which, despite the passage of thousands of years, retain their significance; and, second, the importance of the Jews for the history of medicine will be shown with reference to the course of world history ("*Gang der Weltgeschichte*"). Wherever they settled, Jews quickly reached "an unprecedented level of service to the healing arts, both in terms of practice and of research and teaching; and this holds true until today [*unverhältnismäßig hohem Grade im Dienste der Heilkünde, sowohl als Praktiker, wie als hervorragende Förscher und Meister bis auf den heutigen Tag*]".[62]

In a 1937 work, *Contribution des Juifs á la Fondation des Écoles de Médecine en France au Moyen-Age*, the French physician Jules Askenasi celebrated the Jewish contribution to the origins of an organized French medicine. "Every author who has dealt with the origins of medical schools in France is unanimous in saying that Jewish medical men played a significant role."[63] This occurred between the tenth and fourteenth centuries. Askenasi made reference to a number of scholarly authorities, including Castiglione, and Robert Anchel, who insisted on the importance of Jews for the transplantation of Arabic pharmaceuticals, as well as other medical arts into France. And he quoted from an address delivered by Max Neuburger at the First World Congress of Jewish Doctors in Tel-Aviv in 1936. Among other things, Neuburger spoke of the transmission and transplantation of ancient medical knowledge by Jews into France: "The Jewish physicians transplanted to France the knowledge they acquired in the Roman Empire, from Alexandria, Byzantium, Persia, living amongst the Arabs.... Their influence is clearest above all at the moment when the Arabs begin to build their world empire." Askenasi then concluded that "the expansion of scientific medicine relies at this time above all on the activity of translators, the Jews who play a considerable role as direct and natural mediaters between the Orient and the Occident."[64]

The Jews, in this scenario, are "natural mediators" and translate the East to the West, and thereby secure civilization for the West. The Jews are not marginal, but, rather, central and indispensable figures in the rebirth of civilization and culture after the European "dark ages." The Europe that is celebrated and treasured would not have been possible without the Jews. The Anglo-Jewish physician and historian of science Charles Singer argued that the Jews were instrumental in the "revival of learning" that occurred in Europe in the thirteenth century: "Without Jewish aid this earlier Renaissance would have been long delayed and would have assumed a different form. Without the earlier Renaissance the more familiar humanist and classical revival of the fifteenth and sixteenth centuries would have been retarded." Christian Europe could not directly absorb the wisdom of the East; there was desire for knowledge, but also fear and repugnance for the Orient. "Such was the stage whereon, during the Middle Ages, the Jewish role was played. These are the conditions under which the Jews acted as intermediaries between Orient and Occident. . . . The Jewish carriers represent perhaps the most continuously civilized element in Europe."[65]

3.

Translation, then, was cast first of all in literal terms. Jews were the translators of Greek and Arabic texts into Latin, and this made possible the great chain of Western medical knowledge. Translation in figurative terms, though, was just as important to the narratives of the Jewish contribution to medicine. By figurative translation I mean the ways in which mythical and historical Jewish figures, most prominent among them Moses, and Jewish law and ritual found in the Torah, Talmud, and medieval Jewish literature are reinterpreted and reinscribed within a medical and scientific frame. Thus, Moses was the great lawgiver, but his law was first and foremost not a religious but a hygienic code. The Torah was a guide to preventive medicine, its rules and regulations intended to ensure the health and survival of the Jewish nation or people. This figurative translation depended in part on the insistence of equivalence: the Torah and Talmud contained medical knowledge and insight that was oftentimes equivalent, sometimes superior to what scientists had only recently discovered and brought to light. Thus, in the introduction to his 1928 work *Ha-Talmud ve-Chochmat ha-Refuah* (*The Talmud and Medical Knowledge*), Yehuda Katznelson celebrated the fact that it was the ancient rabbis, and not the Greeks, who first understood anatomical pathology. The Greeks believed that external forces caused disease; the rabbis understood that disease was the product of changes internally, to the organs and the physical system. The rabbis articulated the correct principles of anatomical pathology, principles that would be fully grasped in Europe only in the nineteenth century. Moreover, "it was not only that the scholars of Israel preceded the scholars of Greece in their knowledge of pathology, but that *most of their* [the Rabbis'] *pronouncements* were also in accord with modern medicine."[66]

In the nineteenth and twentieth centuries especially, variations on this argument were put forward in hundreds of scientific and popular books and articles. The interpretive tradition of ancient Judaism as hygienic code gained great force especially towards the end of the nineteenth century, as advances in germ theory, bacteriology, and the understanding of disease transmission led physicians and public officials to place even greater emphasis on sanitary or hygiene practices. Vigilance in the home, in the workplace, in public places, and especially in the care for one's own body and mind, were touted as the way to health. Disease could now be prevented, and not just treated, if people could be made to understand the causal connection between germs or bacteria and disease.[67] Moses, many argued, had indeed understood the principles of sanitary science thousands of years ago, and had given the world the first and best code of personal and communal hygiene. In large measure Jewish collective survival had depended on following these laws, whose significance, again, lay not in their religious nature but in the fact that they prescribed and proscribed a host of practices that created the conditions for individual and collective health.

As a rather large body of scholarship has clearly demonstrated, the nineteenth century witnessed the emergence of a full-blown discourse that constructed a racialized and diseased Jew who was the antithesis of and menace to healthy civilization. Jews themselves, to some extent, participated in and contributed to this. It is nonetheless significant that we find an alternative set of ideas and images, produced by non-Jews and Jews, that linked health to civilization, and insisted that the Jews were and remain the supreme representatives of both. Thurman Rice, a professor of public health and eugenics at Indiana University, celebrated the Jews in such terms. The Jews, he argued, offer the best example of the effects of eugenic principles. More than any other people, they have concerned themselves with racial and sexual hygiene, and ensured their collective purity and survival. The practical result of this race purity, according to Rice, has been the contribution Jews have made to every realm of civilization: "In every line of progress the Jew stands at or near the head of the list and has done so for forty or more centuries." Science and medicine, philosophy and literature, music and art, politics, business and finance – all have been made better by Jewish participation. "There is no better argument for the universal practice of the principles of eugenics than the marvelous success of the Jewish race – the only race to put a rational race hygiene to the test, and probably as a consequence the only race of importance to have a history of progress extending over a period as long as a thousand years."[68] It's worth noting that here, in a text that racializes the Jew and Jewish history (in 1929), the Jews are inscribed within the arc of world history. A racial history of the Jews, ironically, undoes Hegel's de-historicization of the Jews; it places Jews and Judaism very near the center of world history, celebrating their past contributions to civilization and holding the Jews up as models for contemporary and future Western civilization.

It is not the case, then, that every racialization of the Jews took place within a negative framework. The Ohio-based physician C. H. von Klein, in a piece that appeared in the *Journal of the American Medical Association (JAMA)* in 1884, also celebrated the Mosaic and talmudic laws in terms of health and hygiene, and linked these to the contributions Jews have made to civilization:

> I will say that the Jews have a superior claim to the respect of society. Statistics speak for them and show that they produce a vast amount less of venereal diseases than any of the civilized or uncivilized nations on the face of the earth. Above all, I believe that the sanitary mode of Jewish life has great tendency to cultivate the brain and mind. The Jewish race appears to produce a greater per cent. [*sic*] of great men (according to their numbers) in every branch of science and art than any other sect or creed on the earth.

By every branch, he means to include music, theatre, philosophy, poetry, business and finance, and of course physicians and medical researchers.

"Medicine appears to be the favorite study, and as a rule, they always maintain a high standing."[69]

Von Klein did not stop there. The Jews had not only contributed to civilization through their own efforts, as impressive as these had proven. Their contribution could also be found in their influence on leading Western scientists. Jews, von Klein wrote, mistakenly remain silent today in Europe and America about the Talmud and its influence, because they fear prejudice and because they fail to understand the real power of the Talmud. The Talmud's value is, ultimately, not theological but scientific: "It is said Galileo read medicine with a Jewish physician who taught him the Talmud, and from which he formed his ideas of astronomy.... They [the Jews] forget that the *Codex Romana* is taken from the Talmud, on which is based all the moral and civil law of all civilized governments." And they forget, of course, the medical and scientific genius of men like Maimonides, Nachmanides, Rashi, Abraham ibn Ezra, and so on. "Those names just mentioned are but a few of the great commentators, whose discourses taken separately would no doubt be approved by the present most advanced minds of sanitary science."[70]

This argument about the nexus of Judaism as hygienic code, the Jews as a healthy people, and their contribution to culture and civilization appears in one of the most widely disseminated apologetic tracts published in the last quarter of the nineteenth century: Matthias Jakob Schleiden's *Die Bedeutung der Juden für die Erhaltung und Wiederbelebung der Wissenschaften im Mittelalter*.[71] While Schleiden's essay ranged over the gamut of the natural sciences, he did pay a good amount of attention to the Jewish contribution to health and medicine. The Jews, he argued, "considered it further a moral duty to attend to public hygiene as well as the preservation of individual bodily health by means of a suitable diet, careful nursing, and general medical treatment of the sick. This explains how the majority of the Rabbis were well acquainted with medical knowledge devoting themselves to the practice of medicine."

In contrast to Haeser, who had elevated the Jews at the expense of the Arabs, Schleiden celebrated the Jews' wisdom while he denigrated Christians. Counter to the normative narrative of the history of medicine, Schleiden insisted that the Jews had founded the great medical schools in Montpelier and Salerno, and before that they were really the only physicians and medical authorities in Europe; the "incomprehensibly ignorant and crude Christians" believed that the Jews were naturally gifted with medical knowledge, and so left it to them. Kings and princes, including famously Francis I, would have only Jewish physicians (even baptized Jews were sent away). Until the sixteenth century, "the most famous physicians were, to a preponderant extent, Jews."[72] A few pages later, Schleiden summed up the relationship of Jews to Christians: "The preceding data should sufficiently prove that the Jews until the thirteenth century were infinitely superior to their Christian contemporaries both in their general intellectual endowments and their practical pursuits in applied science."[73]

As Ulrich Charpa has recently noted, Schleiden's essay was widely circulated, and beginning in the 1870s, with the economic crash and rising anti-Semitism in Germany and Austria, became a critical text for Jewish apologetics.[74] According to Charpa, Schleiden's intervention into the debate about the Jews and *Kultur* should be understood as a response to Theodor Billroth, professor of medicine in Vienna, and his "defamatory book" *Über das Lernen der medizinischen Wissenschaften an den Universitäten der deutschen Nation* (Vienna, 1876). Billroth had attacked Jewish medical students as a collective in his work, and by the late 1870s had become "a leading figure of academic anti-Semitism in the German-speaking countries. . . ."[75] As with so many other racialist thinkers of his day, he drew parallels between the plant, animal, and human realms, and extended his own convictions, as a realist, about the world of nature to that of the human: there are clear boundaries within the plant world, and so there ought to be clear boundaries in the realm of the "races." Billroth wrote of the need to maintain *"rein deutsches and rein jüdisches Blut* (pure German and pure Jewish blood)."[76] Thus, Jewish medical students did not belong in the same class, or even in the same universities with their Christian German counterparts. Boundaries and categories were real and had to be maintained.

Schleiden, Charpa argues, was more of a nominalist, comfortable with a certain "conceptual vagueness" and a blurring of boundaries and categories. Like Billroth, Schleiden moved methodologically and epistemologically from the plant and animal worlds to the human. But he drew very different conclusions. Schleiden embraced intermixture, representing it as both inevitable and healthy. In the case of the Jews, he argued that it was just such intermixture that helped to account for progress in medicine. Charpa reproduces a remark of Schleiden's from the *Bedeutung* that for some reason had been excised from the English translation: "If Prof. Billroth...takes pleasure in digging up his old prejudice (Auerbach has obviously failed to reprimand him strongly enough), that is his business. But how can a teacher in a university reveal such a boundless ignorance about the history of his own science at the same time? He is evidently not aware of the immense importance of the Jews for medicine and has not realized that without the Jews there would probably be no Professor Billroth." Charpa comments: "This sounds amusing, but it contains a remarkable idea. For Schleiden, the appropriate attitude toward Judaism is a consequence of the correct attitude toward scientific progress."[77] Schleiden understood the Jews to be an essential link in the chain of scientific knowledge, an inextricable component of "the history of epistemic dependence." Whatever reliable knowledge we possess today we owe in some degree to the efforts of those who came before. "Consequently, it is appropriate to acknowledge other people's contributions to 'the preservation and revival of learning'."[78] Ultimately, Charpa argues, Schleiden's reasons for defending Judaism and the Jews lay in his belief that anti-Semitism was founded on "false convictions." That is, he did not condemn it out of any fondness for Jews per se, or out of moral beliefs. "His argument was not *pro bono, contra malum,* but *pro vero, contra falsum.*"[79]

Surely part of the reason for the popularity of Schleiden's text had to do with its content. But more than this, as even commentators at the time noted, it was the fact that Schleiden was not a Jew that gave his arguments whatever force and influence they carried. (In this, Schleiden was similar to Hermann Strack, whose work will be discussed in Chapter 2.) In the preface to the British edition of Schleiden's text, Rabbi Hermann Gollancz insisted that the genuine value of the work was that it was the product of "a non-Jewish author, writing in a spirit of independence and from conviction."[80] In his introduction, the text's translator made the same point. The brief book was remarkable, Maurice Kleimenhagen wrote, but not because it contained anything new or startling in the way of subject matter.

[What] characterizes it as highly remarkable is the fact that its author was a Christian Professor of Science, who wrote and published this essay at a time when the battle of Anti-Semitism in Germany and Austria had reached its culminating point; when that execrable movement had assumed threatening proportions, not stopping short at the disfiguring of historical truth, trying to rob Judaism of its reputation in the world of letters and learning, which it had well earned by generations of gifted scholars, whose work had left its mark upon the development of almost every field of human research and knowledge. It is difficult to understand how historical, bibliographical, and even encyclopedic works could omit to mention names of the first order, such as Maimonides, or accord them but the merest passing notice.[81]

Schleiden may not have offered his readers anything startlingly new, but his enthusiastic and hyperbolic celebration of the Jews' contribution more than made up for any lack of originality: "I have shown how during the whole of the Middle Ages, while all European Nations stood still or retrograded, or, like the Germanic People, had scarcely advanced at all, the Jews stepped forward energetically on the path of mental progress, and developed every side of scientific life, and how much of their acquisitions had been transferred to the various nations who were commencing a new intellectual life by the end of the Middle Ages." The "ignorant Christians" could not, of course, understand the languages that the knowledge of the old world had been communicated in. So the Jews had to step forward and translate. "Had the Jews not done good work as translators, the darkness of mediaeval life would not have been lifted from us for a long time."[82] Schleiden mentioned the Arabs, but they, too, owed their knowledge to the Jews, who translated and interpreted Greek literature for them. Over the centuries Jewish scholars had translated theological, medical and natural scientific works into Arabic, or into Latin so that it could then be translated into Arabic.

In the end, Schleiden made the Jews responsible in large measure for the preservation and transmission of all of Western civilization. During the "intellectually dark and slothful Middle Ages," the Jews preserved agriculture, and "all large industries"; international trade that was so vital "to the well-being of all the nations." The Jews "left no branch of science or learning untouched, ever searching and developing," and then transmitting this to the Christians, who could only then begin the arduous process of awakening from their intellectual slumber. The Jews were the founders of systematic philology, their fruitful modes of textual interpretation contrasted with the "narrow mindedness and ignorance of the Christian clergy." The Jews alone cultivated freely the study of philosophy, and especially ethics and practical morality: "We find again that it was a special object of research with the Jews to elaborate a methodical and scientific study of medicine."[83] Schleiden concluded by quoting another Christian scholar, Ribeyra de Santos, from the work *Memorias de Litteratura Portugeuesa* (1792–1814): "We are largely indebted to the Jews for our first knowledge of philosophy, botany, medicine, astronomy, cosmography, no less than for the elements of grammar, the sacred languages, and almost all branches of biblical study."[84] Even if, as discussed in Chapter 2, the fullest elaboration of this theme of Jews, science, and civilization came from a Polish Jew working in Paris, it is imperative to note that Christians, too, disseminated an apologetic argument that identified the Jews with all areas of valuable and necessary knowledge, and granted them a central role in the development of culture and civilization.

2

Moses the Microbiologist

Alfred Nossig's *The Social Hygiene of the Jews*

I.

In 1894 Alfred Nossig, a 30-year-old Polish Jewish writer, artist, and social scientist, published a history of "the social hygiene of the Jews and ancient Oriental nations" (*Die Sozialhygiene der Juden und des altorientalischen Volkerkreises*).[1] Born in 1864 in Lvov (Lemberg), Nossig studied natural sciences, medicine, law, and philosophy at the universities of Lemberg and Czernowitz, and received a doctorate in law from the University of Czernowitz in 1888. He moved to Vienna in 1892, and then to Paris, where he completed the research and writing of his book on social hygiene.[2] Nossig wanted to contribute, as he told his readers, to the current debate in European parliaments and in the press over questions of public health and policy.[3] Through descriptive analyses of the ancient law codes of China, India, Persia, Egypt, and predominately Israel, Nossig sought to show how these systems had resulted in the five nations' superior biological and moral qualities and how they might, in turn, serve as models for contemporary states and societies. According to Nossig, these law codes were not religious in nature; rather, they were rules of hygiene intended to maintain and advance the health of the individual, family, nation, and race.[4]

Nossig, like others discussed in this book, took advantage of the decline of the long-standing idea that Egypt was the origin of philosophy and science even as he sought to challenge the notion that the Greeks deserved this honor. Jews and Judaism were now being offered as the ultimate source of civilization, if by this one meant not only, or chiefly, the invention of monotheism but also, or even more so, the science of health and hygiene. Nossig's view is evident first of all from the very structure of his book. He begins with a two-page discussion of the Chinese; he devotes six pages to the Indians and five to the Persians. To the Egyptians he gives over nine pages. The remainder of the work's one hundred and fifty pages is devoted to the Jews.

As we saw in Chapter 1, the task that Nossig and others had to perform if they were going to make a viable case for the Jewish contribution to civilization was to separate the Jews and Judaism (or the ancient Israelites) from the Egyptians and other ancient Oriental peoples and link them with Europe. At the same time, they had to deny the main arguments of those who insisted on the racial and cultural superiority of the Greeks/Aryans. This was the role that medicine and science could play, once the Mosaic code and the Talmud had been translated into works of health and hygiene.

Nossig defined social hygiene in the broadest terms, including matters of environment – air, water, earth, public and private space – which had been fundamental to public sanitation movements since the early decades of the nineteenth century.[5] However, he also extended the definition to matters that, by the end of the century, had come to be considered questions of "national" or "racial" health. Social hygiene, in Nossig's words, "encompasses not only the familiar rules of public sanitation, but all things which influence the health and life of a people: its morals, its marriage customs, its sexual life."[6] In the ancient world and into the present, social hygiene's primary goal was "the preservation and advancement of the physical well-being of the nations. 'Physical well-being' – says [Rudolf] Virchow – 'is the foundation of all cultivation and freedom [*Bildung und Freiheit*]'; it is, we should add, the foundation of prosperity [*Gluckes*], of the development and the perseverance of the Nation."[7]

The Jews, Nossig argued, had survived and developed as a nation over thousands of years because they had adhered to the laws of hygiene set down for them in the Torah and its rabbinic and medieval commentaries. This system enabled the Jews to maintain their purity (*Reinheit*) as a nation. Moses, the rabbis of the Talmud, Maimonides, and other Jewish luminaries were first and foremost physicians (*Ärtze*) and men of state – the equivalents of modern medical authorities and sanitation officials – whose task was to preserve the physical and moral health of the *Volk*. In this regard, and in their knowledge of the science of medicine and hygiene, these "wise men" had already achieved, and in some cases surpassed, gains made by modern states and societies.

Nossig made the same point about the other four nations and their leaders. In discussing ancient Egypt, for example, he pointed to a number of areas in which modern notions and practices of health were either equaled or surpassed: The Egyptians' moderation in eating and drinking was similar to "today's vegetarians"; already thousands of years ago the Egyptians could boast of specialized medicine and state-supported physicians. "The Egyptians in all important points concerning public health service already reached a height which present-day hygiene designates as an ideal goal: the position of physicians was state-supported, the physicians were servants of the state in the realm of national health, therapies were regulated so as to prevent incompetence." Regarding ancient Israel, Nossig argued similarly that the Pentateuch contains a "highly developed social hygiene system. We find a place for state physicians – the priests of the tribe of Levi – whose task it is to investigate every suspicious case" of leprosy and other skin diseases.[8] These comments about an ideal interdependence between physicians and the state reflect developments in Europe, and particularly Germany, during the last half of the nineteenth century (and we will discuss a similar development in Great Britain and America in Chapter 3). Very generally, the problems of industrialization and urbanization allowed unparalleled growth in the power and prestige of doctors and health officials; in Germany, more than elsewhere, the power and prestige were tied to state and bureaucracy.[9]

Nossig's work presents an emphatically positive image of historical and contemporary Jewry constructed out of the language, ideas, and assumptions current throughout the Europe of the time. Science (*Wissenschaft*) is the overarching and unquestioned authority. Religion, Nossig asserts, is obscurantist, at least until it is reinterpreted and given its true meaning.[10] Science validates the history and literature of the Jews once their rituals and laws are shown to be, ultimately, scientific and not religious in nature. At the same time, the myriad scientific and medical ideas and practices that had come to prominence in the latter half of the nineteenth century – social hygiene, bacteriology, social Darwinism, and racial anthropology – are reinterpreted as ancient and, in particular, Jewish discoveries or innovations. Modern medicine and science are reconceived as ancient Jewish law, and this scientific tradition is, in turn, used to validate and celebrate Jews and Judaism.

A close reading of Nossig's work, which I undertake here, offers the opportunity to explore in greater detail the interpretive tradition of "the healthy Jew," and also, in turn, to explore the ways in which Jews responded to changing ideas about science and medicine in the last quarter of the nineteenth century and the pertinence of these intellectual shifts in the social and political realms. In part, Nossig's text must be read as a response to an anti-Semitic movement that had appropriated the language of science and medicine; it was also one attempt of the many he was to make to lend scholarly, scientific support to Zionism – a movement with which, by 1894, he had been involved for over seven years. Nossig's interpretation of the relationship between Judaism and social hygiene challenged the negative image of the Jews as inferior and dangerous with counterclaims of their physical and moral superiority. And it equated Jewish law and tradition with all that was believed healthy and good in modern society. By writing Judaism and Jewry into the center of the story of Western civilization and progress, Nossig rejected the idea of Jewish marginality, of the Jew as outside the European drama. By linking the Jews, through traditional religious law and custom and its greatest interpreters, to science – and more specifically to medical knowledge – he sought to dispel at least two related contentions of fin de siècle anti-Semitism: first, that in biophysical terms Jews were agents of disease and degeneration; and second, that Jews were culturally parasitical, able to "barter" in ideas, but unable to create and genuinely contribute to Christian European civilization. Jews, in other words, were facile at imitation but incapable of original contributions to culture and science.

By reinterpreting Jewish law as modern medicine, Nossig might also establish Judaism's potential relevance, not only for Jews but also non-Jews. As already mentioned, he understood his work in part as a demonstration of how the ancient codes – most especially, the Mosaic code – could serve as models for contemporary societies; this at a time when elites throughout Europe were deeply concerned about national and racial health, and increasingly haunted by the fear of demographic decline and physical (as well as cultural) degeneration. The collective survival of the Jews for thousands of years, and their contemporary health and vitality (demonstrated empirically through vital statistics) suggested that nations interested in survival, in staving off decline and disappearance, might do well to look to the Jews.

Moreover, by demonstrating the biological, as well as the historical and cultural reality and unity of the Jewish people, Nossig could provide a theoretical underpinning to Jewish nationalism.[11] His counter-narrative denied the liberal "assimilationist" definition of *Judentum* as a community united solely by religious belief (*Glaubensgenossenschaft*), substituting instead a definition constructed around the concepts of *Volk, Stamm, Nation*, and *Rasse*. The history of Judaism as hygiene was, simultaneously, the "history" of the formation and preservation of the Jews as a *Volk*. This does not mean that every, or even most, of the scholars who recast Moses as a sanitarian or touted the health benefits of Jewish laws were Zionists. I am not arguing for any natural affinity between a particular interpretive tradition and a Jewish ideological position. Elsewhere I have addressed Nossig's interpretation of Jewish history and law as a developing intellectual and ideological strategy, a contribution to the evolving discourse on Jews, health, and disease that informed the "Jewish Question" and that aided Nossig in formulating a position in support of Jewish nationalism based on social science.[12] While I will address both anti-Semitism and Zionism as forces at work in Nossig's thinking about Jews and hygiene, my chief interest here is with exploring his book as the fullest expression of the interpretative tradition of Jewish law and history circulating at the time and after, the translation of Moses into a microbiologist.

2.

That Moses stood on scientific grounds, and that his elevated, penetrating intellect was not clouded by religious delusion, this is a statement which only a thinker who is intimate with the fact of the development and progress of science can accept; a statement which fundamentally differentiates Mosaic legislation from all other ancient Oriental systems and affirms its eternal youth and vitality.[13]

Like other thinkers encountered in Chapter 1, Nossig asserted that the Mosaic code of law was both "Oriental" and yet distinct and superior to all other ancient Oriental systems. Judaism could be seen to have originated in the Orient, but it did not suffer the same fate as those other systems. Its "eternal youth and vitality," which points to and will largely explain the vitality of the Jewish people, means that, contra Hegel and others, Judaism remains within the realm of history, in a symbiotic relationship with science, progress, and civilization. This is so because the laws of Moses are not religious but scientific in nature. However, one must be able to understand the ancient laws in the correct way, in the "deep sense" (*"tiefe Sinn"*) as Nossig writes elsewhere.[14]

The opposition between progressive science (*Wissenschaft*) and regressive religion, enunciated by Nossig, was a familiar theme in the late nineteenth century. The intellectual challenge of bringing Jewish thought and law into line with current, paradigmatic philosophical systems reached back centuries. Beginning in the first half of the nineteenth century, Jewish elites faced the task of making Judaism consonant with the demands of Enlightenment rationalism and civic emancipation, with reforming the Jews and Judaism according to the standards of Europe. The degree to which the nineteenth-century *Wissenschaft des Judentums* was impelled by the goals of reform, regeneration, and integration is well known.[15] Jewish nationalists, Nossig among them, rejected the ideal of social and cultural assimilation; nonetheless, they too embraced the goal of reform and regeneration. Social hygiene offered one way of accomplishing the task of reconciliation between Judaism and European civilization, and at least the potential of aiding the reform of Jewry. It represented both a thing in itself and a code for something much greater.

At the outset of his work on hygiene, Nossig stated categorically that social hygiene would come to be one of the leading sciences (*Hauptwissenschaften*), in fact the "darling science" (*Lieblungswissenschaft*) of the twentieth century. He proceeded to link social hygiene to the great achievements of natural science – physics, chemistry, physiology, pathology, and, finally, technology – and then with the process of civilization itself: "There are as many epochs of hygiene as there are civilizations, and where we find a civilization emerging we find a theoretical and practical system of hygiene."[16] Social medicine, then, was a series of limited concepts and practices that produced health on the individual, social, and national levels. Yet it also represented modernity and progress, in both the material and moral spheres.[17]

The translation, therefore, of ancient Jewish law and ritual into modern European medicine potentially achieved at least two things. First, it "redeemed" the Jewish tradition by demonstrating that it is not religion but science. Judaism could therefore still be embraced – if not necessarily traditionally observed – by the non-observant (including Zionist) as well as observant Jews. At the same time, by equating Judaism with modern hygiene and medicine, Jews and Judaism were transformed into something vital, even essential, to the European present and future. Both the anti-Semitic charge that Jewry was responsible for the degeneration of Europe as well as the image of the Jew as dirty and diseased – or, in fact, as disease itself – are directly refuted by Nossig's narrative. Purity and health, progress and freedom are all linked inextricably to historical and contemporary Jewry.

Nossig accomplished this through the strategy of translation or equivalence. While he explicitly called his work a history and stressed the importance of development over time, he repeatedly collapsed the distinctions between ancient and modern: "We find expressed in the Pentateuch all aspects of modern social hygiene: the hygiene of earth, water, and air; laws against contagious diseases; the hygiene of habitation and clothing; food hygiene, the hygiene of cosmetics, of sexual life, and national life." Each of the founders of the great cultures of the ancient Orient in fact – Confucius, Manu, Zoroaster, Menes, and, above all, Moses – were "men of state and physicians," concerned with the purity and health of their nations. Solomon and the later kings were all "doctors"; Ezra and Nehemiah possessed an "exact pharmacological knowledge"; and a type of "collegium of physicians" existed in the Temple of Jerusalem.[18]

Nossig extended this narrative of the Jews and medicine into the Middle Ages, when the luminaries, in his view, were all men of science and medicine. Rashi was a surgeon, Abraham Ibn-Ezra well versed in medical works. The ideal of preventive medicine, central to the modern social hygiene movement, was already enunciated by the Jewish philosopher Isaac Israeli in the tenth century: "The most important task of the physician is to help avert illness." Nossig then proceeded to ask rhetorically: "Is it not as if the voice of a Skoda, a Nothnagel, a Virchow [all prominent in nineteenth-century public medicine] had been heard here? We see that Arabic-Jewish medicine has subscribed to a point of view already in the tenth century which the progressive part of today's medicine has once again taken as its own: the healing power of nature, the importance of diet, the prevention of illness as the actual goal of medicine." Maimonides, according to Nossig, was a "modern spirit" who transcended his time and was responsible for saving medicine and science for the West. Like Heinrich Haeser, on whose work he relied, Nossig elevated the Jewish contribution to Western civilization by degrading that of the Arab; yet, like Matthias Jakob Schleiden, Nossig also assumed the degeneration of Christendom, so that Judaism alone was able to fulfill the task of transmitting civilization. Maimonides, Nossig wrote, was blessed "with the insight of a prophet." He understood that Arabic civilization was descending into a period of degeneration, that the Christian West was sunk in ignorance and superstition, and that the scientific knowledge passed down over the centuries was in danger of being lost. Maimonides lived in an epoch of "deep intellectual derangement" (*geistliche Umnachtung*), yet succeeded in preserving and renewing Jewish social hygiene. He spoke "almost with the words of the modern hygienist" about the detrimental effects on public health of putrid air, infected waters, and earth overflowing with refuse. Already in the twelfth century, Maimonides concerned himself with "almost all the sources and causes of life-shortening diseases which [occupy] modern medical research."[19]

Nossig discovered in the traditional Jewish law code a theory and praxis of racial hygiene comparable to that of the modern era: "Mosaic legislation, consciously through the rules of sexual life, seeks above all the health of its descendants and the strength of the race." Moses sought to make the entire nation pure, to keep the Jews from mixing their blood with the impure blood of other peoples: "He understood that herein lay the decisive point: that the law of strict national separation of the Hebrews constituted the cornerstone, whose shattering would bring with it the collapse of the entire boldly erected structure." The Talmud extended the biblical rules of sexual hygiene into more stringent laws of "racial and national separateness." Nossig referred to talmudic rules of purity as "*sozialhygienische Politik der Gemara*," echoing the contemporary German term for social policy. He then proceeded to claim that "modern science must approve of the principles of *Seder Taharoth* [rules of purity]. . . . The modern hygienist must be astounded at the insights and observations of the Talmud."[20] The Bible and Talmud are transformed here into vehicles of biological purity. The ritual law retains its meaning and significance because it mirrors contemporary European ideas and goals. This is the source of its power in the modern age.

Nossig also introduced contemporary debates over eugenics and social Darwinism into his discussion of Jewish sexual laws. The Mosaic law, he argued, rejects the "struggle for existence" (*Kampf um Dasein*) based on the State's preservation of "the lives of only those best equipped, most powerful and gifted," and elimination of those poorly equipped for life (*die schlechter Ausgestatteten vernichten*). The law rejects the "selection of men" as if this were the "selection of cattle."[21] In a section entitled "The Causes of Biological Superiority of Contemporary Jews," Nossig again rejected the notion that the struggle for existence should be militaristic. Taking up a common theme of nineteenth-century writings on Jews, he referred to the Jews' loss of military abilities after the disappearance of state and sovereignty. However, contrary to the widely held view that this was a physical and moral detriment, Nossig presented this as a positive virtue biologically. Independence from military service meant the absence of the harmful military selective process, which, in turn, meant that the "strongest and healthiest individuals were not snatched away during those years when they were in the bloom of reproductive activity; the health capital of the nation and the number of male new-born (in relation to female) would therefore be higher."[22]

Elsewhere in the work, however, Nossig appeared far more ambivalent about harsh measures undertaken to strengthen the nation and race. As part of the effort to prevent venereal disease among his people, Moses forbade marriage and sexual relations with foreign women ("*Ausländerinnen*"). Nossig quoted the biblical verses from Numbers (31:9–18) in which Moses sees that the Israelites have killed all the men of Midian but have taken women prisoners back to camp. He orders all Midian women who have had relations with Israelite men killed. According to Nossig: "One sees what determined measures Moses will take when it is a matter of preventing a significant danger to the health of his people. Overall, there is no more radical means for the prevention of venereal diseases than the killing of mass numbers of human beings [*gesammten Menschenmaterial*] who can cause infection."[23]

It is unclear what conclusions Nossig wanted his readers to draw about contemporary social policy from this example. What is evident, however, is that he read current debates over positive and negative eugenics back into the Bible and antiquity. As we shall see in Chapter 4, Nossig was far from alone in understanding biblical and post-biblical law, and Jewish historical experience, within the frame of Darwinism and eugenics.

3.

Nossig's transformation of Moses into a sanitarian and proto-eugenicist represented, of course, a fairly new interpretive turn; it hinged on recent developments in the medical and natural sciences. However, the translation of Moses through embellishment and interpretation of the biblical text was not a recent or modern practice; nor was the image of Moses as a master of knowledge and wisdom. This sort of translation of Moses occurred already in the ancient Hellenistic world. Artapanus, an Egyptian Jew writing sometime in the second century BCE, offered up Moses as the inventor of a sizeable part of Egyptian culture and civilization. Among Moses' inventions and contributions to Egyptian civilization were "ships, weaponry, stone-lifting machines and irrigation systems (vital for Egyptian agriculture) all of which made him dearly loved by the people and popular with the king."[24] Ezekiel, most likely an Alexandrian Jew who lived in the late third or second centuries BCE, composed a play called *Exagogue (Exodus)* that imagined Moses as a Hellenized rather than Egyptian Hebrew, and sought to demonstrate the commensurability of Jewish and Greek culture. For Ezekiel, Moses was the model of the "educated and religious Jew" who at the same time was "fully conversant with the Greek civilization – precisely the 'ideal' which Ezekiel himself embodied with his intense loyalty to the Jewish people intricately combined with his Hellenistic training."[25] Here, Moses is no longer the inventor of civilization but its inheritor. He had been, as Luke has Stephen tell it in the Book of Acts (7:22), "instructed in all the wisdom of the Egyptians."

This is the Moses who appears repeatedly in texts produced by Hellenistic Jewish authors. Ezekiel's *Exagogue* transmits the idea that Moses learned at the Egyptian court; Josephus also includes this in his *Antiquities* (2.236). Philo, in his *Life of Moses* (1.21–24), sets out the various realms in which Moses was instructed by "learned Egyptians": Moses has mastered geometry, arithmetic, astronomy, rhetoric, music, and the philosophy of symbols (i.e., the esoteric wisdom concerning the gods and their worship conveyed through hieroglyphs, which included animal

worship).[26] Early Christian writers, such as Luke, and the early Church
Fathers, reinscribed Moses into their own narratives for their own particular theological and polemical purposes.[27] The image of "Moses the
magician," derived from the Exodus narrative of Moses' competition
with the Pharaoh's priests and magicians, circulated widely in the ancient
world among both Jews and non-Jews. It was such a popular image that,
according to John Gager, Philo and Josephus felt it necessary to compose
texts that countered the idea by emphasizing Moses the philosopher and
lawgiver, and making Moses' power qualitatively different from that of
the Egyptian priests.[28]

One notable point, within the context of this discussion, is that
medicine and the healing arts are absent from Philo and from the other
Hellenistic Jewish authors.[29] Moses was philosopher, lawgiver, magician,
even inventor of ancient arts and sciences. Moses as physician or healer,
however, does not seem to have been a common image. And yet for the
Greeks, one of the celebrated components of the "wisdom" of the Egyptians was the healing arts. Homer defined the unparalleled wisdom of
the Egyptians in part with reference to medicine. Herodotus, in his *Histories*, called the Egyptians the wisest of all men and credited them with
a host of cultural and scientific inventions and achievements that influenced the Greeks. Among these was their "medical expertise; they do
not even have generalists but instead specialists for every single disease"
(Book 2:84). Diodorus Siculus and others followed Herodotus in assign-
ing to the Egyptians a genius for healing.[30] Jan Assmann, in his work
Moses the Egyptian, has noted that diseases such as plague and leprosy
figured prominently in a number of ancient narratives – or what Amos
Funkenstein has called counter-narratives – about Moses and the origins
of the Jews. In the texts of Manetho, Hecataeus of Abdera, Lysimachor,
and Chaeremon, Moses stands at the head of a marginal group of diseased misfits who must flee Egypt and who end up creating a state and
cultic religion that was the negative inversion of the Egyptian.[31] Other
narratives, such as Pompeius Trogus' *Historicae Philippicae*, cast Moses
not as an Egyptian, but as the son of Joseph. Moses leaves Egypt in
possession of Egypt's wisdom and sacred objects, and sets up his cult
in Jerusalem as an extension of "*sacra Aegyptia*."[32] But here, too, the
cause of Moses' departure was plague and sickness. We are closer here

to a "hygienic" explanation for the Exodus, to Moses as a healer in the tradition of Egyptian wisdom, and to the notion of the Mosaic code as a system of hygiene and health.

Moses was seen at times as a healer or "physician" in rabbinic literature. One midrash, for example, comments on the biblical story of Miriam, Moses' sister, who was struck with a terrible skin disease after criticizing her brother's choice of an Ethiopian wife. The midrash, in the words of one medical historian, "relates that Moses went before God and said, 'You taught me the art of medicine and now I am a competent physician; I would prefer that you heal my sister, but if you refuse I will do it on my own account.'"[33]

Thus, the Moses of modern medical narratives, including Nossig's, is just one Moses out of the many imagined over the centuries. Indeed, he is merely one of the various Moseses imagined in just the past two hundred years. Arnold Band has written about four different modern Jewish thinkers and their conceptions of Moses. The Jewish *maskil* Naftali Hertz Wessely published a six-volume epic poem in Hebrew, *Shire Tiferet*, about the life of Moses. According to Band, Wessely's Moses is a "fusion of the traditional Jewish Moses with the reasonableness of Nathan from Lessing's play *Nathan der Weise*.... He is portrayed as the reliable intermediary between God and his people, firm in his opposition to Pharaoh and all other 'sinners,' but striking in his rationality." Wessely had evinced a profound and long-standing interest in the Apocryphal "Wisdom of Solomon," and so in his poem, the Torah and Wisdom (*Chokhmah*) too become fused. "Moses is thus really a projection of Wessely's version of the desired enlightened Jew.... the rational instructor who leads his people into a world of rational illumination."[34] Wessely, then, was the latter-day incarnation of Moses: an enlightened leader of his people. Band goes on to discuss Nachman of Bratslav, whose Moses was a mystical, messianic figure; Ahad Ha'am, whose Moses was the biblical prophet prepared to lead his people out of slavery and exile, but whose demanding righteousness ultimately proved too much for his own people; and, of course, Sigmund Freud's Moses. With Freud we encounter the Moses of Michaelangelo, a Christian and Renaissance Moses, and the Moses of psychoanalysis.[35] And these are only five of the many Moseses that Band could have examined.

4.

Thus, when Nossig (along with the other scholars and writers whose works concern us) makes Moses into a leader possessed of extraordinary knowledge valued by the nations, he is participating in a much older intellectual tradition. At the same time, the medical frame is decidedly recent. It gains its power, in large measure, from the ongoing concern with infectious diseases, the heightened consciousness of germs, and the marked recognition, even celebrity, of researchers such as Robert Koch and Louis Pasteur. Indeed, the most straightforward examples of Nossig's strategy of equivalence derive from his discussions of bodily disease and disinfection. Germs and microbes figure prominently in his reinterpretation of disease in Jewish law. Moses, we are told, possessed a knowledge of diseases and the means of their transmission commensurate with modern pathology. Nossig quoted the French physician Noël Guéneau de Mussy, whose *Étude sur l'hygiene de Moïse et des anciens Israelites* constituted a major source for his own work (as well as for many other writers on Jewish health whom we shall consider later):

> The idea of parasitical and infectious illness, which occupies such a conspicuous place in modern pathology, appears to have actively occupied Moses; one can say that this idea dominated all of his hygiene proscriptions. One need only take a word "impure" – which over the centuries has acquired a moral connotation – in a medical hygienic sense, and one would be able to read modern sanitary rules in the Bible.

Nossig then continued in his own words: "The recognition of pathogenic germs or microbes, and the fear of their effect – or as Guéneau de Mussy expresses it: *cette intuition prophétique des microbes à travers les siècles* – is the basis of Mosaic 'soil-hygiene' [*Bodenhygiene*]."[36] The Israelites make a place outside camp to relieve themselves and then bury the excrement (Deut. 23: 12–13), demonstrating the "common knowledge," Nossig concluded, that typhus and dysentery are mainly caused by non-disinfected waste matter and infected air.[37]

The Hebrews, in Nossig's view, understood that germs can be passed along through clothing and can attach themselves to the walls of one's residence. Moses' knowledge of microbes thus led him to order the burial of contaminated clothing and the intermittent inspection of housing. "The writer of the Bible understood the anatomy and physiology of microbes as well as possible without a microscope." Nossig reinterpreted the purification ceremony involving the ashes of the red heifer as a medical practice of disinfection based on Moses' "modern" understanding that a mixture of water, vegetable, and animal ash is a powerful purifying agent. "So we know," he summed up, "that the Hebrew lawgiver had knowledge not only of natural elementary means of disinfection (earth, water, air, and fire), but also artificial or synthetic [*künstlich*] means, which we today refer to as *Karbols*."[38]

Knowledge and concern over germs and disease explain Jewish dietary laws as well. As many physicians had already made clear, Nossig noted, all those animals prone to parasitical disease were excluded from the Mosaic dietary regime: "The intention of hindering the transmission of disease from the animal body to the human organism accounts for the rule that the fat, surrounding the abdominal organ, must be burnt; this, precisely because this fat contains lymph ganglia, in which parasites reside."[39] The talmudic laws of *shechitah* (ritual slaughtering according to Jewish ritual) "often bring reproach on the Jews from less educated circles";[40] however, customs of ritual slaughtering undoubtedly lead to better hygiene. The rabbis understood, as did Moses before them, that germs and disease in many cases reside in the blood. They prescribed the draining of all blood from the animal and the salting of the flesh in order to ensure complete removal. This also prevents rapid decomposition of the meat.[41]

Modern science, Nossig asserted, delights unreservedly in the Jewish laws of sanitary inspection of slaughtered animals. He reviewed inspection procedures for the lungs, entrails, liver, and spleen, which most effectively reduce the risk of disease transmission. The lungs cannot be "nicked"; a lung must be puffed up with air and then checked for tears that would indicate impure flesh. In order to avoid all chance of error, the lung must be immersed in water in order to detect a rupture.

What extraordinary foreknowledge!" exclaimed the French physician Dr. Guéneau de Mussy. "The contagiousness of tuberculosis has only been demonstrated a short while ago. The transmission of this disease through food is still not granted by everyone – but note that Jewish law, which preceded modern science by some thousand years, contains in its regulations prophylactic measures against tuberculosis. If," Dr. Guéneau continues, "one can attribute a nick in the sidewalls of the lung to other causes, tuberculosis remains the most frequent cause. One can find a nicked lung without tuberculosis, but almost never tuberculosis without a nicked lung."[42]

The significance of narratives of tuberculosis for the interpretive tradition analyzed here will be taken up in far greater detail in Chapter 5. At this point what bears emphasizing is that Nossig's focus on germs and disease – the desire to transform Moses into a microbiologist – was impelled by the discoveries in germ theory and disease transmission identified with Koch in Germany and Pasteur in France, and the cultural value this knowledge quickly assumed.

In the last two decades of the nineteenth century, researchers isolated the bacilli responsible for anthrax, tuberculosis, typhoid, and diphtheria.[43] State and military authorities strongly supported institutional research into bacteriology at the level of the private laboratory, university, and public health ministry.[44] And bacteriology was quickly taken up by many of those interested in social and racial biology. Germs that infected the individual body, it was argued, contaminated the national body as well. Concerns over falling birth rates, declining economic production, waning military capabilities – everything that could be made into a sign of "degeneracy" – fueled hygienists' interest in germ theory and research. Certainly, a number of different epidemiologies emerged at this time, competing for the allegiance of politicians, scientists, and physicians. However, as Paul Weindling has convincingly argued, bacteriology had an enormous impact on both the scientific and public imaginations. Moreover, it affected directly how people behaved and interacted.

Darwinism and bacteriology transferred problems of health from the geographical and social environment to the microscopic level of germs. The achievements of bacteriology impressed the public, which rapidly contracted "bacteria phobia," and generally enhanced the authority of scientific medicine. There was a borrowing of medical imagery by antisemitic extremists. This was evident in phrases such as "the Jewish bacillus," which became a stock-in-trade slogan of antisemites. Serum therapy raised the issue of purity of blood, which could also be popularized by ideologists of racial purity. [45]

The power of the microbe, the germ, the parasite as metaphors for a perceived threat to the social and political body lent, in turn, significance and relevance to the claims made by Nossig and others that Jewish hygiene reduces or eliminates this threat.

As is well known, by the 1890s the image of the Jew as parasite or germ and the links between Jews and disease were firmly established in anti-Semitic discourse. Jews were defined as "vermin" or "pests" and as "parasites." This imagery drew much of its force from the power of medicine and science and from concerns over individual and public health. "With the infiltration of natural scientific ideas and methods in the social sciences, the concepts 'parasite,' 'parasitism,' and 'sponging' were taken over by the human sciences in their new biological sense."[46] The metonymic use of "parasite" proved particularly powerful, for it helped the anti-Semite describe a political and social reality and danger. An organism that exists at the expense of others, the parasite oftentimes utterly destroys the invaded life form; the Jews, then, were the parasitic race, living among the healthy and productive nations and drawing the blood and life force out of them. This was a view common on the political and social Left as well as the Right.[47] The French socialist Pierre-Joseph Proudhon, for example, writing in 1858, described the Jews as born to a "mercantile and usurious parasitism," living since the time of Jesus "at the cost of others." "*Le Juif est resté Juif, race parasite, ennemi de travail.*"[48] As the embodiment of capitalism and finance for both socialists and conservatives, the Jews were believed to stand in opposition to everything healthy and nurturing; they were, in the words of Mikhail Bakunin, "an exploiting sect, a nation of leeches, a singular devouring parasite" (*eine ausbeuterische Sekte, ein Blutegelvolk, einen einzigen fressenden Parasiten*). In addition, the Jews were described as bacilli and trichinae – literally as alien life forms that introduce disease and death into a healthy organism (the community or social body). In 1892, offering a critical appraisal of contemporary European anti-Semitism, the Italian physiologist Paolo Mantagazza wrote the following in the pages of the widely read Viennese newspaper, the *Neue Freie Presse*:

> [The Jews] are not members of our European body, not sinews of our flesh, not veins of our blood, but tubercular growths, tumors, swellings, which are dispersed all over and hinder the free circulation of our life juices and

powers. They are, in a word, the most corpulent and audacious parasites
in European life.[49]

Blood, like the parasite, was central to the anti-Semitic imagination.
The Jew, as an infection introduced into the national and social organism,
polluted the blood, the life force of the community; he clotted the "free
circulation" of European life. A social and political metaphor, drawn
originally from the language of biology, was transformed into a bio-racial
"reality," completely conflating the biological and the social. Moreover,
this image of blood and of the danger of the Jews was reinforced through
the blood-libel charges and trials throughout Central and Western Europe
in the final decades of the nineteenth century.[50] We need only refer to Hermann Strack's fascinating work *Das Blut im Glauben und Aberglauben
der Menschheit*, first published in 1891 and reprinted eight times by 1900,
to gain a sense of the power and resonance of the connection between
the Jews and blood.[51]

Strack, a prominent Protestant theologian and Orientalist at the University of Berlin, set out to disprove the centuries-old myth of the blood
libel. His work detailed, among other things, the public debate he carried on with the press and other theologians – most notably the Church
theologian and professor of Semitic languages, August Rohling – over
the veracity of charges against the Jews. In the 1880s and 1890s, dozens
of works appeared, based upon Rohling's model *Der Talmudjude*, seeking to prove that throughout history Jews, following instructions in the
Talmud, ritually murdered Christian children and used their blood for
religious ritual purposes.[52] Strack attempted to show that in fact blood
was central to popular folk and medical beliefs and practices in Christian
Europe into the nineteenth century. Jews did not eat and drink blood;
Christians did – though he was careful to point out that this was not
due in any way to adherence to Christianity. If some "mentally unsta-
ble" Jews at times believed in the power of blood, this was due to the
influence of the wider culture in which they lived, and not to Judaism
itself.[53]

It is important to note that Strack, like Matthias Schleiden, was an
eminent Christian scholar. The power and influence of his apologia for
Judaism was due not only to the strength of the argument but to Strack's
identity as a Christian, a theologian, and a professor. Moreover, the

content of Strack's work itself provides ample evidence of the way in which the Talmud and such Jewish practices as circumcision and ritual slaughtering are implicated in the blood libel. It is the "Talmud Jew" who commits the horrific deed, who requires the blood of Christians to fulfill religious obligations imposed by the Talmud. So it is the Talmud that places the Jew outside the realm of civilization, outside the bounds of humanity. The ritual murder is referred to as *"rituelles Schächten,"* connecting it to the prescriptions for slaughtering animals. Elsewhere, it is linked to the ritual of circumcision.[54]

In sum, blood, disease, Jews, and Judaism were intimately interconnected in anti-Semitic discourse. Jewish law and ritual were at best obsolete or irrelevant; more commonly, they were believed to be responsible for inhumane acts perpetrated by the Jews against Christians and Christianity. In other words, Judaism either exists outside the flow of history and progress or stands as the antithesis of all culture and civilization. And the Talmud – emblematic of a dangerous, barbaric Judaism – was central to this representation.

Nossig's narrative, in contrast, establishes the Talmud's fundamental importance as a source of national and racial purity and health and as a positive force for the progress of civilization. Its elaborate system of social hygiene – a "pure medical knowledge" far exceeding that in the Bible – builds on the scientific tradition developed by Moses and extends it to meet the changing needs of the Jews. So, whereas Nossig narrowed historical differences equating ancient and modern knowledge of health, he also pointed up historical development within the Jewish tradition. And this, too, served particular polemical purposes.

Playing on the well-known "chain of tradition" found in the *Pirke Avot*, Nossig argued for a secret oral tradition of medical and scientific knowledge passed down from Moses to Aaron and the Levites, through Joshua, the kings and prophets, to the rabbis, and finally to Yehuda ha-Nasi, who set it down in writing in the second century CE. At the same time, he presented this tradition as both superior to that of the Greeks, and as prior and equivalent to modern achievements: "The Talmud contains in [the mishnaic] tractate *Oholoth* a complete osteology, in tractate *Berakhot* elements of physiology, tractate *Hullin* and other tractates, a knowledge of pathology, all of which exceed in scope the Hippocratic school." Nossig rewrote the normative narrative of the

history of medicine and science and placed the Jews at the center. In
fact, throughout the work he minimized the role of the Greeks in that
history: "One commits a great injustice by equating the history of hygiene
with the Greeks, and dismissing the achievements of the Oriental peoples
with a few phrases. This is particularly true of the social hygiene of the
Jews." The Greeks constitute just one link in a long historical chain of
medical development, which began with the ancient Orient ("the cradle
of civilization") and ends in Europe.[55] The normative understanding of
"civilized" and "uncivilized" is hereby overturned, at least in part (since
Nossig's reinterpretation still depends in the end on the notion of Europe
as the teleological endpoint of civilization, and thus the ultimate valida-
tion for the Jews as healthy). The "Orient" – the foreign and dangerous,
the antithetical "Other" for the Christian West (as well as for the majority
of Central and Western European Jews) – becomes the origin of precisely
that which the West now defines as *the* force of civilization.

We can see Nossig's assertions in part, then, as a response to historians
of medicine who counterposed the rationality of Greece with the magic
and superstition of "the Orient."[56] Just as important, his contention
reflected and contributed to the debate among anti-Semites, Jewish assim-
ilationists, and Zionists about the historical and cultural value of the Orient and the definition of the Jews as an Oriental people. Modern Central
and Western European Jewish identity was constructed to a significant
degree in contrast to *Ostjudentum* (Eastern European Jewry).[57] Russo-
Polish Jews, in the image of many in Central and Western Europe (and
the United States), were physically, intellectually, and morally degenerate;
by the 1880s, they were firmly established as the "bearers and symbols
of *Unbildung*," mirror opposites of Western "refinement, *Kultur*, and
Reason."[58] Orientalizing the Jews meant identifying them with Arabs,
Turks, and Muslims, and with the Near East, an exotic "place" that
for centuries had been for Europeans both profoundly intriguing and
horrifying.[59] For our purposes, a number of interrelated images are of
particular interest: the Eastern European Jew as dirty and diseased, and
as ignorant and impoverished, all in large part because of continued
adherence to talmudic Judaism.

As is well known, the large-scale immigration from East to West that
began in the 1870s produced heightened anxiety among many "native"
non-Jews and Jews in the West, evident on the one hand in an intensified

anti-Semitism, and on the other in a heightened effort within official Jewish communities to assimilate these Eastern Jews. There was, however, also a reevaluation of the *Ostjude* on the part of some Jews in the West, part of a broader Western romanticization of the "Orient." Zionists, in particular, challenged the traditional Western image of the Eastern Jew. The ghetto Jew was transformed into the embodiment of a "genuine" or whole Judaism, in contrast to the fractured and inauthentic Judaism of the assimilated bourgeois West. Ideas of healthy and degenerate were transposed in this reevaluation; the purported "uncultured," "unrefined," "irrational" character of *Ostjudentum* was held up as an ideal, as a potential regenerative healing power for the impaired modern bourgeois sensibility.[60]

In a quite general way, we might view Nossig's reinterpretation of Judaism as one instance of this explicitly antirational and antibourgeois romanticization of the East as the source of *Kultur* and civilization. For many Zionists, embracing the "ghetto Jew" meant rejecting the ideal of emancipation and especially assimilation into liberal, middle-class Western society.[61] Nossig, however, celebrated scientific rationality and bourgeois values. The ancient laws of the Bible and Talmud shaped a people whose values and practices were in full accord with those of the nineteenth-century Western European bourgeoisie. In this, Nossig's *Sozialhygiene* was in complete comport with the interpretive tradition of the "healthy Jew" in general. The impulse of Jewish nationalism can indeed be identified in this work; however, the *embourgeoisement* of Jews and Judaism, the making of Jewry into a model of hygiene and respectability, united Nossig's work in a more profound way with the myriad other writings produced in Europe and America in the main by individuals with no discernible ties to Zionism. If there is a politics to the interpretive tradition of the healthy Jew, it is this desire and need to transform the Jews and Judaism into something clean and respectable, in their own eyes as well as in the eyes of the Gentiles. In this, and despite the profoundly anti-historicist nature of the enterprise, books like Nossig's reflected the impulse and aims of the nineteenth-century *Wissenschaft des Judentums* movement.[62] This overriding concern on Nossig's part with the rationality and bourgeois respectability of Judaism becomes evident when we examine in greater detail his ideas about sexuality and purity and place them in the context of nineteenth- and early twentieth-century medicine – particularly as social thinkers and public officials became increasingly concerned with national and racial health.

5.

Issues related to sexuality and marriage were crucial to the health and hygiene movements in Imperial Germany, France, England, and the United States. A nation's strength, in both industrial and military terms, depended on the "healthiest" individuals being encouraged or compelled to produce children in the greatest numbers. Statistical studies on birth and death rates supported the widespread belief in every country that its healthy (that is, productive and respectable) classes were disappearing, while its "degenerates" were reproducing in unprecedented numbers. Prostitution and venereal disease were viewed increasingly as threats to the biological, as well as the moral, health of the nation. Degeneration theories, rooted in notions of heredity and natural selection, linked sexual immorality with criminality, insanity, and alcoholism in a discourse of "social disease" in which the biological and moral health of the nation were under constant siege.[63] This widespread belief that society and culture were under attack from a sexual immorality, and that this signaled a more fundamental decline in the fabric of state and society, was strengthened in the minds of many by the emergence of the feminist and homosexual rights movements. This, in turn, led to an organized moral purity campaign that sought to retard these social movements, strengthen the existing laws against "immorality" – especially section 175 of the German penal code, outlawing sexual relations between two males, and bestiality – and reinforce a commitment to "respectable" sexual mores.[64] The representation of a Jewish sexual morality that was healthy because it repudiated not only prostitution and bestiality, but homosexuality and sexual relations outside of marriage, aligned Jews and Judaism with dominant, even reactionary notions of normalcy and abnormality. In some cases this alignment was implicit, in others attention was drawn explicitly to Judaism's agreement with and anticipation of contemporary moral standards.[65]

In his treatment of sexuality, Nossig took great pains to demonstrate that Jewish ideas and practices fit contemporary bourgeois notions of health and purity. Judaism discountenances all forms of sexual "perversion" or deviation: prostitution is taboo, as are adultery, premarital sex, free love, and incest. Jewish communities have no one who suffers from venereal diseases, which result in "the production of entire degenerate families," and no young married men who "sow their oats" and "have only contempt for their family and race." The chastity (*Keuschheit*) of young women before marriage, according to Nossig, is one of the fundamental principles of the Mosaic system. Young Jewish men and women realize, when they come to sexual maturity, that "there is no other way to satisfy their impulses other than marriage." For Nossig, the ultimate goal of the Mosaic rules of sexual hygiene is "the certitude of a chaste and fruitful marriage," for this is fundamental to "the increase and preservation of the race" (*Vermehrung und Erhaltung der Rasse*).[66]

Rituals related to sex, seemingly religious in nature, are in fact hygienic precepts. Circumcision, for example, functions to "dampen" perverted expressions of sexuality by "weakening the organ," a common medical notion at the time, but one that Nossig might very well have taken from Maimonides.[67] This limitation of sexual inclination is particularly necessary for peoples of hotter climates, who are given over to "a type of excess of sexual energy, an overpowering reproductive urge; the temperature makes this sort of person inclined to love and sexual excess." This diminution of the sexual drive through circumcision "facilitated the historical process whereby the idea of a chaste and pure nation [*Volk*] was embodied [*verkörpern*] by the Jews. And this is the deep meaning [*tiefe Sinn*] of the words, that the circumcision will be as a sign of a covenant between the Creator and the people of Israel."[68] In touting circumcision, and linking it to individual and national/racial health, Nossig was participating in a long-standing debate among physicians, theologians, and others over the health benefits of the practice. By the last half of the nineteenth century, circumcision had been medicalized, and claims by medical authorities about its ability to cure and prevent a wide array of disabilities and diseases, from masturbation (widely considered to be both an illness itself and the cause of other maladies) and paralysis to syphilis and numerous forms of cancer were being endorsed or challenged.[69] Interestingly, Nossig accepted the commonly held notion about "oriental" sexuality put forth in scholarly and popular works of anthropology and race. The juxtaposition of "peoples of hotter climates" and "excess of sexual energy" recalls the analysis of earlier centuries that looked to geography and other environmental factors to explain ethnic or racial traits.[70] Yet Nossig used it to reverse the evaluation of Jewish sexuality. He domesticated Jewish sexual habits by aligning them – as he did with law and ritual in general – with respectable European sensibilities. The Jews (as Orientals), he argued, were prone on account of climate and geography to excessive sexual urges. Their laws, however, civilized them. Moses had already condemned, thousands of years ago, every degenerate tendency felt to be threatening European society at the end of the nineteenth century. The bourgeois ideals of virtue, chastity, faithful marriage, and healthy reproduction were *literally embodied* in the Jewish nation. The religious, metaphysical truth of the covenant between God and Israel, symbolized by the circumcision, is transformed here into a purely physical truth. The "deep meaning" (and, for Nossig, the true meaning) of this act lies in its biological function; it is a sign of physical health and superiority.

This *embourgeoisement* of ancient Jewish laws regarding sexuality offered a counterpoint to the real and imagined sexual dangers posed by Jews to bourgeois sensibilities. Prostitution, for instance, was a genuine political and socioeconomic problem for European Jewry at the end of the nineteenth century. Jewish involvement in the white slave trade was widely acknowledged and condemned by official Jewish communities and addressed by international committees and conferences. Of course, this issue proved highly valuable to anti-Semites who sought further proof of Jewish immorality and degeneracy.[71] The healthy Jew, and a Judaism that not only echoed modern European values but antedated them by millennia potentially countered the real and imaginary challenges to European middle-class sensibilities.

Alfred Nossig was not a social hygienist but a poet and sculptor, a political activist and writer on the "Jewish Question." If he was indeed serious, as he claimed in the introduction to *The Social Hygiene of the Jews*, that he was motivated in the main by a desire to reform European society as a whole, he did little in the wake of its publication to further this goal.[72] He was known as somewhat of a dilettante, and his attentions quickly turned elsewhere.[73] By 1900 he was living in Berlin, and over the next few years his prodigious energy would be devoted to organizing a Jewish statistical movement. Nossig's 1894 work was, rather, an attempt to counter the image of a diseased and degenerate Judaism and Jewry by offering up an alternative set of images as the historical bearers and beneficiaries of a scientific knowledge of health and purity. At the same time, this "demonstration" of the biological and moral purity of the Jews was an attempt to prove the truth and viability of the Jewish nationalist project. In this sense, his work was part of a broader effort, carried out by a great number of individuals and groups throughout Europe and Anglo-America, to wed medical knowledge to power and to render social science useful to the nationalist cause.

At the same time, his work on social hygiene cannot be reduced to either a response to contemporary anti-Semitism or a handmaiden of Jewish nationalism. Intellectually and culturally, it constituted one example, albeit one of the most comprehensive, of a particular interpretive tradition, one that was not tied to any one ideological position, nor, as we shall see in Chapter 3, limited to continental Europe.

3

Healthy Hebrews, Healthy Jews

The Bible as a Sanitary Code in Anglo-American Medical Literature

I.

In November 1893, a year before Alfred Nossig's book on social hygiene appeared, the Chief Rabbi of Great Britain, Hermann Adler, gave a public talk, "Sanitation and the Mosaic Law," to the Church of England Sanitary Association. The talk was later summarized and analyzed in the pages of Great Britain's most prominent journal of medicine, the *Lancet*. Adler, according to the *Lancet*, "proposed to make it clear that, as a sanitarian, the great Jewish law-giver [Moses] was not only well ahead of his time but in many respects abreast of ours, and to show that the Jewish 'tradition' – i.e., the two parts of the Talmud – supplemented or even surpassed the teachings of Moses in this respect."[1]

The editors of the journal fully endorsed Adler's argument (which had also been made earlier by Sir Benjamin Ward Richardson) that the Mosaic law and the talmudic laws are, in their practical effect, "largely sanitary." On other realms affecting the community or society, such as criminal law, the Mosaic code is quite scanty. But with regard to those laws and rituals concerned with sanitary or hygienic matters, the code is full of detail, and the two realms, the religious and the medical, are inextricably intertwined: "There can be no doubt that the Jews under Moses' direction were far in advance of the nations around them in sanitary matters, and that whoever kept the letter of the Mosaic law would enjoy immunity from infectious disease, as well as that high standard of health which results from personal care and cleanliness."[2]

This is a striking example of a "non-Jewish" authority – the *Lancet* – doing the sort of work usually associated with Jewish apologists (such as the Chief Rabbi). While discussing Adler's arguments, the editors endorse the equation of Mosaic law with sound sanitary policy, and make the case for the health and the normalcy of the Jews. For the most part, the journal's editors wanted their readers to know that Jews who follow the laws of Moses are permitted to eat just what their non-Jewish fellow citizens usually consume; what they are forbidden is not that different from what is forbidden the rest of the "civilized world." The editors note that the great exceptions are, of course, pork and shellfish. There is really nothing very onerous about the laws of *kashrut*, according to the *Lancet*. *Kashrut* – and, by extension, the Jews who obey its rules – are, at least potentially, de-exoticized here. The *Lancet* translates the ancient religious laws into contemporary medical and scientific measures, thereby linking the Jews with modern notions of health and hygiene. We should add that, at least implicitly, the *Lancet*'s editors repudiated the Christian theological notion of the "deadliness" of Jewish law. At least at the physical, material level, if not at the moral, Jewish law literally saved the Jews from, rather than condemned them to, misery and suffering. Nor should it go unmentioned that Rabbi Adler delivered his talk in an explicitly Christian setting.

The *Lancet* explicitly situated Adler's discussion of Mosaic food laws within the context of the contemporary debate in England over kosher slaughtering practices, and the movement to outlaw kosher slaughtering because of its alleged cruelty to animals.[3] The journal's editors were scornful of such attempts, seeing it as a side issue. They referred to Adler's assertion that *shechitah* (they used and explained the term) is the least cruel and most humane method of slaughter, and they endorsed that view. Adler invoked Rudolf Virchow, one of the leading lights of German medicine, and the *Lancet* quoted Virchow at length on this matter.

The article concluded, however, on a far more ambivalent note. The *Lancet* congratulated Adler on his "eloquent championship of the Jewish code," and noted that hopefully this would retard some of the prejudice, born of ignorance, of Judaism's detractors. Then it added that responsibility for such attacks had also been the result of "the backsliding of such a large number of his own people. This latter he himself admits, and with our knowledge of the habits of the Russian, Polish, and German Jews, to say nothing of those of the Jews who multiply in the East-end of our own metropolis, we can see that he could not do otherwise. It is obvious that the possession of an admirable set of regulations will not keep a nation cleanly and healthy, although the observation of those regulations might do so."[4]

Yet, despite this ambivalence about contemporary Jewish immigrants, the editors of the *Lancet* nonetheless presented Jews and Judaism as both normal and healthy, even if they remained at some level a people discursively and physically apart. Something similar characterized the representation of Jews and Judaism in the United States. In both professional and popular media, Moses was recast in the role of hygienist, the Mosaic laws were understood as sanitary regulations, and the positive impact on the Jews historically and in the present was duly noted. In many cases, as we shall see in Chapter 6, Gentiles and their governments were urged to follow in the footsteps of the Jews and adopt those rituals that physicians believed were preventative or curative of disease.

In this chapter I extend the discussion of the strategy of translation and equivalence to the Anglo-American realm. My focus here will be on the United States, and to a lesser extent on Great Britain, and on the question of why in the period of roughly 1830–1940 the desire to transform Moses into a medical authority proved so attractive to many physicians and medical writers, both Jewish and Christian. Unsurprisingly, Jewish physicians and writers on medicine produced much, though by no means all, of the literature that celebrated the conjunction of Judaism, Jews, and health and hygiene. Relevant texts appeared in books and articles with a "Jewish" provenance. However, it is significant, and bears emphasizing, that many of the articles on Jewry and hygiene written by Jewish physicians were published in general medical journals in both the United States and Great Britain; this included the leading journals in both of these countries, the *Lancet* and the *Journal of the American Medical Association* (*JAMA*). Moreover, Jews were by no means alone in advancing this set of ideas and images about Jews, Judaism, and health. Christian authorities, too, took up the idea of Moses as "founder of preventive medicine," as one non-Jewish British writer put it, and teased out the implications of this concern with health for the history of the Jews.[5] In reconstructing and analyzing the main contours of these medicalized narratives about Jewish sacred literature and history, I draw as much as possible on articles published in the general medical and popular press in order to emphasize this point about the Christian participation in this intellectual process.

One of the chief purposes of this chapter is to demonstrate that, contrary to what the scholarly literature might suggest, Jews and non-Jews in America and Britain engaged in a medicalized discussion about Jews, and that this was not uniformly negative in its imagination and representation of Jews and Judaism; and that this representation, though it first appeared earlier in the nineteenth century, circulated more widely during the decades of mass immigration (1880–1930), at the same time as an undeniable heightening of hostility towards the Jews in both Britain and the United States was occurring.

The healthy Jew and a hygienic Judaism were widely circulated notions during the same decades in which the images of the dirty and diseased Jew appeared with greater frequency in scientific and popular forums. In his 1910 celebration of the Jewish contribution to civilization, the Protestant theologian and preacher Madison C. Peters paid tribute to the fact that, among numerous other enviable traits, "the Jew is extremely fond of soap and water under all circumstances; especially has he a fondness for the latter. Whenever he has an opportunity to take a bath he takes one."[6] In June 1913, the *Washington Post* ran an article, "Mosaic Laws Sanitary," which informed its readers "that the sanitary laws of Moses were not only on a line with the modern rules of hygiene, but in some cases in advance of them." Nor was this limited to Moses. The Talmud was celebrated for introducing slaughtering methods acknowledged today "as the most sanitary," and which "pointed out the danger to man from tuberculosis in cattle," and this, thousands of years before "Koch gave to the world the results of his researches [*sic*] in bacteriology. . . . " Moses also understood the importance of isolating those with contagious diseases, and burying the dead outside the walls of the city: "These hints the Gentile world did not fully accept until a century or two ago."[7] The *Post* article was a summary of a longer piece on the wisdom of Jewish law and ritual that ran in *Harper's Weekly*. Obviously, there is no sure way to determine how many people at the time glanced at or read these articles, and, if they did, what if anything they took away from them. These were two articles among thousands published (though, as we shall see, they were far from isolated or idiosyncratic). Yet, the same could very well be said about the articles published by nativists and anti-Semites, articulations of a hostility to Jews and immigrants that are more often than not taken as representative of the period. How, then, apart from by actions (i.e., policies such as the 1924 Johnson Act in the United States) do we determine when a particular period is "anti-Semitic"?

There were, then, representations that celebrated the Jews and Judaism as healthy and hygienic circulating at the same time as denunciations of Jews as dirty and dangerous. Nonetheless, even the affirmative evaluations of Jews still marked them as different. I am not arguing that such positive representations of Jews and Judaism refrained from identifying the Jews as different, even racializing them; they certainly did that. Jews, in fact, like all other "white" minority and immigrant groups, participated in the process of such a racialization, as this allowed them to become over time "Caucasians," and thus to attain full integration.[8] After all, the very idea of assimilation seemed to assume that the Jews were in some fundamental way both racially as well as culturally different enough to require reformation, and yet "white enough" eventually to become part of the American or British political and social body. As one leading American racial thinker wrote in 1927, "most of the immigrant stocks [and this included the Jews] are racially not too remote for ultimate assimilation"; they won't disturb the "racial make-up" of the country enough "to endanger the stability and continuity of our national life."[9] This did not apply, it should be noted, to non-European immigrant groups such as the Japanese, Chinese, or others defined racially as non-whites.

But the narrative that presents the discourse about Jews and race in the United States and also Great Britain in the unrelenting terms of perceived inferiority, dirt, disease, and danger is incomplete, just as it is with regard to continental Europe. It may very well be accurate to say, as Matthew Frye Jacobson has, that "[W]herever 'difference' was cast as race, certainly, the weight of the culture in general tended most often toward negative depiction."[10] But, as Jacobson himself acknowledges, difference was not always inferiority. Analyses of anti-Semitism and nativism can, albeit unwittingly, produce a monochromatic picture of this past by bringing together figures such as Madison Grant, Lothrop Stoddard, Edward A. Ross, Prescott Hall, and other American nativists and white supremacists (or their equivalents in other countries) in order to reconstruct the reigning image of the Jew in the period before 1924. Again, it is not that these writers and activists should not be brought together; nor should we minimize the import of their ideas. It is only to suggest that there circulated at the same time, in scientific and popular venues, alternative images and ideas about the Jews. In the most important respects, judged by the implementation of government policy and its very real impact on the lives of Jews and millions of others deemed inferior and dangerous, the eugenicists and nativists succeeded; their ideas won out. In 1924, the United States passed highly restrictive immigration legislation that effectively blocked Jews, along with others from Southeastern and Eastern Europe, from entering the country. In Great Britain, restrictivist legislation had been passed in 1905 and then again in 1919. But there were other ideas and images out there competing for the attention of politicians and the public, and this fact must necessarily complicate the story historians tell.

That the Jews were different, everyone could agree upon. But just what that difference signified remained open to debate. When the non-Jewish authors of the 1904 work *The Science of Eugenics and Sex Life* insisted, sounding very much like Alfred Nossig, that "The Jews as a race are singularly free from the contaminations arising from the sexual diseases," and that this was due to "the law of Moses on sex-hygiene,"[11] the narrative assumed the Jews to be a race and inscribed them in the narrative as such. But the moral or historical judgment to which we have been accustomed – that to racialize the Jews was to find them inferior and dangerous – is absent here. Indeed, a central motif of anti-Semitism is directly contradicted: Jews are not agents of syphilis, and the reason for that can be found in Judaism itself.

2.

When Jews appear in narratives of Anglo-American health and disease, it is usually when the story reaches the 1880s and the beginnings of mass immigration of Eastern European Jews into the United States and Great Britain (as well as, of course, into other Central and Western European countries). Yet, Jews were a part of the Anglo-American medical imagination decades before that. In his 1830 article, "On the State of the Medical Art Among the Jews, as Recorded in the Bible," the physician J. K. Walker argued that while the Levitical code had as its main purpose the division of the Jews from their idolatrous neighbors, it was also "the wisest [set of rules] that could have been enacted for the preservation of the health of the people."[12] Walker's discussion was firmly embedded in a Christian theological interpretive framework. The laws of Moses were given to the Jews to secure their physical and moral well-being, but when they disobeyed the Lord, they were threatened and indeed struck down with a host of physical maladies: "The Lord shall smite thee with a consumption, and with a fever, and with an inflammation, and with extreme burning." Walker then adds, "How awfully the above denunciations were executed, the reader of the Jewish history will find too frequent proofs in the sequel of Jewish apostasy [sic]."[13]

Walker moves back and forth indiscriminately between ancient Israelites and Jews, so that in the end the two are interchangeable. At the same time, he speaks of the Jews in a more mundane, though still not wholly de-theologized, way, situating them within a normal or natural frame. Jews, he insists at one point, were not immune to the normal diseases that affect every other nation; but "so long as they maintained inviolate the great truths confided to their care, human affairs seemed to take their ordinary course...."[14]

Walker, then, makes a case for the "healthy Jews" as the normative condition; only when they desist from keeping the Mosaic laws regulating hygiene – he stresses diet (including the prohibition of consuming blood), cleanliness, and frequent bathing – do the Jews risk disease and untimely death. Walker also sought to make the case for the link between Jews and health by tracing medicine itself back to the Jews. We've seen that this sort of argument was common in Jewish apologia; it also had its place in some Christian narratives. In Chapter 1 we saw that Walker believed that much of medicine derived from the ancient near East, and from the Jews in particular. The Arabs, more than many would believe, derived their knowledge from the Jews, as did the Greeks. Thus, modern medicine owed far more to the Jews than is commonly acknowledged; to accept the Greek's own account of this history and their central role within it was a mistake. Moreover, the Mosaic laws anticipated modern medical insights, and this helped account for the health of the Jews. Walker ended his article by insisting that the whole point of his piece was to demonstrate "the advanced state of our art [i.e., medicine] among the Jews."[15]

As we've seen, a central element in counter-narratives produced by Jewish authors was this notion of ancient Hebrew law and ritual as the unacknowledged source of medicine, and the Greeks as owing more to the Jews than was commonly acknowledged. But, as Walker's text demonstrates, Christian writers also advanced this idea. In 1847, John M. B. Harden, writing in the *Southern Medical and Surgical Journal*, dismissed the idea advanced by previous historians of medicine such as Parr, Broussais, and Le Clerc, that Hippocrates was the first physician, and modern medicine found its earliest incarnation in the ancient Greeks. If one is looking for the first instance of healing as a profession, Harden insisted, rather than the propagation of medicine as a philosophy, then we must look not to Hippocrates and the Greeks, but to Moses and the Jews.[16]

This counter-narrative of the relationship between Jewish and Greek knowledge survived well into the twentieth century. It can be found in a 1940 article by the eminent (Jewish) scholar of Jewish medical history Solomon Kagan. Writing in the journal *Medical Leaves* on the subject of talmudic medicine, Kagan found evidence of a remarkable level of medical and scientific knowledge in the Talmud, based on "tradition, observation, experiment or training in the offices of experienced physicians." The rabbis possessed an advanced knowledge of pathology and hygiene, and had "evolved a system of studying not only the symptoms of diseases and their treatment, but also pathological anatomy as well as personal and public hygiene."[17] According to Kagan, the rabbis of the Talmud performed experiments and laboratory tests, "many of which are of great interest to medical science and some are in accordance even with the methods of modern research." They contributed new methods of "medical research, diagnosis and therapy...[And] this fundamental knowledge of pathology was 1500 years later independently confirmed by modern investigators."[18]

Kagan did his best, therefore, to turn the rabbis of the Talmud into physicians and medical researchers. In some cases the rabbis were medical innovators, making discoveries that would later become accepted wisdom in the general world of medicine. Like Yehuda Katznelson before him, Kagan insisted that "the sages of the Talmud were the first to state that the symptoms of diseases are merely manifestations of internal changes in the tissues of the body, and that pathological changes in the body are the result of external favorable factors."[19] In this, they went in intellectual directions that the Greeks failed to go. Kagan cited the work of Dr. Fielding H. Garrison, *An Introduction to the History of Medicine* (1922), in which Garrison wrote that, in Kagan's words, "the autopsies performed by the ancient Hebrews upon slaughtered animals to determine which was 'kosher' . . . and which was '*trepha*' [ritually unclean] . . . threw much light upon the pathologic anatomy, the study of which the ancient Greeks never took up."[20] It is difficult to avoid the conclusion that the attraction of Garrison's argument for Kagan lay not only in the point it made about the superiority of the Hebrews over the Greeks, but that this point was made by a non-Jew, whose voice might therefore carry greater conviction in this matter.

Kagan used Garrison's particular point to universalize the idea that the rabbis were indeed far ahead of the Greeks in terms of medical knowledge:

> *Humoralism* (Hippocrates), *Solidism* (Asclepiades), and *Pneumatism* (Galen) were the main doctrines of Graeco-Roman medicine. There were three different ways of explaining disease, as disturbances of the liquid, solid or gaseous constituents of the body. These three theories have prevented the scientific study of pathological anatomy for many centuries. *Structural alternations* [sic] was the Hebrew doctrine on disease based on observation and experimentation. This was in conflict with that of the Greek and Roman theories and it actually conformed with the theories advanced by modern medical research.[21]

For some it was not the Greeks who received too much credit, but the Egyptians. The French author Noël Guéneau de Mussy, in writing about the health benefits of circumcision, believed that the Egyptians were probably influenced by the Israelites in this regard, and not the other way around as commonly believed. The translation of Guéneau de Mussy's article, in which this particular argument appeared, was published in the *New York Medical Abstract* as "The Hygienic Laws of Moses."[22] His writings on Moses and hygiene were widely cited in both American and British writing on Jews and health, and so are not out of place in a discussion of Anglo-American discourse.

Guéneau de Mussy's work does double work for us: in both its French and Anglo-American contexts, it demonstrates the fact that the debate over Jews, Judaism, and health and disease was not limited to the Central European context. And it provides another instance of a non-Jewish authority, in this case a widely disseminated voice, who largely celebrated the health and hygiene of Judaism and Jewry. At the outset of his article, Guéneau de Mussy collapsed history, as the ancient Hebrews and modern Jews were, for him, one in their "prodigious vitality." And this, he said, was and is due less to "the primordial physical qualities of the race," than to "the legislation of Moses, a legislation as admirable from a moral as from a hygienic point of view."[23] Moses, according to Guéneau de Mussy, was a pathologist: "The idea of parasitical and infectious maladies which has acquired so large a place in modern pathology strongly preoccupied him; it dominates all of his hygienic ordinances."[24]

There is no doubt, it should be noted, that Guéneau de Mussy was working from a Christian perspective. Towards the end of the article he wrote that the best proof of Moses' continued power and relevance is the fact that it "has now become admirably completed in the ordinances of Christianity." Though Moses' laws might have started out in an "exclusive or restricted" context, Christianity (and Islam) universalized them.[25] At the same time, Guéneau de Mussy granted the relationship between Mosaic law and the Jews a legitimacy, an autonomy, and a continued relevance apart from Christian history. "In its primitive form," the Mosaic law "still exists, and those who live by it, dispersed according to the prediction of the great legislator to the four quarters of the earth, have drawn from it a force and a vitality which has enabled them to triumph over all obstacles and over the persecutions of which they have been the object."[26]

Guéneau de Mussy minimized the contributions of the ancient Egyptians to medicine. More often, though, the Egyptians were given credit for a high level of knowledge about science and medicine, and their influence on Moses was admitted. J. K. Walker, as we saw, was a fervent advocate of the idea that the Greeks and Arabs owed their knowledge of medical science to the Jews. Yet he also granted that Moses, and hence the Bible, derived medical knowledge from the Egyptians. Moses "was versed in all the knowledge of the Egyptians ... " Walker wrote, obviously echoing the Book of Acts.[27]

However, other medical authorities were unwilling to grant the Jews this central role in the development of medical knowledge. W. C. Bitting,

speaking on "Biblical Medicine" before the 1891 annual meeting of the
New York State Medical Association, told his audience that "medicine
never was a science among the Hebrews. Semitic minds have given religion and poetry to the world, but not science. No organized knowledge of
any sort came from Abraham's descendents before the Christian era."[28]
A bit later on, Bitting spoke again of the "essentially unscientific character of the Semitic mind."[29] There is an echo in Bitting's remarks of the
common anti-Semitic trope that the Jews were not true creators or pro-
ducers, but consumers, living and thriving off the efforts of others, that
the Hebrews relied to a great extent on acquired knowledge from numerous sources: "While not launching into the pregnant world of experiment,
the Israelites absorbed the results of others' industry with avidity," the
Egyptians first and foremost.[30] Egypt was known the world over for its
physicians, for medical specialization, for advanced medical knowledge
(embalming, dentistry). Later, the Jews absorbed the knowledge of the
Greeks, so that, by the time of Jesus, the Jews shared in the larger world's
knowledge of medicine created by Greek science and spread by empire.

Yet nonetheless, even in a text such as Bitting's, which is less celebratory than most produced on the subject of the Bible and medicine,
the fundamental hygienic value of the Mosaic law is put forth. The
ancient Hebrews may have little to offer in the realms of anatomy, pathology, obstetrics or pharmacology. But in the realm of hygiene, "Mosaic
medicine is superb.... We might venture to ask some of our modern
health officers and street cleaners to read attentively the utterances of
Moses, who could be their teacher in more ways than one." Ultimately,
Bitting offered up a highly ambivalent image of the relationship between
Judaism and Jews; in his text, healthy Hebrews confront dirty Jews. The
celebration of ancient Hebrew hygiene and purity became at the same
time an explicit attack on contemporary immigrants, which of course
included Eastern European Jews.

What was inflammable must be bathed in fire to cleanse it, and everything
else had to be washed in water. These men were high protectionists in the
interest of health. Our government could do nothing better than apply
at Castle Garden and Ellis Island these same tests to the hordes of great
unwashed immigrants and their baggage. Such things as our filthy streets,
bungling scavenger work, foul and disease-breeding tenement-houses, and
numerous pest spots, could not have existed in Moses' day. We have

evolutionized backward in this matter. O for a modern Moses at the head
of our health department![31]

While hardly an endorsement of immigration, this was a far cry from
the racialized anti-Jewish and anti-immigrant texts that are the mainstay of the historiography on nativism and American and British anti-
Semitism. There is no suggestion in Bitting, or the many other non-Jewish
writers who wrote in a similar vein, of an inherent or immutable inability
of Jews and other immigrants to embrace health and hygiene. Rather, it
is a matter of evolution and devolution of mores, of an approximation
or falling away of a Jewish ideal. "When we examine the Mosaic laws
regarding food and water, bathing and waste removal, we realize that
the Hebrews ought to have been the cleanest people on earth."[32] And,
again, it was Moses and the ancient Israelites who gave the world these
ideals of cleanliness and health.

The influence and importance of the Egyptians exercised writers on
Jews and medicine throughout the decades under discussion. The Jewish
physician Max Danzis, writing nearly forty years after Bitting, was still
insisting that the Jews took nothing from the Egyptians. The scientific
principles of preventive medicine and hygiene, he wrote, were already
to be found in the early books of the Bible, and these were the product
of Moses' genius: "The real early Jewish contribution to medicine is
found in the book of Leviticus, where sound and rational laws are laid
down governing the prevention of certain diseases, and isolation and
disinfection are thoroughly discussed."[33]

At the same time, Jewish physicians and writers could be just as
adamant in insisting that the ancient Hebrews and the rabbis of the
Talmud owed whatever medical and scientific knowledge they possessed
to other nations and cultures. Benjamin Lee Gordon, in an article on
"medicine among the ancient Hebrews" in *Annals of Medical History*,
explicitly countered the claim that the Hebrews possessed a medical tradition comparable to the modern West's. Characterizing the whole Mediter-
ranean region in the period between the second century BCE and the
fourth century of the present era, Gordon noted that "Independent observations, rational thinking, and practical skill are rare. Pathology, or the
study of structural, functional and chemical changes resulting from disease, is *terra incognita*." Disease and physical calamity were understood
as Divine punishment.[34] Yet, again, if Gordon, like Bitting and others,

was unwilling to subvert the dominant narrative regarding the relationship of the Jews, Egyptians and Greeks, he nonetheless still asserted the
superior hygienic value of Mosaic law:

> If the ancient Hebrews [in contrast to the ancient Egyptians] left no illu-
> minated path in the art and practice of healing, they greatly excelled in
> the knowledge of hygiene and sanitation. Their laws pertaining to social
> hygiene, disinfection, isolation of those suffering from contagious diseases
> and ablution of those who were in contact with them, were far in advance
> of the times.... [I]t cannot be doubted that in the light of modern hygiene,
> they were both scientific and practical.[35]

Gordon extended this overwhelming concern with cleanliness to the
rabbis of the Talmud; no other subject so preoccupied then as did hygiene.
They took a deep interest in water and bathing, in the positive effects
of pure air and exercise, and above all, in the impact of food and
drink on levels of health. Moreover, Gordon strongly suggested – albeit
implicitly – that the rabbis understood the modern notion of germs, and
the relation of germs to disease. And he did assert, explicitly, that most of
the hygienic precepts found in the Talmud "are in harmony with modern
science."[36]

3.

If Gordon hesitated to claim a full equivalency of medical knowledge
between ancient Jewish authorities and contemporary science, many
others were hardly reluctant to do so. "So far as we know," Edward
T. Williams wrote in 1881, "Moses was the creator of preventative
medicine, an idea thought to be peculiarly modern."[37] Over half a century later the same idea could be found in prominent medical journals.
"Among the Hebrews health was cult," Dr. David A. Stewart wrote in
Annals of Medical History in 1935. "Their ritual at the killing of animals for food was the beginning of modern meat inspection. The ritual
of cleanliness prepared for antiseptic surgery. The Hebrew law of cleanliness anticipated the laws of Pasteur and Lister."[38]

The argument was taken up and integrated into larger synthetic narratives of Jewish history. James Hosmer, for instance, the British (and
non-Jewish) author of *The Jews: Ancient, Medieval, Modern*, made the

hygienic value of Mosaic law part of his longer discussion of the nature of the Torah and Talmud. Calling explicitly on the work of Guéneau de Mussy, Hosmer argued that "the idea of parasitical and infectious maladies, of which we now hear so much, occupied also the mind of Moses." Moses, "with great wisdom," identified those animals that were clean, and those liable to parasites; he mandated that all blood be removed, and the fat burned – "it has been established that it is precisely the blood and the fat which are most liable to retain parasitic germs and carry infection." The liver, lungs, and spleen must be carefully inspected, as these are the organs most given over to disease. Moses concerned himself with the hygiene of clothing and dwellings. He mandated the observance of a day of rest because it brings with it great health benefits; and "even circumcision can be defended as an excellent sanitary expedient." In several respects, Hosmer concluded, "the Mosaic Law is declared to have anticipated modern science by several thousand years."[39]

While such assertions appeared in forums that seem relatively unsurprising, such as histories of the Jews, it is more significant in certain respects that they also found their way into general medical journals and academic treatises. Even those articles written by Jews take on a different status and import when they appear in such forums (rather than self-identified Jewish publications). The potential audience would be different, and the transmission of a particular sort of knowledge different in its reception. When Nuphtuli Herz Imber published a piece on "The Medical Science of the Talmud" in the *Denver Medical Times* (1900), or Lester Levyn, a physician in upstate New York, published on the susceptibility and immunity of Jews to particular diseases in the *New York Medical Journal* (1913), they probably had little to teach their fellow physicians about hygiene.[40] Yet they likely would be instructing many of them in the basic facts of Jewish ritual laws and aspects of Jewish life, and presenting these in a quite favorable light. Mark Blumenthal, writing in the *New York Journal of Medicine*, explicitly framed his discussion of "The Sanitary and Dietetic Laws of the Hebrews, as Related to Medicine" in practical terms of instruction (what we today might call sensitivity training). Blumenthal was at the time (the late 1850s) a resident physician at the Jews' Hospital in New York City. He was concerned that his non-Jewish colleagues were not suitably or sufficiently knowledgeable about Judaism, and this at times interfered with their task as physicians. In New

York, "where the Israelites form a large and respectable part of the community, and among whom every practicing physician has patients," it is perhaps advisable "to direct him [the non-Jewish physician] in his conduct and advice when treating a Hebrew...."[41] Blumenthal repeatedly framed his remarks in terms of "toleration and liberality" – physicians may not be aware when treating Jews of things that can offend. Out of benign ignorance doctors may suggest or recommend treatments or actions that run contrary to Jewish beliefs and rites. And "would not every conscientious physician and gentlemen of education and refined feelings prefer not to take the responsibility of ordering anything forbidden, or wittingly to wound the feelings of any one?"[42] Note again the language of respectability. The Jews already possess this quality, as of course do the physicians to whom Blumenthal speaks. Blumenthal's colleagues are men of refinement, and their actions with regard to another respectable community ought to reflect that.

4.

Jewish and Christian medical and religious authorities, writing in the nineteenth and twentieth centuries in American and British professional journals and popular forums, propagated equivalence between ancient Jewish laws and rituals and modern forms of scientific medical knowledge. These writers, consciously or not, contributed to a particular (and peculiar) medicalized biblical hermeneutics or midrash. How can this hermeneutic, this translation of Moses and the rabbis into modern medical men, be explained in the Anglo-American (but also European) contexts? What functions might this interpretive tradition have played for those who took it up and advanced it? There were, at least, three general contexts, heuristically distinct though interrelated, in which this medicalized biblical hermeneutics emerged. One, referred to a number of times already, was the intellectual-cultural context of the growing significance of preventive medicine and hygiene in the last half of the nineteenth century, and especially the popularization of knowledge about germs and bacteria, disease transmission, and the importance of public and personal hygiene. A second context was that of the professional or institutional realm, and concerns about the status of physicians and "mainstream" medicine. A third was that of the shifting and dynamic relationship between religion and science, and the status of religious leaders vis-à-vis scientists and doctors.

We can begin with the obvious. Rabbis could and did invoke the hygienic benefits of Jewish law and ritual in order to convince their congregations of the wisdom of following these laws. Rabbi Maurice Fleugal, speaking (in German) in May 1880 at Temple B'nai Israel in Kalamazoo, Michigan, informed his audience that, regrettably of course, the longstanding pattern of health and longevity among Jews was in the process of being undermined. "American Israelites" now suffered even more than did Christians from diseases such as cholera and yellow fever; disregard of the Mosaic laws was bringing about higher rates of mortality. Rabbi Fluegal reminded his audience that the well-known longevity and immunity to disease among Jews was due in large measure to adherence to the Mosaic laws.

None of this is surprising. Calling Jews back to ritual observance is, of course, part of the modern rabbi's task. What is surprising, or at least illuminating in the context of our discussion, is how Rabbi Fleugal framed his admonition. He began by assuring his listeners that "we want to be modern; we believe in science and progress." But this faith in science, he quickly reassured the congregation, is perfectly compatible with continued religious observance. To prove his point, Rabbi Fleugal called on the authority of Dr. Minor, a non-Jewish British physician, whose recent article in the *Lancet* lauded the health effects of the Mosaic laws. Dr. Minor, according to Fleugal, was "not a rabbi, not a ritual slaughterer, not a Jew, but a practicing physician and a man of science [*Wissenschaft*]."[43] The doctor had celebrated the health of the Jewish people, noting that they were the most cosmopolitan of races, and arguing that this trait had allowed Jews to acclimatize to whatever environment in which they found themselves. Jews were free of all congenital, degenerative diseases; they were immune to the plagues of the Middle Ages. Rabbi Fleugal called on the authority of a Gentile expert in order to convince Jews of the continued relevance of Jewish law and ritual. At the same time, he touted the Mosaic laws of health and hygiene as of likely benefit to Christians, who could increase their longevity and decrease the likelihood of illness through observance of these laws.

Again, a number of themes traced throughout this book appear in the rabbi's sermon: first and foremost, Fleugal's translation of religion into science, and the acceptance of science as the authoritative and legitimizing frame of reference; the participation of non-Jewish authorities in this celebration of Mosaic law and its health benefits, and the image of a healthy and vital Jew disseminated in these "Gentile" narratives; the invocation of these non-Jewish voices by Jews in order to give force to the argument about Jewish cultural achievement; and finally, the notion that the observance of traditional Jewish laws of hygiene would be beneficial not only to Jews but also to Christians. The British rabbi Hermann Gollancz, in a sermon on "The Dietary Laws," also invoked not the authority of religion but of science. Touting the health benefits of *kashrut*, Gollancz told his audience that modern science confirms the particulars of Jewish dietary rules; more generally "the wisdom of the laws of health prescribed ages ago for the guidance of the Hebrew people is becoming acknowledged day by day."[44]

In the Central European context, the translation of Moses and Mosaic law into modern medical terms functioned, *inter alia*, to legitimize the power and authority of physicians vis-à-vis an entrenched rabbinate that had until the nineteenth century enjoyed a high degree of autonomy. This is evident, for instance, when we look at the struggles in the nineteenth and early twentieth centuries over the issue of circumcision. Whether one was for or against the procedure, it was medicine rather than theology that increasingly shaped the terms of the debate. The physician, rather than the rabbi or *mohel* (ritual circumciser), had the authority to speak about the legitimacy of particular procedures such as *metzitzah* (sucking the blood from the circumcised penis), and about the benefits or dangers of the circumcision procedure in general.[45] The circumcision debate was part of the emancipation and integration process whereby the autonomy of the rabbinate was increasingly limited and much of its traditional power assumed by the state.[46] Social hygiene and health policies were an integral part of the nineteenth century state's assertion of power over individuals. Realms of Jewish life that before emancipation had come under the control of religious authorities now were the province of representatives of the state, and sanitation officials and physicians came to speak in the name of the secular state.

This struggle over Jewish communal and rabbinical autonomy as part of the emancipation process did not occur in a similar way in either Great Britain or the United States. While the rabbinate's position and status were and remain very different in Great Britain and the United States, in neither country was the power and authority of the rabbinical establishment ever as significant as in Continental Europe.[47] Thus, rabbis in Britain and America might be expected to gain in prestige by aligning themselves with scientific authority, including the authority and power of medicine. Gollancz and Fleugal are examples of a legitimation process that was unidirectional. Modern science and medicine validated religious practice.

Ironically perhaps, when physicians and medical writers analyzed the relationship between Jewish laws and health, they engaged in a reciprocal legitimation process between religion and science.[48] Certainly, when the laws concerning *kashrut*, circumcision, and family and sexual purity are juxtaposed with empirical research on the importance of diet and health, or the relationship between circumcision and rates of cervical and penile cancer (as well as a host of less severe genital disorders), the value and status of Jewish ritual is ostensibly raised. But when we look at the representation of Moses, the Temple priests, and the rabbis of the Talmud as rational, enlightened health officials, we can see the ways in which contemporary medical ideas and institutions could be legitimated through reference to this sacred past.

When N. D. Stebbins, a Detroit physician, set forth his defense of natural medicine in the 1850s, he argued that the model for natural, or what Stebbins also referred to as "rational," medicine is "the plan laid down for the Jewish priests" in the Old Testament.[49] Stebbins spent a good amount of space examining biblical passages related to leprosy and its treatment. Indeed, leprosy received a great deal of attention from physicians and medical writers in the nineteenth and early twentieth centuries. Since leprosy itself was no longer of any real concern for most Americans or Britons, why were the biblical passages concerning leprosy of such interest to physicians? Of course, a host of skin diseases did continue to preoccupy physicians, and the connection between race/ethnicity and skin diseases remained a valid subject of medical research.[50]

There did exist a far older intellectual tradition, reaching back to ancient writers such as Manetho, that linked Jews with leprosy. Voltaire and other eighteenth century Enlightenment figures incorporated this notion into their works.[51] So it is possible that the nineteenth and twentieth century texts under discussion here were in dialogue with this older tradition, and can be seen as a repudiation of this belief. The major concern in these narratives, however, was not leprosy per se, but the authority of the priesthood, and their role as health officials. The ancient Hebrew priesthood was identified as the only caste within society empowered to recognize and diagnose diseases properly. Thus, for Stebbins,

> the Jewish priests were [when it came to cases of possible leprosy] . . . obliged by their law to watch the changes [of the skin] and their character. These, as we have said, are pathological changes. . . . We argue from this that it is the duty of a physician to study the pathological changes of all diseases, and certainly these changes involve the living principle in such a manner, that a knowledge of physiology is necessary, to be fully competent to the task of correctly judging of disease; and it would not seem necessary to argue the case, to show that the physician ought to use every possible help to make himself the master of these branches of medical science.[52]

Ultimately, it is God himself who has determined that physicians deserve an elevated place in the hierarchy of men: "The importance of physicians and medicines for the interest of man is esteemed so great in the mind of the Lord, that He frequently, in figures of speech, enforces in very strong terms the necessity for their aid for the cure of disease."[53]

One of the functions of this discourse on hygiene, to call forth the authority of the medical professional as such, is particularly clear, then, in the case of leprosy. But it is no less valid when it comes to the more relevant or immediate diseases or illnesses that concerned the doctor and medical authority. The discourse on Moses and medicine was concerned with authority and power, and this did not necessarily have anything to do with the Jews per se. That is, the authority of the physician and medical researcher was reasserted through these "Jewish texts" and the implications for Jewry might have been negligible or non-existent for the authors of these texts. At the same time, we cannot cut these texts loose completely from their content and from what they represent once they are produced and disseminated. They could, in fact, function as both assertions of medical authority and power, and as interventions in the ongoing question about the nature of Judaism and the Jews.

For one British authority, writing in the early twentieth century, Moses was the chief health official and overseer of an entire sanitation system. Possessed as he was of a complete knowledge of infectious diseases, and of the principles of preventive medicine, Moses asked himself the question "that is still being asked in the twentieth century: if preventable, why not prevent it?" And he set about doing that. "He appointed the necessary personnel"; he entrusted the priests with tasks of inspection, isolation, etc. "Each priest thus became a state medical officer, a medical officer of health in fact. Aaron was appointed chief medical officer of health with his sons as his deputies." Moses set forth basic principles for the control of infectious diseases: "These principles were notification, isolation, frequent inspection, quarantine, and disinfection."[54] If in some contexts science can be seen to have empowered religion, in others religion could empower science – as long as the translation process had occurred.

The reinterpretation of Moses as a sanitarian and physician, and the ancient Jewish ritual laws as a hygienic code, provided one way to cement further a developing collective identity around the notion of special knowledge or wisdom. In addressing the question of the function or *sitz im leben* of the ancient Jewish image of Moses as both "god and king," Wayne Meeks suggests that at least one clear function of the tradition was "as a guarantee of esoteric tradition."[55] A community may organize itself around a notion of specialized knowledge, secret wisdom unavailable or beyond the reach of ordinary others. Such a community has access to "a higher order of truth," and this relationship to a special sort of knowledge and wisdom is constitutive of identity. By emphasizing the *origins* of this special sort of knowledge, and linking it with a semi-divine figure such as Moses, the community becomes its guardian. A chain of tradition is created that reinforces the chosen community's legitimacy as elite and powerful. Science, including medicine, does not explicitly construct itself of course around a notion of secret or esoteric knowledge. Rather, its practitioners pride themselves on the transparency of method and truth. Nonetheless, medical authorities certainly understood themselves as guardians of a specialized type of knowledge, and of a profession whose boundaries needed to be clearly defined and protected.[56]

It is not only religion or ancient Jewish law that is legitimated or given a greater status through such an analysis, but modern medicine, physicians, and health officials. Their role in society remained ambiguous, as the medical profession sought in the last half of the nineteenth century to professionalize, to establish its exclusive control over matters related to hygiene and health. This included identifying expertise and professionalism vis-à-vis "quacks," midwives, folk medicines, and other alternative forms of healing.[57] Ronald Numbers, a historian of American medicine, has outlined the crisis of status and authority medicine began to suffer in the mid-nineteenth century.[58] Doctors were undereducated and undertrained in medicine; even those with no degree and only a minimum number of hours of instruction called themselves doctors and set up practice. Medicine itself was increasingly factionalized, as sectarians advanced alternative forms of treatment such as homeopathy and botanics. The disagreements and infighting that quickly developed between sectarians and regulars produced an increased skepticism about medicine among the general public, and a loss of reputation and prestige for the profession.[59]

Thus, doctors had to establish and re-establish the status of normative medicine, and their status as professionals and authorities. One component of this process, albeit a very minor one from the perspective of medical history, was the strategy of translation and equivalence between ancient Jewish and modern medical worlds. The process entailed, first and foremost, translating Moses and the other ancient Jewish authorities into hygienists and physicians, equipped already three thousand years ago with an understanding of preventive medicine and disease transmission equivalent or superior to that of modern science. Already in 1847, John Harden, in "Notes on the Medicine of Moses," argued for physicians as a distinct profession already in biblical times.[60] In a paper originally read to the first meeting of the Ohio State Sanitary Association, and subsequently published in *JAMA*, William Morrow Beach invoked the Mosaic code to draw attention to the shortcomings of his own profession.[61] Physicians and health officials have failed to convince lawmakers and the general public of the need for stricter sanitary laws and regulations. After providing a cursory review of the plagues and epidemics that ravaged communities throughout history, Beach asked what might be done to prevent such disasters: "The sanitary laws of Moses (Levitcus xiii)," he told his audience, "contain the most that is necessary to be known concerning the sanitation in leprosy even to this day."[62] Invoking the Mosaic code in this context helped Beach make his main point, that given governmental resistance to sanitary reforms, medical authorities needed to do a much better job of convincing the public of the need for such measures; that is, the authority of medicine needed reinforcing. Then, politicians will know that if they do not do this, their political status and jobs will be in jeopardy. Again, in this case the ideal of the ancient acted as a possible spur to an imperfect present.[63]

The New York physician Herman Bendell, in an article entitled "The Physician of Sacred History," represented the ancient Hebrew or Jewish world as immersed in medical and scientific research and interest. Old Testament and rabbinical figures were described as physicians, surgeons, and medical specialists, and compared to modern heroes of bacteriology and immunology.

> A Talmudical remedy against the ill effects of a bite from a mad dog shows that an injury of that kind was not supposed to be followed by immediate ill consequences, and leads us to believe that the germ theory of Pasteur, Jenner and Koch was anticipated by these pre-Aescolepian writers. "For twelve consecutive months," says the Talmud, "let the bitten person drink only through a copper tube," doubtless to bring about a cure by means of the supposed chemical action of water on copper.[64]

Bendell's point here was not only that the rabbis understood germ theory to a degree akin to Pasteur and Koch, but also that in ancient as in modern times a professional class of experts existed and it alone should have the power to direct health policy. His explicit ire was directed at medical quacks, who could be found in ancient Jewish sources as much as in contemporary society. Here we have an example of a sort of negative equivalence: No sooner have the medical authorities whom Bendell compares to Pasteur, Jenner, and Koch spoken, than "the quack comes along and offers up his kabbalistic cure for dog-bite."[65]

The strategy of equivalence usually focused on ancient Jewish figures – Moses, the rabbis – and at times extended into the medieval period (Maimonides, etc.). However, this translation process also reached into the modern period. At times, the ancient Jewish milieu became the modern Jewish ghetto, and the need for the expertise of medical authorities posited through such an equivalence. One of the more elaborate examples of this sort of legitimation can be found in an article by the British Jewish physician John Snowman. In April 1896, Snowman published an extended piece on Jewish law and sanitation in *Medical Magazine*; the piece subsequently appeared in pamphlet form as *Jewish Law and Sanitary Science*. Snowman began by calling attention to the relatively recent emergence of hygiene and preventive medicine as a distinct scientific realm of research and practice, and this despite the fact that hygiene was now recognized as the most important branch of medicine.[66] Since so much disease can be prevented with "human foresight," the significance of hygiene cannot be overestimated. And yet, sanitarians agree that the general public has greeted the knowledge about disease prevention with "callousness and listlessness," that the response has fallen far short of the appeal.

The Jews, according to Snowman, can serve as an example to contemporary British society because Judaism is a totalizing system; it "does not stop at the synagogue or temple," but regulates every aspect of a Jew's life – food, clothing, housing, sexual and family relations. "It is a religion which holds forth immunity from disease as one of the rewards of a faithful adherence to its tenets, a religion which represents God as the physician of His people, whose laws are life giving in a physical as well as a spiritual sense." Ultimately, the Mosaic laws are "calculated to preserve the national health."[67]

Snowman, it must be noted, felt it necessary to deny the validity of the notion of the equivalence of ancient and modern knowledge. "It cannot be too strongly insisted that there was no anticipation of subsequent discoveries in hygiene, and the value of the quasi-sanitary laws of the Pentateuch must not be gauged from modern standpoints. . . . The relation between the religious and the scientific is at best indefinite."[68] And yet, his entire work resists this explicit denial and he ends up, in fact, making a case for the anticipatory power of Mosaic law.[69]

When Snowman sought to provide an image of ancient Jewish town life – life centered or built upon the "courtyard" (*chatzar*) – he described in fact a contemporary ghetto (London's East End or New York's Lower East Side) and transposed it to ancient times. The ancient Jewish town, built around a collection of courtyards, was "a densely populated hive of industry, with shops, dwelling houses, stalls, schools, small factories reverberating with sounds indicative of every variety of industrial activity." Noise was omnipresent, emerging from multiple sources: the clanging hammers, the grinding millstones, the "cries of the petty salesmen," the comings and goings of everyday citizens, and, above all, the "shrill prattle of the schoolchildren at their lessons." Snowman quotes an unnamed author: "Scenes of confused buying and selling, and endless variety of action in sounds, colours, and things. The ground is paved with broad unshaped flags from which each cry and jar and hoof-stamp arises to swell the medley that rings and roars up between the solid impending walls."[70]

This sort of environment demanded that the rabbis, as legislators, pay attention to the health effects of such crowded and cramped circumstances. At one point Snowman discusses the rabbis' views on what constituted nuisances and dangers to the health of the town's citizens, and refers to these as the rabbis' own "Public Health Act." Thus, the ancient rabbis become nineteenth-century British social reformers. But if Snowman intended to elevate talmudic rules and de-exoticize ancient Jewry in the eyes of contemporary readers, he also used the example of ancient Jewry to legitimize further the growing control of medicine and hygiene, to normalize the power of medical authorities to legislate over the lives of everyday people. "Rabbinical control" was the theme of Snowman's discussion. The strategy seems to have been to demonstrate that "it was ever thus." If you imagine, he seems to be saying, that the municipal government of London today is doing something radically new in regulating homes, workplaces, and public spaces with a view to health and hygiene, then know that already in the Bible we can find this sort of nexus of health and power.

Snowman engaged in an extended discussion of what constituted, in the eyes of the rabbis, adequate or safe housing: the structure of walls and floors, ceiling height, courtyards, waste disposal, neighbor relations, and so on. Arguing through implicit analogy, he sought to make a case for both reform of tenement or working-class housing and for the legitimacy of strengthening the authority of medicine and science to make decisions about how men and women will live and work. Thus, in the middle of his discussion of the rabbinical regulations regarding housing he writes:

> We find the same principles of law and order applied to communal life, many of which recall the duties of the modern district surveyor and sanitary inspector. The duty of the townsfolk to attend to those aspects of town-life which tell on their health is enforced. No wise man would dwell in a town which did not possess a medical officer. . . . All were compelled to contribute to the expenses of the municipal arrangements on behalf of the welfare of the inhabitants.[71]

The translation of Moses and the rabbis into health authorities, and the equivalence drawn between ancient purity laws and contemporary practices served potentially to heighten the cultural capital of both science and religion. This was not a one-way street, with Judaism, and religion in general by extension, gaining relevance and prestige by linking itself with science and medicine. It was that to be sure. But medicine, as a profession in the making, yet still uncertain in its status, also had a great deal to gain by aligning itself with Scripture. Modern medicine benefited by linking itself, more specifically, with notions of authority, hierarchy, and the rule of "priests" found in the Bible. If doctors were not yet "gods," they were certainly on their way. The first step was to become priests, a select group within society that possessed valuable and esoteric knowledge and employed that knowledge for the good of the whole.

This theme of Moses and the rabbis as men of science and medicine survived well into the twentieth century, long past the period in which physicians found it necessary to legitimize professional medicine. In the 1930s and beyond, the discourse remained more or less unchanged, but the contexts, and therefore the meanings, changed. As I mentioned in Chapter 1, narratives produced in the 1930s and 1940s about Jews and medicine, Jews and their contribution to health and hygiene, would more than likely have been intended and been read as explicit responses to German and European anti-Semitism and to the physical danger in which Jews in Europe now found themselves. That they continued well past this period and into the present testifies to the continuing fluidity of boundaries when it comes to notions of legitimate and illegitimate medicine, continuing popularity of alternative or nontraditional forms of healing, the ongoing question as to the efficacy of Jewish rituals vis-à-vis health and disease prevention, and the resurgence of questions about the relation between biology, genetics, and Jewish identity.[72]

5.

Nancy Tomes, in her fascinating cultural history of germs and germ theory, has linked what she has called "the gospel of germs" directly and unequivocally to cultural modernism, to the "cult of the new" that emerged in America and elsewhere in the Progressive era.

> This rising consciousness of the germ coincided with the emergence of a new style of cultural modernism. . . . The gospel of germs offered a vision of hygienic modernism that was perfectly suited to this 'cult of the new' and

its 'perfectionist project,' as historians William Leach and Jackson Lears have respectively termed it. . . . The cult of the new and the gospel of germs were but two facets of the same enthusiastic pursuit of modernity.[73]

Without doubt, the hygienic movement celebrated modern science and medicine, lauded recent discoveries in bacteriology and disease prevention, and made heroes of scientists such as Pasteur, Koch, Lister, and others. Yet, along with this cult of the new, hygiene and medicine constructed a cult of the ancient. When we begin to explore the extent to which the "ancient," in the guise of the Mosaic laws and even post-biblical Jewish literature, appeared in the hygienic literature, and became a chief source of pointing up the lacunae or failures of the modern health movement, Tomes' notion of a "cult of the new" within sanitary science seems to require emendation.

If modern medicine and science served to validate the ancient, to counter the disparagement of religion by redefining it in medical and scientific terms, the status and legitimacy of modern medicine was also buttressed by linking it with the ancient biblical tradition. A reciprocal process of legitimation was at work in the strategy of translation or equivalence. One of the impulses and effects of this process, as I have argued, was to imbue physicians and public health officials, and their efforts, with a greater aura of sanctity by equating them with Moses and his law code. This was achieved mainly through the representation of Moses and the rabbis as medical men, possessed of knowledge equivalent or superior to that of modern authorities.

Yet another effect – and at least when it came to many, though by no means all, authors, another impulse – of this medicalized discourse was the representation of Judaism and the Jews as healthy and vital. Again, this construction of the image of a healthy Jew was undertaken by Jewish and non-Jewish writers alike. And it was achieved in the main through discussions of particular biblical and post-biblical laws and rituals that had a direct impact on the individual and collective Jewish body: the dietary laws (*kashrut*), the laws of family and sexual purity (*taahrot ha-mishpokah*), circumcision, and the laws regulating the communal environment.

"Filth," according to Judith Leavitt and Ronald Numbers, "was the premier public health problem in the nineteenth century."[74] Health

experts paid increasing attention to garbage, waste (both human and animal), sewage, and contamination of water supplies, food supplies, and
air quality. This interest in public or community hygiene was matched
by concern with personal hygiene: diet, living and working conditions,
sexual practices and mores. In the last half of the nineteenth century,
hygiene and preventive medicine emerged as one of the chief avenues
of dealing with disease. Crisis heightened the belief that personal and
public cleanliness were directly linked to levels of disease and mortality.
Cholera, typhus, and yellow fever epidemics were instrumental in bringing public health – issues such as purity of water supplies, proper waste
disposal – to the forefront of American and British attention. Wars also
served to impel public health activities. America's Civil War, for instance,
was transformative in this regard. More soldiers died of dysentery than
of wounds incurred in battle. Health activists, mainly women inspired
by Florence Nightingale's example during the Crimean War, organized
to improve conditions in military camps and instruct soldiers in the basic
principles of hygiene. After the war, this organized effort at public and
personal hygiene migrated to the cities, which were seen as similar to
the army camp with regard to conditions of health and disease.[75] As we
shall see in Chapter 4, it will be the urban environment that becomes,
in the last half of the nineteenth century, the locus of concern not only
in debates over general health and hygiene, but also over more specific
debates about the health of Jews and Judaism.

4

From Ghetto to Jungle

Darwinism, Eugenics, and the Reinterpretation of Jewish History

I.

How to account for survival and preeminence in civilization? How to account for empires, and how to ensure their survival? Is every nation and empire akin to an individual, fated to be born, grow, and then inevitably decline and die? Or is the easy analogy a mistake; is intervention possible, decline and death avoidable? Such questions preoccupied nationalist, racialist, and eugenic thinkers at the turn of the twentieth century.[1] At the other end of the spectrum, at the level of local communal existence, the questions were equally pressing: what sort of environment was most conducive to individual and communal health and survival? What effect did urban life have on individuals physically and mentally? And how did this translate into the health of the nation, the *Volk*, the ethnos or race? For many who considered such questions, the millennia-long survival of the Jews as a collective – a race, a *Volk*, a nation – along with their purported longevity and health as individuals, provided a key.

Structurally, the narrative on the Jews and survival mirrors in important ways the apologetic discourse on the contribution of Jews to medicine and civilization. Both reify the collective, and both depend on a notion of agency that credits "the Jewish people" with particular achievements – the translation of texts, transmission of knowledge, survival over millennia. The notion of agency, of course, does not really mesh with a strict Darwinian explanation of survival and transmutation based on natural selection. Yet, the academic and popular writers whose works I explore in this chapter were hardly consistent in their deployment of Darwinian theories. Notions of personal agency and environmental causality (what at the time would have struck many as neo-Lamarckism more than Darwinism) could be found together with natural selection as explanations for aspects of Jewish history and Jewish collective behavior and traits. Still, physicians, scientists, and theologians interested in Judaism, Jewish history, and the nature of the Jews employed Darwinian ideas to understand all three, even if their commitment to consistency was often incomplete. Moreover, there was a concerted effort that began at the turn of the twentieth century to establish an equivalence between Judaism and eugenics, to demonstrate that the ancient Jewish authorities – the patriarchs, Moses, and the rabbis – were as concerned with national and racial health as were contemporary Europeans and Americans.

In the post-Holocaust literature on eugenics and Social Darwinism the Jews are most often portrayed, understandably, as victims of this set of ideas and governmental practices. This is true whether we are talking about the history of Germany, Great Britain, or the United States. The particular histories of the Jewish communities in these different countries vary widely, of course; nonetheless, at a fundamental level, the Jews are understood first and foremost as victims: objects of research and then, in the case of Europe at least, objects of an increasingly radical policy. Yet, as important as this understanding of the historical relationship between Jewry and racial science is, it is only part of the story. In Germany, prominent members of the *Rassenhygiene* movement in the pre-Nazi period such as Alfred Ploetz and William Schallmayer praised the Jews in eugenic terms and disavowed anti-Semitism (even if they also insisted on the ultimate superiority of Aryans, and more or less embraced Nazism in the 1930s).[2] Non-Jewish eugenicists in the United States and Great Britain were also celebrating the Jews, and this during the period identified by historians as a time of peak hostility to the presence of Jews in these societies. Again, in no way am I seeking to minimize the hostility. But I am arguing for a more complex and ambiguous picture of that period, and more generally, suggesting that this more complex picture involve a greater scrutiny of certain assumptions about anti-Semitism, especially a purported causal relationship between anti-Semitic texts and anti-Jewish actions.

If Darwinian and eugenic ideas were undoubtedly significant for the construction of the image of the diseased and degenerate Jew, they also figured in the construction of the healthy Jew, and in the reinterpretation of Jewish history as an illustration of the principles of natural selection and survival of the fittest. My interest in this chapter is not with the concerted effort on the part of Jewish theologians to respond to Darwin's ideas, and either reconcile the biblical and post-biblical notions of creation with Darwinian theories, or reject the attempt as futile and dangerous.³ Rather, it is with the attempt to translate Abraham, Moses, and the rabbis into ancient versions of Francis Galton and Charles Davenport, to name only two of the most prominent eugenicists of the time, and apply evolutionary and eugenic ideas to an understanding of Jewish history and Jewish survival. In an essay on "Deconstructing Darwinism," the historian of science James Moore commented on the fact that "little effort had been expended by historians of science in tracing the proliferation of Darwin-related vocabulary and interpreting its function in public discourse."⁴ This chapter is an attempt to show how a Darwin-related vocabulary contributed to the construction of an interpretive tradition about the Jews and Judaism, and suggest how it might have functioned as a counter-discourse in public debates.

2.

Of all six hundred and thirteen commandments in the Torah, the Anglo-Jewish physician William Feldman wrote in 1939, "reproduction is the most important." Feldman asserted this at the outset of his discussion of the "eugenic principles of the ancient rabbis," which in turn was part of his article on "ancient Jewish eugenics."⁵ The ancient Hebrews combined "judicious selective mating with intelligent antenatal and postnatal care," and thus "succeeded in rearing a race, not indeed of supermen, but one which is probably the most virile that ever lived, and which has survived at times when many other apparently stronger races, not subjected to anything like the same persecution and physical as well as mental stress and torture, have perished." Judaism, Feldman proudly wrote, was and remains so committed to eugenic ideas that "it is permissible for a woman to be sterilized if she is likely to bear children who are going to be tainted with physical or mental disease."⁶ Feldman was also a lecturer on hygiene and pediatric physiology in London, and the author of *The Jewish Child: Its History, Folklore, Biology and Sociology.*

In his introduction to that book, James Crichton-Browne diplomatically praised the work and its author. Granted, he wrote, that it contains "a good deal of archaic physiology, doubtful anthropology, and ethics, not in accord with existing notions." Nonetheless, Feldman's work clearly demonstrates "how Rabbinical and Talmudic precepts anticipated many of the hygienic teachings of today, and linking [sic] Oriental imagery with statistics and mathematical analysis."[7] Crichton-Browne was at pains to point out that while Feldman, following the Anglo-Jewish geneticist and racial thinker Redcliffe Salaman, wanted to make a strong case for "nature," or the influence of biology, heredity, and racial eugenics, his work in fact demonstrated the extraordinary effects of environment and "nurture." It is the lessons of Jewish "nurturing," the power and influence of the Jewish mother and the ideal of motherhood, rather than the understandably biased claims for the "prepotency" of the Jewish race, that Crichton-Browne hoped and expected the English reading public would take from Feldman's work.[8] Thus, in a monograph from 1939, we encounter a Jewish scholar insisting on a "hard" genetic approach to the history and anthropology of the Jews, including a celebration of negative eugenics, and a non-Jewish scholar seeking to counter these claims with an environmental or cultural approach. Both, however, agreed on the vitality of the Jews and sought to explain this with reference to Judaism.

When Thurman B. Rice invoked the Jews at the outset of his general guide to eugenics and race, it was, like Feldman, to celebrate the conterminous natures of Judaism and eugenics, and the racial hygienic value of the Jewish people.[9] Rice was an associate professor of bacteriology and public health at Indiana University, a lecturer on eugenics there, and the chairman of the Indiana Eugenics Committee. In his book *Racial Hygiene*, under the subheading "Race, Culture, and Religion," he remarked on what he considered a strange phenomenon: Many religious people oppose eugenical theory and practice; and yet, "a great number of these same [eugenical] teachings are identical with the principles set forth in Holy Writ. The chosen people of Israel are the most spectacular and successful of all experiments in human race culture. The principle of keeping the race pure is nowhere better illustrated than in the history of the Jewish people; sex hygiene began with the Jews; race hygiene was almost a fetish with them."[10] The result of this fetish is the remarkable persistence of the Jewish race, the continuity of language, religion, tradition – a "race consciousness and solidarity" that is remarkable given their "jumbled national history." Races, Rice concluded, "rise and fall, but Israel is immortal."[11]

Rice insisted that his enthusiasm should not be mistaken for a "eulogy of the Jew." The Jews as a race display many negative qualities, though the contempt for the Jew is more often than not born of prejudice than reason. Rice was not arguing that the Jews are a pure race or the best race, only that they have been an extraordinarily successful race in eugenic and Darwinian terms, and therefore worthy of study, admiration, and emulation.

The issue of the Jews' survival was of course not new. Jews and non-Jews had been wondering and theorizing about the collective existence of the Jewish people for more than two millennia. But after Darwin, and particularly as the nineteenth century drew to a close, the issue came to be addressed in another and different way, with a new set of terms drawn from the world of biology, evolution, genetics, and eugenics.[12] Consider the remarks of Dr. Mark Blumenthal, delivered at the New York Medical Union in February 1859, in the same year that Darwin's *On the Origin of Species* appeared. Blumenthal was at the time resident physician at the Jews' Hospital, New York. Speaking on the topic of "The Sanitary and Dietetic Laws of the Hebrews," he at one point spoke of the ghetto, of the oppressive conditions in which Jews lived, and of their vitality despite such conditions: "During the dark ages, the Israelites, if at all tolerated, were compelled to live in the most crowded state and confined to the lowest localities in the various cities of Europe, under conditions undoubtedly every way favorable to the production of miasma, fever, and pestilence. They nevertheless preserved their innate vigor of body and mind as their history, as well as their present state abundantly testifies."[13] Over fifty years later, in an essay titled "Jewish Eugenics," the American rabbi Max Reichler asked the question that so many had asked before him: "Who knows the cause of Israel's survival?" But the rabbi's answer reflected the turn in the interpretation of the Jewish past and present, a turn that had taken place over the preceding quarter century. Jewish survival, according to Reichler, could be explained by the Jews' adherence to the "Law of Life," or eugenic principles, and to their success in the Darwinian "struggle for existence."[14] Blumenthal, too, believed the key to understanding the Jews' survival and vitality resided in their adherence to Mosaic law.

He, too, sought to reinterpret Jewish law and ritual in terms of hygiene and preventive medicine. Religion and health, he argued, are inextricably connected: "the tendency of the religious laws is conducive to the physical and spiritual welfare, the vigor of mind, and strength of body of the Israelites."[15] But in 1859, Blumenthal did not (could not) argue for a confluence of Judaism and eugenics; and while he noted that Jews had over the millennia experienced both persecution and epidemic disease, he did not frame his discussion in the language of the Darwinian or Spencerian struggle for existence.[16] The Jews, in Blumenthal's narrative, survive and thrive *despite* persecution and disease, not because of them. Yet, as the nineteenth century went on, Jews and non-Jews would have at their disposal a new language and set of ideas with which to analyze the historical persecution of the Jews, the impact of disease, the "spectacular" survival and vitality of the Jews as a people, and the role of Judaism in this.[17] For many Jewish and non-Jewish thinkers, the Jews had survived not despite the suffering and persecution but *because* of them.

3.

Just as ancient Jewish texts and practices were reinterpreted in terms of hygiene and preventive medicine, so, too, Jewish and non-Jewish writers re-framed the Torah and Talmud in light of eugenics and Darwinism. This use of eugenics and Darwinism to help explain the Jews and their survival as a collective was a particular interpretative moment in Jewish historiography,[18] framed not by any new revelations about the Jewish past per se, but by revolutionary shifts in understanding and practice in the world of science and medicine.

When the language of eugenics came to be seen as both legitimate and necessary for analyzing issues of collective identity and survival, and the central role of medical authorities and the state in ensuring these goals was recognized, Judaism could be – some argued even had to be – reinterpreted along these lines.[19] The key element in this was the same strategy of translation or equivalence that I have examined in previous chapters: in this case, Moses as the Francis Galton of the ancient world, and the Torah and Talmud as a eugenic code. The millennia-long survival of the Jews and their national and racial vitality were the result of this code. "If eugenics be the study of the conditions under human control which improve or impair the inborn characteristics of the race," the *Jewish Chronicle* in Great Britain declared in 1910, "then Moses, the Lawgiver, was the first and greatest of all eugenists, for, as Sir Francis Galton...agrees, the indirect influence of the hygienic regulations of the Mosaic Code in preserving the Jewish race 'fit' has been great. The whole Law of Moses is, in fact, a remarkable body of eugenic effort – a wonderful comprehensive code for the building up of a strong and 'fit' people."[20]

The *Chronicle* reminded its readers that Galton's call for "parental responsibility" had already been a watchword for Jews for millennia. The sins of the fathers shall be visited upon the children for generations: "No warning as to the seriousness of parental responsibility ever smote the ears of mankind with such irresistible force and penetrating brevity." This brief celebration of Galton and eugenics, and its confluence with traditional Jewish practice, called readers' attention to the interview with Galton in the same issue of the newspaper. The editors introduced the interview by referring to eugenics as Galton's "high ideal," and proceeded to argue that "from the days of Moses Jews have been 'eugenists'. . . . "[21] The interviewer asked Galton whether or not he believed "that the hygienic regulations of the Mosaic Code have contributed to the fitness of the Jewish race?" He responded that yes, he could believe that the Mosaic code had played its part. Galton was asked about the impact of historical persecutions on the Jewish race, about the effect of migrations, and about the relationship between eugenics and religion (he insisted that religious institutions have an important role to play in eugenic health). Galton's polite answers are less illuminating than the interviewer's insistence that Galton the eugenist give his blessing to Judaism and Jewish history. The *Chronicle* was, clearly, deeply invested in making Judaism and Jewry harmonious with eugenics and racial health.

Rabbi Max Reichler, too, made a point of citing Galton, the founder of the eugenics movement, and other eminent non-Jewish authorities such as the leading American eugenicist Charles Davenport, on the historical connection between Judaism and eugenics. Reichler explicitly lauded the opinions of these non-Jewish authorities, arguing that their status as non-Jews demonstrated the unbiased truth of their claims. In making such an argument, Reichler appears to have accepted, consciously or not, a common claim made about Jews and science in these decades. Non-Jewish eugenicists and race scientists in the United States, Great Britain, and Germany often argued that Jews could not be objective when writing about race and eugenics precisely because they were Jews. Thus, like the opinions of Schleiden and Strack in Germany, those of Galton, Davenport and others – many of whom were far more ambivalent about Jews than their comments about Judaism and eugenics would indicate – meant so much because these authorities were not Jewish.

"The Jews," in the words of one such non-Jewish authority invoked by Reichler, "have always understood the science of eugenics, and have governed themselves in accordance with it; hence the preservation of the Jewish race." Eugenic principles were to be found in the earliest biblical accounts; it was just a matter of rereading the biblical and post-biblical literature through the prism of eugenic and Darwinian theories. According to Reichler, "The very founder of the Jewish race [Abraham] recognized the importance of certain inherited qualities." Hence, Abraham insisted that Isaac's wife come not from the Cannanites, but from "the seed of superior stock."[22]

Rabbi Reichler embraced the racial identity of the Jews and the idea that they had been "preserved" racially over thousands of years through a eugenic and Darwinian-like selection process. He did, however, qualify the above statement by arguing that eugenics "as a science" could not have existed among the Jews in ancient times. However, "many eugenic rules were certainly incorporated in the large collection of Biblical and Rabbinic laws."[23] In the end, the thrust of Reichler's work was aimed at demonstrating that Judaism and eugenics shared the same ultimate goal: "Indeed there are clear indications of a conscious effort to utilize all influences that might improve the inborn qualities of the Jewish race, and to guard against any practice that might vitiate the purity of the race, or 'impair the racial qualities of the future generations' either physically, mentally, or morally."[24]

Other medical writers were less hesitant than Reichler in making the argument of equivalence. In a series of articles on Judaism and hygiene published between 1910 and 1918 in the well-regarded journal *Hygienische Rundschau*, a Wiesbaden physician, identified only as Dr. Ratner,[25] sought to demonstrate that ancient Judaism had been preoccupied with precisely those same issues that preoccupied contemporary physicians and policy makers – marriage and the quality of offspring, sexual perversions and prostitution, and their impact on society and social welfare – and that ample evidence existed to show that a eugenic or racial hygiene system already existed in ancient Israel.[26] Ratner, like every other physician we've encountered, read the Hebrew Bible literally; thus, he employed a medicalized hermeneutics that assumed the biblical narrative is a straightforward historical record, and that an analysis or diagnosis of motives or condition reveals something about the actual status of ancient Jewry. The eugenic principle, for instance, can be found already in the narrative of Abraham, when he sends his servant Eliezer out to find a bride for his son (Genesis 24: 3–4). Abraham commands his servant to look not among the Cannanites but among "the house of my fathers." According to Ratner, "He [Abraham] did not want a daughter-in-law from among the daughters of the other, culturally inferior races/tribes [*Volksstämme*], but from his own tribe [*Stamm*]. He was already compelled by 'eugenics,' if one may be permitted to express it thus."[27] We might easily assume that, given the celebratory nature of Ratner's interpretation, Ratner was a Jew. Yet, Ratner's case is illuminating precisely because he cannot be identified for certain by means of the content of his writings (we will encounter another example of this in Chapter 5). Both Jews and non-Jews argued in this vein about Jews and Judaism during these decades. The healthy Jew, a product of a Judaism finely attuned to eugenic as well as hygienic principles, was not solely the creation of Jewish scholars.

Ratner offered numerous other examples taken from Genesis before pronouncing that "This runs through the earliest history of the Jewish people like a red thread: racial selection and eugenic breeding for the purpose of maintenance and survival of the race" (*"So zieht es sich wie ein roter Faden durch die Urgeschichte des jüdischen Volkes: Rassenzuchtwahl und eugenische Auslese zur Festigung und Erhaltung des Stammes"*).[28] And, Ratner continued, this proved true as time went on. Any marriage or sexual union that might prove harmful to the Jewish race was absolutely forbidden, and punished in the harshest terms (e.g. Exodus 39: 11–15). Since we are quite familiar from the Bible with all of the perversions that the ancient pagans engaged in – magic, child sacrifice, sodomy, adultery, pederasty, rape, etc. – is it any wonder, Ratner asked, that the Israelites were commanded as they were? "How extreme was the vengeance taken on miscegenation [*Blutvermischung*], so that the higher race could be saved from inferiority, even extinction?" ("*Wie würde sich also Blutvermischung bitter rächen, wie würde sie die höher stehende Rasse zur Inferiorität, vielleicht auch zum Aussterben hinführen?*").[29] Ratner then moved on to discuss eugenics in the Talmud, insisting that very stringent customs regarding racial unity and ancestry were maintained; this is designated as "*Jichus.*" The rabbis forbade marriage to anyone from families judged to be physically or intellectually inferior. "Both physical and mental qualities are inherited," according to the ancient Jewish sources. "When a woman is married off for money, unworthy children are the result" (*Pesachim*, 49b). "Intellectual attributes are inherited," Ratner concluded; "this is precisely what the fine young science of Galton teaches!"[30]

For the British physician William M. Feldman, Jews in the ancient world had a clear-cut understanding of the principles and significance of eugenic thinking. Jews were highly concerned with remote as well as proximate genealogy, and thus "foreshadowed Galton's law of ancestral heredity." Ancient Jews maintained special pedigree books or scrolls "in which the genealogical trees of people were recorded." And the Bible, of course, records genealogical tables "of such minuteness of detail as would rejoice the heart of the most ardent eugenist."[31] Max Danzis, speaking in Temple B'nai Abraham of Newark, New Jersey, in 1930, told his audience: "The Talmud, as well as the Old Testament, has many interesting and valuable eugenic lessons. Talmudic sages were early to recognize the effect of a clean, moral life upon preservation of the race. Sex, hygiene, and eugenics, almost modern in its sense, received careful consideration in the Talmud." Danzis' talk later appeared as an article in the *Journal of the Medical Society of New Jersey*, thus potentially finding its way to a much broader audience than that in the synagogue.[32]

There were, it should be noted, a few gestures towards a recognition of eugenics' brutality, and an insistence that fusing eugenics with Judaism meant that the latter had humanized the former. Alfred Nossig argued that the Mosaic code rejected the idea that "the selection of men" ought to be equivalent to the "selection of cattle."

The Hebrew lawgiver recommended to his people unrestrained procreation and forbade the murder of infants in the strongest terms. He employed a far more humane system of racial selection [*Rassenzüchtung*] than Lycurgus, whose system was based primarily on the goals of war. [Moses] rejected that noxious influence which modern research has designated as "militaristic selection."[33]

Judaism, according to Nossig, approved of positive eugenics, of practices that encouraged the union of healthy individuals and the reproduction of healthy infants. But Moses and Jewish law were not heir to the more toxic elements of eugenic thinking and practice embodied by the Spartans, what came to be called negative eugenics. William Feldman granted that the rabbis of the Talmud almost certainly adopted "much of the eugenic wisdom of their Greek and Roman predecessors," but also amended it in important respects. The Jews "infused a humanitarian spirit" into their eugenic system; "eugenics with mercy" as Feldman called it in 1939. According to this view, Jews, unlike Greeks and Romans, did not practice or condone infanticide; they did not advocate, as did Plato, the abandonment of the chronic invalid to die; unlike the Spartans, the Jews recognized the complexity of human personality and development. Thus, while the Spartans "reared a people that were preeminently fitted for war, the Jews aimed at cultivating a race that was fitted both for peace and for war."[34] Isidore Simon, a French medical doctor and founder of the *Revue d'Histoire de la Médecine Hébraïque*, made much the same point ten years later. Unlike the Greeks, who clearly understood the laws of eugenics, heredity, and selection, and employed "radical methods" to insure "*l'amélioration de la race*," the Hebrews "did not approve of 'selection' or rather, the suppression of the weak and feable..." (*n'admettaient par la 'selection' ou plutôt la suppression des faibles...* "). Nonetheless, their sacred writings demonstrate an intense interest in matters "that we today would call eugenics and heredity."[35]

On the other hand, there were those like the German Jewish social scientist Arthur Ruppin, writing in the first years of the twentieth century, who could bemoan the un-Spartanlike nature of Jewish eugenic practice. In the context of a discussion of comparative death rates between Christian and Jewish Germans, Ruppin commented on the overall favorable statistics that demonstrate that Jews live longer. The decrease in Jewish death rates, however, he said, does have its negative side. Ruppin's argument drew directly on the general eugenic notion that the developing welfare state was intervening in the process of natural selection and keeping alive those whom nature would eliminate. Those weak individuals, Ruppin argued, who have survived through painstaking care, would never have reached adulthood without the intervention of the state: "From the purely economic point of view, one can ask whether the saving of these physically weak individuals is of benefit for the Jews, since these individuals do not live long into adulthood, even if they do survive childhood."[36] Writing in 1917 on "Jewish racial selection," the leading American social scientist of the Jews, Maurice Fishberg, wrote glowingly of the eugenic impulse found in Judaism (I'll return to this aspect of Fisbherg's article later in this chapter). Nonetheless, he did feel obliged to point out that the marriage laws and social customs that structured ghetto life also contained strong and effective anti-eugenic tendencies, which made possible the reproduction of the physically and intellectually defective.[37]

In this traditional Jewish culture, Fishberg argued, echoing what by this time was already a cliché, only intellectual qualities mattered. Thus, physical qualities were deemed unimportant, and the physically unfit survived and reproduced. The most significant anti-eugenicist practice, according to Fishberg, was the institution of "*hachnassat-kallah*" [the communally raised dowry for impoverished brides]. This communal care for the poor Jewish bride meant that everyone was married off, so even those with physical and intellectual deficiencies were allowed to procreate. Blind men were often paired off with lame girls, for example, and degenerate descendents were the inevitable result. Western and Eastern European Jews continue to make this a duty of theirs, Fishberg argued; that is why one finds a higher number of degenerate individuals among wealthy Jews than among wealthy Christians. Jewish charity was also a major factor in degeneration. Charitable organizations in Berlin, London, and particularly New York, he said, supported the "less worthy" ("*minderwertigen*") members of society, and allowed them to reproduce; this was "frightening" when one considered that most of the offspring were intellectually and physically deficient. Fishberg also noted, as did so many other social scientists at the time, that there were relatively few alcoholics among the Jews. In the context of eugenics, this was of course a cause for celebration. The relative absence of alcoholism among Jews was often invoked as one major cause of Jewish health. Nonetheless, in certain respects Jewish culture and eugenics clashed with respect to alcoholics. They were not disqualified from assistance by the Jewish community; they were considered "unfortunates," and given aid. In addition, the absence of alcoholism, particularly among women, reduced the rate of infant or child mortality (*Kindersterblichkeit*.) All of this contributed to the increase in the number of biological and social defectives. According to Fishberg, the "*gute jüdische Herz*" ("good Jewish heart") will always assist the defective. Then, sounding like a Jewish version of Oliver Wendell Holmes Jr., he lamented that "the chain will remain unbroken."[38]

4.

For the most part, however, writers on Judaism, eugenics, and Darwinism felt no compulsion either to celebrate or bemoan Judaism's relative humaneness vis-à-vis the weak and unfortunate. The main task was to make the case for a correspondence or affinity between Judaism and eugenics, and the positive impact of this on the condition of the Jews. This, in turn, established a correspondence or affinity between Jews and Judaism, and the modern state and a bourgeois culture of respectability. The discourse on eugenics and hygiene allowed elites to demonstrate both that Jews and Judaism anticipated the modern state's central interests when it came to questions of its population's quality, and that Jewry posed no danger to the state's and society's vision and interests in this crucial matter.

Yet social Darwinian and eugenic ideas and images were compelling for a variety of reasons. The most common explanation centers on the rise of a racialized anti-Semitism in the last quarter of the nineteenth century, and the crucial role Darwinian and eugenic thinking played in this. Many of those who felt compelled to respond to this new sort of attack on Jewry believed that the most efficacious way to do so was to utilize the scientific language, images, and arguments that had been deployed against the Jews. Yet, as powerful as the need to respond to the new scientific racial anti-Semitism was, this explanation alone is not nuanced enough to capture the power that science, including racial, evolutionary, and eugenics-based science, possessed for Jews and non-Jews alike. Biology and medicine more and more influenced social thought in the last half of the nineteenth century, and the demand to reinterpret Jewish sources and Jewish practices came as a result of the excitement about these new scientific ideas as much as from the challenge of anti-Semitism. In a 1905 article on the "idea of the chosenness of the Jews in the light of biology," Alfred Nossig argued that in order to truly understand the Jews, one must first comprehend that the personal God of the Bible is identical to the highest abstraction of Being, and that his will is identical to the general laws of nature. Thus, the moral legislation of the Jews coincides with the laws discovered by natural science: "Their history is not the product of divine will, but of their relation with natural laws." The Jews and Judaism cannot be fathomed outside of the realms of biology and the natural sciences.[39] If all history and culture now had to be comprehended within the framework of biology and evolution, how could Jews and Judaism remain exempt from this reinterpretive process?

"I am convinced," the American Max Levy wrote in a 1905 piece called "Jewish People and the Laws of Evolution,"

> that the relation of the Jew to his surroundings and environment will follow laws that have been found to be universal in their application. I see no reason why the Jews, any more than any other man or animal, should be above the conditions which govern the development of species. The influence of the environment upon the origin and development of species has been clearly set forth by Spencer, Huxley, Darwin, and other exponents of the theory of evolution, and the same class of considerations that effects the physical development of species is clearly shown to exert an equally powerful influence on the development of civilization.[40]

Levy was not a professional social scientist, but an inventor, best known at the time for his involvement in photographic technology. His article, like that of Rabbi Reichler's, testifies to the popular appeal of evolutionary and eugenic theories among interpreters, both scholarly and popular, of Jewish history. Writing twenty-five years later, on the "biologic interpretation of Jewish survival," the physician Hyman Morrison, of Tufts College (later, Tufts University), inquired into the "key to the riddle of our [Jews'] survival?" The answer could be found in the Darwinian principles of evolution and natural selection. "We are a chosen people only in the sense that because of naturally inherent traits, physical as well as cultural, we were able to adapt ourselves to various environments and so have survived."[41] Through natural selection "only the sturdiest individuals of the group survived; pruning and engrafting added to its strength." Jews, like other organisms, quickly learned to adapt and survive hostile environments. And the "shifting of the population through expulsion and economic migrations was in fact transplantation to new and fresh environments." Thus, today "in spite and because of centuries of terrific suffering, natural selection is the reason for our unusual ability to resist infectious disease, and for our longevity."[42] Morrison was convinced that scholars of Jewish history and society would be well-advised to do some adapting of their own, to begin to think and speak of the Jewish past and present in natural scientific terms. "At this stage of human intellectual development ... our survival ought to be expressed in terms of the general laws of natural evolution which are more or less equally applicable to plants, animals and human beings."[43] Published in 1940, Morrison's polemic would seem to suggest that little reconsideration of Jewish history in the light of the laws of natural selection had occurred. Yet, if such a reinterpretation had not become the dominant, let alone the only, valid way of looking at Jewry, Morrison nonetheless severely underestimated the extent of the work that had already been done.

5.

The idea of the ghetto as a place of isolation, poverty and oppression, of physical and spiritual debility, has been central to the modern Jewish imagination.[44] The *maskilim*, or Jewish enlighteners, made the intellectual and cultural isolation of the ghetto the focus of their program of self-reform. Jewish nationalists, beginning in the late nineteenth century, identified the modern ghetto, now the equivalent of the eastern European *shtetl*, as both cause and effect of Jewish degeneration (even as some of them, following the Zionist philosopher Ahad Ha'am, could also identify a spiritual nobility that accompanied physical deprivation). Most commentators agreed that the physical conditions in Eastern Europe were abominable, characterized by overwhelming poverty, dirt, disease, and misery. One Austrian Jewish physician compared the *Ostjuden* (Eastern European Jews) to "chained dogs," the least fortunate group of people in all of Europe. This physical impoverishment left its mark on the Jewish mind and body, creating a diseased, abnormal Jew.[45] The immigrant communities in the major Central and Western European cities and in the United States were commonly represented as *loci* of overcrowding, crime, and disease – oppressive physically and morally.

The language of Darwinism offered an alternative way of interpreting the conditions of the ghetto and the condition of the Jews. In the Darwinian interpretive frame, persecution and oppression produced strength and vitality, and accounted for the continued survival of the Jewish people. In this view, the disease and misery of the Jews, their historical isolation and suffering, produced in the end health and the ability to survive the struggle for existence. This was lachrymose history with a twist.

Thus, the Italian Jewish physician and eminent criminologist Cesare Lombroso could explain the Jews' profound involvement in progressive ideas and movements in terms of the natural selection process. From Moses and Jesus to Heine, Lassalle, and Marx,

> the Jew has been the teacher of doubt; all revolutions have been channeled through him, either secretly or in the light of day. The Jews, like the Arabs, populated the universities of Toledo, Cordova, Salerno and Montpellier. We have them to thank in large measure for our knowledge of philosophy, botany, medicine, astronomy and cosmography, as well as fundamental notions of grammar and dialectic. The Jews exceeded or transcended not only the level of [the other] Semitic races, of whom it is usually denied that they can reach the same intellectual levels as European peoples . . . but they have raised themselves at times above the Aryans and produced things of significance equal to them.

Note how Lombroso attempted to undermine the racialized anti-Semitism that would define the Jew as antithetical to intellectual achievement by raising the Jews above other Semitic races and making them at least equal to the Aryans. This was no denial or rejection of racial thinking on Lombroso's part, only a rejection of the exclusion of the Jews from the accomplishments usually assigned solely to Aryans.

What reasons, then, did Lombroso give for the inextricable nexus of Jews and progress? He discussed the power of racial mixing and environment, and then invoked Darwin and the notion of natural selection through the struggle for existence: "The constant centuries-long persecutions functioned, as one would say following Darwin, as a selecting factor for the race as well as the individual; this represented a force for progressive development. Only through craftiness, industriousness, and the appearance of wretchedness, which later truly became miserliness, could the Jews hope to protect themselves from the most extreme persecutions. . . . "[46] In his seminal work, *Die Juden der Gegenwart*, Arthur Ruppin offered a similar argument. Ruppin accepted the common notion that Jews were predisposed to capitalism, and he employed the language of biology and evolution to describe and explain this phenomenon. He followed the well-known German national economist Werner Sombart in tracing this talent back to ancient times.[47] But Ruppin also believed that this particular trait owed something of its power to the Jewish historical experience in Europe. During the Middle Ages the economic talents of the Jews increased, but so too did the pressures and persecutions. These persecutions acted as a "selection process" (*Auslese*), eliminating the less cunning Jews, and leaving only the smartest, those most capable of dealing with the most difficult economic conditions.[48]

The Jews no longer survived as a people despite the persecutions endured in Europe but because of them. History combined with nature to strengthen the Jews and place them on the victorious side in the struggle for existence. Writing in *Die Zeitschrift für Demographie und Statistik der Juden*, the official journal of the Jewish social science movement, the racial theorist Leo Sofer summarized a recently published study by Dr. Albert Reibmayr on the reasons for the Jewish immunity to contagious diseases. According to Reibmayr, the explanation resides in Jewish history. "In the course of its history the race, through its endurance and survival of contagious diseases, had acquired hereditary immunizing power, and through in-breeding strengthened and passed it on." Jews, it seems, acquired this resistance in Egypt and Palestine already in biblical times; they carried it with them in their wanderings through Europe. This power to resist disease allowed them to withstand the plague during the fourteenth century (a very popular notion in the medical and scientific literature). Had the Jews not possessed this capacity, "they surely would have succumbed to the plagues in their dirty and unhygienic ghettoes." They were not immune to cholera, yet they quickly became so, while other European nations became enfeebled and lost their resistance. This loss of resistance was due above all to racial mixing, a temptation that until now the Jews, because of the isolation of the ghetto and adherence to ritual laws, had succeeded in resisting. However, "in those places where the Jews have ceased practicing strict endogamous marriage, or in-breeding, they too have lost their biological advantage." According to Riebmayr, Jews could give up all other customs and practices related to Orthodoxy, but if they continued to in-breed they would retain their bio-statistical advantage.[49]

The big question, of course, was how to account for the survival of the Jews. Within this, though, there were other, more specific questions that Darwinism and eugenics might help to answer. The Scottish racial theorist Caleb Saleeby, for whom collective survival and vitality were intimately linked with the power of empire, wondered how the Jews had managed to survive without such an empire. Paradoxically, he offered the Jews as the best case for demonstrating the general principles about natural selection and collective survival. Precisely because they lacked land and power, and yet survived and maintained a distinct racial identity, the Jews were emblematic of eugenic health. Saleeby was a physician, a Fellow of the Obstetrical Society of Edinburgh, and a member of numerous eugenics organizations in the U.K. He did not devote a great deal of space to the Jews. They figured in his broader discussion of "race culture and history," and when they are first invoked in his monograph on eugenics it is within the context of Saleeby's repudiation of what he called "the fallacy of racial senility."[50]

Saleeby's larger concern was working out how empires (i.e., the British empire) survive. Natural selection is the key, but civilization is at odds with the natural selection process, as comfort and ease lead to a reversal of the healthy process of removing the weak and diseased. Thus, no empire in history has yet figured out how to maintain itself once its early period of struggle has been won and it enters into the phase of success. Despite the fact that the Jews were not an imperial people, they fascinated Saleeby, since their survival appeared to hold the secret of racial survival in general and to offer a valuable lesson in the wages of success. The "most conspicuously persistent of all races in the historic epoch, the Jews have survived one Empire after another of their oppressors, but have never had an Empire of their own."[51] He saw the Jews as the prime example of a race that persisted over thousands of years and continued to struggle for existence. In a subsection devoted to "the survival of the Jews," he set forth his argument that the Jews were the supreme illustration of the historical selection process: "It has been asserted that that race or people decays in which selection ceases or is reversed; that in the absence of selection of the worthy for parenthood, no species, vegetable, animal or human, can prosper – much less progress. Now the Jews, the one human race of which we know assuredly that it has persisted unimpaired, have been the most continuously and stringently selected of any race, I suppose, that can be named." The Jews have been persecuted and repressed by almost every people among whom they've lived. Other people have grown prosperous, and their

> struggle for existence has abated; it was, so to say, as fit to be unfit as to be fit – with the inevitable result. But this has never been the case for the Jews. They have always had to struggle for life intensely; and their unexampled struggle has been a great source of their unexampled strength. The Jew who was a weakling or a fool had no chance at all; the weaklings and the fools being weeded out, intensity and strength of mind became the common heritage of this amazing people.[52]

And yet, the Jews did appear to be physically debilitated, even if their mental abilities were usually granted; the Jews were weaklings, though not fools. It did not escape the attention of most commentators that there existed a disparity between the largely negative physical image of the Ashkenazik Jews and their purported vitality and longevity. So here was another riddle that physicians, eugenicists, and other scholars felt compelled to address. "Why should the Jew," as one medical authority asked, "physically inferior to his Christian brethren, ward off with more potent factors the onslaught of disease and emerge from the conflict with a lesser mortality?"[53] Lester Levyn began his analysis with apparent negatives – the physical inferiority of the Jews, their anthropological disadvantage: "There is no race that appears less strong"; however, there is also "none that can so well resist misfortune." The reason for this is a selection process "that has lasted two thousand years, and has been the most severe and most painful which living beings have ever had to endure." A "puny, sickly, pale and shrunken" body hides an indomitable spirit and soul.[54]

Physical impoverishment left its mark on the Jewish mind and body, creating a diseased, abnormal Jew.[55] These negative traits were accompanied, however, by a host of positive traits: longevity, immunity from a number of illnesses, moderation in food and drink, a devotion to family and to learning rarely seen in the general population. Social Darwinism was invoked to help explain both the negative and positive conditions of Jews in the ghettos of the East, but also their descendents in the West. This ambiguous image of the Jew, and the ghetto as the site of a Darwinian process of adaptation appears in perhaps its fullest articulation in the 1928 work *The Ghetto* by the Chicago sociologist Louis Wirth.[56] In evaluating the enormous influence the ghetto exerted on Jews and Jewish history, Wirth made full use of Darwinian language. The history of the Jews in the diaspora, he writes early on, is the history of isolation in the ghetto. It "has put its imprint, not only upon the manners of the Jew, but upon his character."

Wirth begins his historical survey of the ghetto in the Middle Ages, and he frames his analysis in Darwinian terms. After noting that the first ghettos in Europe were voluntary havens and not the product of external force or pressure, Wirth invokes the concept of "adaptability," and this becomes one of his central interpretive concepts. In the realms of commerce, trade, and moneylending, the Jews found a "niche" in the rigid structure of medieval society; this allowed them to adapt and survive.[57] It would be a mistake to read Wirth's work solely through the lens of Darwinism. As a sociologist, he was uncomfortable reducing everything to the power of nature and biology. At different points in the text, other historical forces such as social structure, culture, and psychology appear as causal variables in Wirth's explanation of Jewish life in the diaspora. Thus, the overall frame of analysis in the first four chapters of the book is sociological rather than anthropological. Wirth is interested there in the ghetto as a social space, and in the functional role played by the synagogue, heder (elementary religious school), and other traditional institutions in creating a sense of solidarity and group identity. In Chapter 5, though, he turns to a discussion of the Jews as a race, and it is here that Wirth employs fully the language of a racial anthropology, Darwinism, and eugenics.

Wirth's was hardly an unambiguous representation of the ghetto and the Jews; his analysis moved at times from the romantic and rosy – prefiguring the extraordinarily influential portrait later set forth by two anthropologists, Zborowski and Herzog, in *Life Is With People* – to the dispiriting and pessimistic. The healthy Jew and the diseased Jew inhabited the same space. Nonetheless, his analysis offers further evidence of the degree to which natural scientific language had come to contribute to framing interpretations of the Jewish past and present. After tracing the origins and development of the Jewish ghetto over the centuries, and then analyzing the institutional structures of the ghetto, Wirth turns to "the Jewish type." He refers to the debate among anthropologists and sociologists over the definition of the Jews: are they a race, a nation, a religious or cultural group? Have they maintained their "purity," or are they a mixture of different races and peoples? Quoting Maurice Fishberg's *The Jews: A Study of Race and Environment* (1911), Wirth argues that the Jews lack any real identifying physical traits: "Among modern anthropologists the notion of 'pure' races is no longer seriously entertained. The Jews are apparently a hybrid people, like all the rest."[58]

And yet: there is an argument that "their peculiar historical experiences have contributed to maintaining a fairly close adherence to the characteristics which they displayed when they first appeared on the European scene, nearly two thousand years ago." Wirth cites the opinion of the well-known American race theorist William Ripley, who wrote of the Jews' pigmentation, their "brunetness," and their "coloration." The Jews appear to have maintained these distinct traits, and many others, despite all migrations and climates. How to account for this? "Ever since Darwin," Wirth continues, "isolation has been recognized as one of the basic factors in the development of biological variations. The Jews therefore furnish a crucial experiment."[59] Wirth then quotes Israel Cohen, a popularizer of Jewish history:

> Behind the walls of the ghetto the Jewish type was carefully protected from the influence of its alien environment, and there it also received a special impress, the product of exile and oppression. The chronic outbreaks of massacre and banishment, the unceasing reign of petty despotism, economic misery, and nervous alarm, have wrought traces upon the organism of the Jew; they have bent and stunted his body, whilst they have sharpened his mind and brightened his eye; they have given him a narrow chest, feeble muscles, and a pale complexion; they have stamped his visage with a look of pensive sadness, as though ever brooding upon the wrongs of ages. But the frame that has endured and survived so much suffering is also endowed with a high degree of resistance.[60]

Analysts of the ghetto translated the historical and contemporary experience of Jewry into evolutionary, Darwinian terms. Thus, nature

becomes human society, and time, human history; the ghetto is the isolated geographic region or niche; oppression (i.e., the persecution of the
Jews by the Christian majority) is the agent of evolutionary change, the
mechanism of natural selection. Survival, therefore, depends on the Jews'
ability to adjust over time to these conditions, to adapt to this environment. The Jews, then, are a "species," (i.e. a race or people), with particular traits or characteristics developed over the centuries in a particular
niche – the ghetto.

Species compete with other species for survival, and individuals compete amongst themselves (intraspecies) for survival. So the strongest individuals survive, and the strongest groups survive. In the words of the
historian of evolutionary biology Ernst Mayr:

> An individual organism competes not only with members of its own species
> but struggles for existence also against members of other species. And
> this process is probably the greatest source of evolutionary progress. Each
> newly formed species, if it is evolutionarily successful, must represent, in
> some way, evolutionary progress. Darwin explained this as follows: 'But in
> one particular sense the more recent forms must, on my theory, be higher
> than the more ancient; for each new species is formed [that is, has become
> successful] by having had some advantage in the struggle for life over other
> and preceding forms.'[61]

Jewish history and contemporary Jewish life could now be analyzed
along these lines. A number of forces or historical factors were repeatedly
invoked: the centuries-long experience of hostility and persecution; the
tendency of Jews to settle in cities, sites of struggle for physical space and
economic resources and security; the restrictions on Jewish economic
activity; and the religious laws and rituals of Judaism. All of these acted
as mechanisms of natural selection, shaping the Jews in a particular way,
forcing them to adjust or disappear. For instance, the *American Hebrew*,
in 1884, invoked the law of the survival of the fittest, connected this with
Jewish ritual laws, and then used this to explain Jewish group identity and
survival: "The law of fittest surviving, aided by the breeding of hereditary
qualities in a pure race, has given the Jews a physiological and mental
superiority which can be perpetuated only by the perpetuation of the
race purity."[62] In a 1901 article published in the *New York Medical*

Journal, the American physician Maurice Fishberg sought an explanation for modern Jewry's negative and positive traits. He granted that other factors such as adherence to the dietary laws and urban life were at work; yet he stressed above all the importance of history and natural selection in the survival of the Jews and in their physical and mental make-up:

> The past history of the Jew explains to us the reason why he has such a wretched aspect. Persecuted and abused for two thousand years, the Jew of to-day has comparatively less physical strength and muscular power, his blood is more diluted, his stature smaller, his chest and shoulders narrower, than those of his non-Jewish neighbors. But notwithstanding all these physical infirmities, the Jew resists misfortune, disease, and even death . . . better than almost any other race. The reason for this apparent contradiction is not far to seek: the modern Jew is, physically and mentally, a product of natural selection, of a process of survival of the fittest which has been going on for two thousand years. Being persecuted, oppressed, and tormented for centuries, only those who were the most stubborn, the most callous, the most energetic, could venture to remain Jews. All those who were too weak, sickly, and infirm, bodily and spiritually, were eliminated from the race either by death or baptism. The modern Jews, are, therefore, possessed of a great 'tenacity of life.'[63]

Fishberg invoked the ghetto in Darwinian terms in order to explain aspects of both the Jewish past and present. One of his chief interests was the question of the Jews and tuberculosis, and he spelled out his understanding of the struggle of existence and the ghetto in articles on this subject. Since I discuss in detail the subject of the Jews and tuberculosis in Chapter 5, here I limit myself to a brief discussion of Fishberg's analysis of the topic with reference to the ghetto and natural selection.

Fishberg began his analysis with a general, universal argument about the devastating effect of tuberculosis and other contagious diseases on rural peoples such as the nomadic Kirghiz Tartars, and the aboriginal peoples of Australia, Polynesia, and North and South America: "We find that tuberculosis was quite unknown before the advent of the white man, who brought to these tribes not only civilization, often in the shape of whiskey, but also the tubercle bacillus" (he might also, of course, have mentioned smallpox, measles, and yellow fever). Rural populations of modern civilized countries, Fishberg argued, are akin to these primitive groups; they never underwent the process of selection that would have killed off those individuals most predisposed to the disease. The Jews, on the other hand, lack

> this class of rural dwellers, not adapted to indoor city life.... [The Jews] have for 2,000 years lived exclusively in cities, and during the Medieval ages were confined in the worst parts of cities, the Ghettoes. Indeed, only rarely was the Ghetto enlarged to meet the demands of a growing population, but the Jews were compelled to accommodate themselves the best way they could in a small area. Under such conditions most of the Jews who were predisposed to tuberculosis succumbed, leaving no progeny. The same process is to-day going on with most other inhabitants of large cities. The Jews have only the advantage of having passed through a process of infection during past centuries. Hence their lower mortality to-day from tuberculosis.[64]

Behind this brief historical narrative of Jewish survival in cities is a centuries-old European discourse on the relationship to urbanity and civility, the city and disease, the primitive and advanced, white and non-white, barbaric and civilized. "Primitive" peoples, history informs us, have no resistance to infectious diseases such as tuberculosis; nor do Europeans who live in rural areas. "Civilized" in the discourse of eugenics and racial Darwinism means the ability to survive the assaults of nature, to adapt to one's environment and pass on traits to succeeding generations. The Jews, as white and European, must be the most highly civilized group in history, as many eugenicists believed, for they had survived the millennia intact as a distinctive group, had adapted to a particular niche – the ghetto – and emerged into modernity stronger and more vital for having discarded those who were weaker and less fit for the struggle. In his representation of the ghetto, Fishberg – like all those who participated in the particular interpretive tradition of the healthy Jew – was countering the older Enlightenment representation of the ghetto as the primary site of Jewish debility. Tuberculosis and the ghetto did not present Fishberg with the problem of the diseased and degenerate Jewish body; nor was Fishberg internalizing a set of anti-Semitic images and then turning them on himself and his own people. Rather, tuberculosis offered Fishberg (and many other medical commentators) another opportunity to insist on the superior health and vitality of the Jews. Moreover, it did the sort of cultural work that Matthew Frye Jacobson and others have explored: it moved, or at least sought to move, the Jews into the category of respectable and acceptable whites at a time when the respectability and whiteness of Jews was highly contested.[65]

After arguing for the historical significance of the ghetto and the Jewish experience with infection, Fishberg brought his discussion into the present. Contemporary New York City, he believed, offered an excellent example of this same selective process. Southern Italians in their native Italy had some of the lowest rates of TB in Europe, but in New York City they suffered at three times their former rate. (And even this statistical difference was misleading, because many of those who died in Italy of tuberculosis were immigrants who had contracted the disease in America and then returned to their native land to die.) The Jews in New York, on the other hand, died at lower rates than any other group, even though they engaged to a far greater extent in indoor occupations – those related to textiles above all – universally believed to be conducive to the contraction of the disease.[66] Unlike the Italians, the Jews moved from one highly congested urban environment to another when they came from Russia to the United States. Thus, the Jew "has paid the price for urbanization already for several hundred years, while the Italian, Syrian, Irish, Slavonic and Hungarian peasant coming to the United States meets with the urban conditions for the first time and must pay an exorbitant price for it in the shape of victims to the white plague."[67]

Fishberg's argument about Jews, history and the struggle for survival reappeared in his 1911 monograph on Jews and race.[68] This work was translated into German and published in 1913 as *Die Rassenmerkmale der Juden*, and thus made its way into the work of German social scientists, including the leading German Jewish social scientist, Arthur Ruppin. While the thrust of Ruppin's research was geared toward demonstrating the abnormal and diseased nature of modern Jewry – the result, he believed, of the advanced state of assimilation among modernized Jews – even he had to bow before statistics and anecdotes that showed that in important ways Jews evinced signs of health. Ruppin sought an explanation, for instance, for why Jews seemed to show a greater immunity than Christians to certain types of disease. He invoked Fishberg's 1913 study and the argument that this greater immunity was due to the natural selection process: "Tuberculosis is predominantly an urban disease. The Jews have been an urban people for two thousand years. Through their tightly crowded living conditions in the cities, the Jews were exposed to the TB infection to a far greater degree than Christians, who lived primarily in small towns and villages."[69]

The idea that two thousand years of city dwelling had strengthened the Jews physically or biologically was a mainstay of social scientific narratives of the time. The German Jewish physician Hugo Hoppe, an authority on alcoholism and disease, listed a variety of afflictions from which Jews had enjoyed immunity: pneumonia, typhus, malaria, cholera, and tuberculosis. "Already during the devastating epidemics of the Middle Ages it was generally observed that Jews were more immune than Christians."[70] Hoppe was repeating an idea that had circulated widely for centuries; yet, he was translating it to a scientific, rather than theological or mythological, context, thus seeking to imbue it with the power science and medicine possessed. Thus, he explained this remarkable immunity in naturalistic terms: greater moderation, especially with alcohol, and the Jews' history of urban living.

Even some of those who explicitly repudiated interpretations of the Jewish past along Darwinian and eugenic lines appear to have felt it necessary to invoke Darwin, and to play upon his ideas to make their point. Thus, the eminent German-Jewish historian Heinrich Graetz, in a speech delivered in London in 1887 to celebrate the Anglo-Jewish Historical Exhibition, called upon Darwin and the idea of the survival of the fittest to help explain Judaism's survival over thousands of years.

> Your great countryman, Charles Darwin, has discovered a terrible law of nature, and won universal acceptance for it. A shudder is produced by the mere name of the law, as given in a formula which sums it up: *The Struggle for Existence*, that rules among the infinite bodies of the universe, as much as among the lowest organisms. The stronger assails and destroys without mercy the weaker in longer or shorter time. Weak peoples are conquered by strong ones, and are eaten up and destroyed, even in the historical sphere. Such is the will of this merciless law of nature, and no one can rescue himself from its influence. This inexorable law reaches its final expression in the formula *Might before Right*. But is there really exception to this fatality? Yes, the Jewish people, or Jewish race, offers a remarkable and imposing anomaly.

Is there anything weaker or more vulnerable than the Jews? Graetz asked. And yet, they exist, an "ineradicable persistence."[71]

It seems at first glance that Graetz rejected a Darwinian understanding of history, and offered the Jews as the supreme example of the fallacy of such an interpretation. Indeed, in his *Geschichte der Juden*, Graetz put forth a supernatural, rather than natural, understanding of historical causality.[72] Yet, in his lecture in England, he not only spoke in naturalistic language, but in the end allowed that, in fact, we are not necessarily faced with an exception to the "iron law of nature, the survival of the strongest" when it comes to comprehending Jewish history.[73] For Graetz, it all depended on what one meant by "weak" and "strong," since supreme strength lies in the "ideal" of the nation. "Spirit," as force, thus overwhelms material strength. According to Graetz, the "ideal" of Judaism is the pure knowledge of God and a higher morality. It is the people of Israel's task, or mission, to spread this ideal throughout the world; hence, their dispersion or diasporic condition. And it is the diaspora that has acted as a mechanism for Jewish survival, since the nation's enemies could never attack the "whole body," only "separate members."[74] Israel's mission, then, requires a presence in the world, requires that Jews go out into the world. "Thousands of years are needed for the work, and Israel must wander in order to be better fitted for his task."[75]

Graetz was faced here with the same paradox as the other thinkers encountered in this chapter: how does one account for the survival and vitality of a group that appears to be so physically debilitated? He answered it by redefining the key terms, and emphasizing that what matters in history is spirit. This is, of course, hardly a Darwinian argument. Yet Graetz did offer in the end a sort of social Darwinian explanation of Jewish survival, even as he clearly rejected the biological for the spiritual. His language is drawn from the world of biology and evolution. The Jews are a body, an organism that must survive under hostile conditions; in order to survive, it must obey certain principles or laws that will allow it to remain fit. Certainly, the sort of interpretation he offered here may owe something to Graetz's presence in England, and a desire to flatter his audience with an invocation of Darwin and his theory. Nonetheless, it testifies to the challenge Darwinism posed that even thinkers fully committed to a German idealist intellectual tradition felt the need to translate Judaism and Jewish history into the new language of evolutionism.

6.

At least two interpretive modes were at work, then, among Jewish and non-Jewish writers concerned with explaining Jewish survival. More often than not they were to be found in the same narrative, though they are nonetheless distinct interpretive strategies. One sought to explain Jewish health and survival, as well as a host of purported particular Jewish traits, as the result of adherence to Jewish law and ritual, and to draw an equivalence between these and modern medicine and science, including the science of eugenics. The second interpretive strategy focused on the ideas of struggle and survival, and reinterpreted Jewish history, especially the medieval period and ghettoization, as a Darwinian process of natural selection. This strategy also entailed a translation or reinterpretation of both traditional Jewish literature and Jewish history.

It was not just that history had made the Jew stronger through disease, persecution, and ghettoization – better able to survive the exigencies or demands of urban life. It was also that the modern world was increasingly urbanized. The Jews may triumph – in the minds of anti-Semites, but also according to the theories produced by Jews and philosemites – because the world was increasingly a place in which Jews could exercise all the acquired traits that allowed them to survive and thrive. There were, to be sure, competing interpretations of the modern Jewish condition, oftentimes even within the same author's work. The ability of the Jews to survive in the city was juxtaposed with the city's negative impact on collective Jewish identity and will: the city as the site of assimilation, of Jewish-Christian social and sexual intermingling, of capitalism's unrelenting attack on all forms of traditional belief and behavior. Like their non-Jewish counterparts, Jewish social thinkers could see in "the Jews" the embodiment of both an extraordinary vitality and degeneracy.[76]

Thus it could be argued that the ghetto had prepared Jews for the Darwinian struggle for existence, and produced positive eugenic qualities. Yet, this argument was often qualified with the insistence that modern conditions had also produced, or were in the process of producing, highly deleterious effects on the Jewish mind and body, that the historical immunity to all sorts of physical and social diseases was being undermined by the powerful transformations underway as a result of capitalism, industrialism, and, paradoxically, urbanization. Jewish narratives could oftentimes sound as if opponents of the Jews had composed them; the images of sickness and degeneracy mirrored or echoed those that filled the pages of anti-Semitic books and pamphlets.

Yet, the differences were important and pronounced. Elsewhere I have analyzed these differences and their significance.[77] Here I want to emphasize that for many Jewish and Christian thinkers the vitality and strength that came historically as a result of persecution, urban and then ghetto dwelling, and repeated exposure to infectious or contagious diseases, was in the main a blessing. Whereas anti-Semitic writers cast this collective strength as a pronounced danger to Christian European society, Jews and their allies of course viewed this as an advantage. But those who celebrated the misery of ghetto dwelling could hardly do so unreservedly, nor could they envision a regenerated future in terms of a return to the ghetto.

Even when scholars denigrated the Jews, there was also a good chance that they would grant a superior degree of health and vitality. "In the slime of the modern city," wrote two non-Jewish American authorities in 1918, "the Jewish type, stringently selected through centuries of ghetto life, is particularly fit to survive, although it may not be the physical ideal of the anthropologist."[78] This sort of ambiguity and complexity was characteristic of much of the discourse produced about Jewish health, by both Christians and Jews. Other non-Jewish authorities offered less ambivalent evaluations of the eugenic value of Jewish tradition. We've already encountered Thurman Rice's opinion of the Jews and their eugenic value. Another Indiana physician, William Shrock, declared in an article published in the *Journal of the American Medical Association* (*JAMA*): "Wherever and whenever the hygienic laws of the Mosaic dispensation were obeyed, there and then do we find marked progression toward a better physical man."[79] This is the preface to his extended celebration of a social Darwinian and eugenic approach to health and hygiene. While he did not elaborate on the idea, Schrock clearly believed that the Mosaic code taught eugenics.

Thus, it was not only Jewish authors and authorities that celebrated the survival skills of the Jews and located this survival in the eugenic wisdom of Moses and other ancient Jewish authorities; Christian writers and public figures also participated in this celebration. And Jewish publications would at times enthusiastically publish these encomiums. As we've seen, the *Jewish Chronicle* in England celebrated Francis Galton's endorsement of Jewish vitality and survival, and identified Moses as the ancient version of the founder of modern eugenics. In the first year of its run, in 1915, the *Menorah Journal* in New York published a number of speeches and articles by well-known Christian elites along these lines. In his speech before the Menorah Society, titled "Yankee and Jew," G. Stanley Hall, president of Clark University, informed his audience that in profound ways Yankees (that is, White Anglo-Saxon Protestants) and Jews were very much alike. Among other attributes, both had a keen appreciation of eugenics rooted in the Hebrew Bible. At present, though, Jews enjoyed one advantage, insofar as "you are increasing in number while we are decreasing."[80] In the following issue, Charles W. Eliot, president of Harvard University, published an essay on "The Potency of the Jewish Race." Eliot understood the Jews as a race, though he attributed their survival and success to "lofty ideals." The Jews had, over the course of their history, "succeeded in competition with other races to a remarkable degree." When they were poor, they were less poor than their neighbors; among free and prosperous nations they became more prosperous than most: "Confined in unwholesome Ghettos, they retain to an astonishing degree their health and vitality, helped doubtless by the dietary and sanitary directions given in their ancient Scriptures."[81] British writers on eugenics and race could also celebrate Jewish survival, and invoke the Jews as the exemplar of eugenic health. As we saw above, the Scottish physician Caleb Saleeby offered the Jews as the best case for demonstrating general principles about natural selection and collective survival.

This debate over Jewish survival and Darwinian-like struggle also found its way into the editorial pages of *JAMA*. In a 1907 piece on Judaism and sanitation, *JAMA* commented on the extent to which Jewish sanitary laws "anticipated and are in accord with the best teachings of modern hygiene."[82] The aseptic methods of modern medicine were introduced by Moses and then enlarged on by rabbinical commentators. Jewish law is also stricter, *JAMA* pointed out, than the laws recently passed by the United States government regarding meat inspection. There could be no doubt then about the overall salutary effects of Jewish laws and rituals. But *JAMA* also asked to what extent Jewish survival and health had been due to particular historical circumstances and environmental forces. To what extent, the editors asked, had "enforced conditions of life" endowed the Jews

> with a certain degree of immunity such as probably exists among most civilized races toward certain diseases which, comparatively mild among them, become devastatingly fatal epidemics when introduced into the virgin soil of savage races. The white race, for example, is probably almost saturated with tuberculous infection, but resistance has been gained which makes it comparatively harmless to three-fourths of civilized mankind. The mass of the Jewish race has been living for hundreds of years under most unhygienic conditions as regards this particular infection, and with this, aided by their religious sanitary observance, they may have acquired a still greater resistance to it than the rest of us. On the other hand, they have acquired a certain neurotic predisposition, a condition apparently not guarded against by aseptic rules, but one, as the late Dr. [Charles] Beard used to claim, accompanied by a certain degree of apparent immunity to some other diseases. Racial peculiarities and their relation to hygienic practices form an interesting subject for study, which has not been very thoroughly worked out even in the case of the Jews.[83]

A racialized medical discourse giveth and it taketh away. The Jews are healthy, and they owe this both to their religion and to their history; but they are also given over to mental illness, which their rituals are powerless to prevent. The Jews are white; they are no savage race. More than other civilized races, they appear to be immune to the devastation of tuberculosis. Yet, again, they are a race apart, with their own "racial peculiarities" that not even researchers into race and health have fully explained.

7.

Central to discussions of Jewish racial or national identity and survival were the rules and customs governing marriage and motherhood, which included the laws of sexual relations and ritual purity. According to many racial and eugenic thinkers, the Jews offered an excellent example of a people who abided by one of the fundamental principles of eugenics: the centrality of marriage and motherhood. In a 1912 piece on the laws of sexual purity in ancient Jewish literature, the Wiesbaden physician,

Dr. Ratner, made his readers aware of just how seriously and stringently
ancient Judaism took the rules meant to ensure the purity and health of
the race. Marriage, he wrote, was a central concern for the Jews, and they
approached the subject from a eugenic point of view. When it came to
marriage, what mattered was "a good family, the ancestry [*Abstammung*]
and intellectual disposition of the nearest relations." Echoing a widely
held notion at the time, Ratner concluded that it was "not money, but the
intellectual/spiritual dowry [that] was crucial" when Jews came to select
mates.[84] In a Yiddish work from 1922 on the Jews and hygiene, the Polish Jewish physician Gershon Levin insisted that Moses, seeking to instill
in the Jews the value of a "pure, healthy family life, free from venereal
diseases," instituted Judaism's laws of marriage. Illicit relations with foreign women were forbidden, an offense punishable by death. Although
he did not use the language of social Darwinism or eugenics, Levin – like
Nossig before him – viewed the slaughter of Midianite women, and the
severity of punishments meted out to those who transgressed the laws
of sexual relations as perhaps the clearest evidence of Moses' overriding
concern with the purity, health, and survival of the Jewish people.[85] Caleb
Saleeby was insistent throughout his book that races and nations were
not doing nearly enough to educate and protect healthy mothers, who
were of course central to the ideal of raising healthy future generations.
Everyone agrees, Saleeby wrote, that Jewish infant mortality is lower than
among Gentiles; that Jewish children are "superior in height and weight
and chest measurement to Gentile children," and this despite the fact that
Jewish children are today raised in environments far more impoverished.
Gentile children may enjoy "a better material environment," but they
suffer from "a far inferior maternal environment." Saleeby concluded
with an encomium that celebrated Jewish mothers, the Jews as a people,
and the power of eugenic selection to create a superior people.

> The Jewish mother is the mother of children innately superior, on the aver-
> age, since they are the fruit of such long ages of stringent parental selection,
> and she makes more of them because she fails to nurse them only in the
> rarest cases, when she has no choice, and because in every detail her mater-
> nal care is incomparably superior to that of her Gentile sister. Given a high
> standard of motherhood in a highly selected race, what other result than
> that we daily witness and envy can we expect?[86]

The American Jewish physician and scholar David Macht not only insisted that Jewish laws of marriage and sexuality corresponded with modern eugenic principles, and that this helped explain Jewish health, but that these facts demonstrated the superiority of Judaism over Christianity. Macht contrasted Judaism's approach to matters of the body and sex to those of Christianity, and found the latter wanting. For the Jews the body is not, as in Christianity, castigated and punished for its urges and needs; in Judaism "all its normal physiological functions are regarded as wholesome and intended for good." In line with racial and eugenic thinking, Macht insisted that when it came to sexuality and procreation, Judaism's interest lay not with the individual, but with the nation and race. The "procreative faculty," when "subserving its true purpose – the rearing of a sturdy race of servitors to God," is a sacred duty.[87]

Such celebratory remarks depended, of course, on accepting unproblematically the racial and eugenic discourse that reduced women to the role of reproducers of the nation and race. As Beth Wenger has noted in her analysis of the American context, the Jewish family came to be seen as the "one indispensable unit whose health and stability were perceived to determine the fate of the Jewish future." Jewish survival was increasingly a matter of Jewish women's behavior, and the regulation of sexuality understood as necessary in this ongoing struggle.[88] Male religious and medical authorities called upon Jewish women to take up the traditional laws of *niddah*, or sexual purity, in order to ensure both their own health – an oft-repeated claim was that regular use of the *mikveh* (ritual bath) and adherence to the laws of marital abstention around the time of menstruation lowered significantly the dangers of uterine cancer – and the health of the Jewish people. Non-Jewish as well as Jewish authorities could invoke the laws of *niddah* to explain demographic discrepancies between Jews and Gentiles. Thus, in his work on Jewish statistics, Joseph Jacobs noted that, among other things, Jewish women gave birth to a greater number of males (Jewish birth rates were higher in general, Jacobs wrote; Jewish marriages were more fecund and fertile than those of non-Jews). He then invoked the French statistician Gustav Lagneau, who in his *Du Dénombrement de la Population* (1882) attributed the greater number of male Jewish births to the observance of *niddah*.[89]

Even if their ideas appear to have been "progressive" in some ways, inverting reactionary, anti-Semitic judgments, these medical and scientific authorities remained firmly entrenched within a familiar world of religious, racial and sexual hierarchy. For some, Jews were superior to Gentiles; nonetheless, the legitimate role of Jewish women was as wives and mothers, and ultimately as guarantors of the future of the Jewish people. As Caleb Saleeby wrote about the role of the mother: "Woman is Nature's supreme instrument of the future."[90]

Unsurprisingly, perhaps, the narratives of male Jewish scholars written in a eugenic vein – texts written by Jews about Jews and Judaism – reflected and participated in the dominant eugenic and racial imagery, save for the oft-encountered derogation of the Jews themselves. Eugenics from the outset was a solidly middle-class ideology, and "Jewish eugenics" was no different. Max Danzis, for instance, touted the fact that Judaism placed the highest value on heredity, "particularly in its relation to marriage." Thus, Jewish law prohibited marriage with epileptics and leprous females; imbeciles were not permitted to marry. A father should marry his daughter off only to a healthy man of learning or wealth: "The unlearned, as it is said, are an abomination, their wives are vermin, and of their daughters it is said, 'cursed is he that lies with a beast.'"[91] In a 1917 German-language article, published in a decennial celebratory volume of the Berlin-based Verein für jüdische Statistik, Maurice Fishberg insisted that "the rabbis had preceded Galton by 1600 years," and one clear indication of this was that Judaism had long ago discovered how to produce superior offspring. Fishberg cited approvingly Caleb Saleeby's assertion that the Jews had been extraordinarily successful in the intensive "struggle for existence" (*Kampf ums Dasein*), and he took the opportunity again to assert that the Jews were a "model sample" for eugenicists. There was an "agreement" between eugenics and Judaism that did not exist to the same extent between eugenics and either Christianity or Islam.[92]

The Jews' way of life, in the Middle Ages and in the ghettos of contemporary Eastern Europe, London, and New York, explained both the strengths and weaknesses of Jewry: "I know of no social, religious, or political community in which the positive eugenic is observed and pursued in such great measure as in the ghetto."[93] Fishberg repeated his thesis, already encountered, that historical oppression and suffering had their profound negative effects, but they also proved beneficial in the Jews' struggle for survival. The explanation for Jewish survival could be located in history, in the oppression and persecution endured by Jews in the past and, for many, the present. This historical explanation was supplemented by reference to the eugenic value of traditional Jewish practices, derived in one way or another from Jewish law. Central to this was the importance Judaism assigned to marriage and motherhood. The learned, as a class, were held in the highest esteem; the wealthy within the community always sought to marry their daughters off to a *talmud bocher*, or student of traditional religious texts. "Honorable" families would never marry off their daughters to ignoramuses; this in contrast to the non-Jewish aristocracy in Europe, who married only according to birth, regardless of talent or knowledge. Gentiles would never marry outside of their caste or class, so they brought forth far fewer intelligent and talented children than did the Jews. For Jews, "the learned man was the aristocrat," what Fishberg called a *Geistesadel*.[94]

Thurman Rice identified the traditional Jewish practice of marrying wealth to intelligence as one of the four main axioms of Jewish eugenic health (the others were the curse of sterility and the blessings of a large family; the resistance to racial intermixture with others through marriage; and early marrriage).[95] Rabbi Reichler, too, found proof of Judaism's eugenic impulse in the rabbinic laws governing marriage: "The Rabbis, like the eugenicists of today, measured the success of a marriage by the number and quality of the offspring."[96] The rabbis warned against unions between certain types of people so as to avoid augmenting less favorable stock. So the "awkwardly tall" were not to marry one another, lest a giant result; two very short people were not to mate lest a dwarf be produced. "For the same reason the intermarriage between blonds or between dark-complexioned people was not countenanced. A number of precautions in sexual relations were prescribed in order to prevent the birth of defectives, such as lepers, epileptics, the deaf and the dumb, the lame and the blind."[97]

Thirty years earlier, in his 1887 work on Jewish statistics, Alfred Nossig stressed the eugenic value of Jewish marriage laws. In offering up an explanation for the overall comparative health of the Jewish people, Nossig stressed the importance of traditional Jewish sexual morality: "The positive consequences of this sexual arrangement show themselves in the biological conditions of the Jewish population, so it is impossible to exaggerate the scarcity of syphilitic sufferers among the Jewish masses

and the significant and beneficial consequences of this to the existence of
the *Volk*."[98] Nossig attributed the sexual morality of the Jews directly
to an adherence to the Mosaic law, and to the conservative way of life of
the majority of the Jewish people. He called special attention to the decisive moral stature of Jewish women. Only in the most seldom of cases
is a Jewish wife an adulteress, even when she knows her husband to
be unfaithful. And Nossig transformed even a seemingly negative social
phenomenon like prostitution into an advantage in the eugenic struggle.
The relatively large number of Jewish prostitutes speaks *for*, not against,
Jewish morality. Almost without exception a Jewish *Mädchen* who has
lost her chastity is cast out of the family and out of respectable society.[99]
Ostracized, she is unable to pollute the reputable members of the community.

Nossig did not dwell long, however, on the immorality within the
Jewish community. He insisted immediately that even the young girl from
the lowest levels of society, who must of necessity be economically on
her own, guards over her purity (*Reinheit*) – unlike, he added, her non-
Jewish counterparts. Thus, adherence on the part of the Jews to the
rules governing sexuality and marriage, and the elimination from the
community of those who violate those rules act to produce a healthy and
strong *Volk*.

Agreement did not always exist on how to evaluate eugenically any
particular practice. Many scholars, for instance, cited the practice of early
marriage among traditional Jews as a factor in their successful struggle
for survival.[100] As just noted, Thurman Rice listed early marriage as
one of the four main reasons for Jewish eugenic health. Rabbi Reichler
endorsed the eugenic value of early marriage, arguing that in this, as in
so much else, rabbinic thinking agrees with modern eugenics. The rabbi
again quoted Francis Galton, who defined eugenics as the furthering of
the reproduction of the "blessed" human protoplasm, and the elimination of the "cursed." The rabbis of the Talmud agreed, seeing in early
marriage one crucial way to achieve this. "The Rabbis, like the eugenicists of today, measured the success of a marriage by the number and
quality of the offspring." Only those who have "scrupulously preserved
the purity of their families," Reichler concluded, "will be privileged to
witness the manifestation of the Holy Spirit" (the *Shechinah*).[101] William
Feldman noted that Jews traditionally encouraged early marriages, and

that in this respect, they were, "from a strictly eugenic standpoint, wiser than the Greeks."[102] Others viewed early marriage as an anti-eugenic practice. Joseph Jacobs, a one-time associate of Francis Galton, linked early marriage to poverty, physical deformity, and hence to a disadvantage in the "struggle for existence."[103]

In some instances the image of the superior Jewish mother and the healthy Jewish child were advanced without the explicit language of eugenics. Dr. William Hall, speaking on "The Influence of Feeding on the Development of Aryan and Semitic Children," argued that Gentile women had lost the natural instinct as mothers to breastfeed their children that Jewish women still possessed. Gentile children, therefore, suffered from a host of diseases, such as rickets and bow-leggedness, that Jewish children did not. Jewish mothers were treated as sacred objects, protected from "alcohol, prolonged labor and insufficient food." This gave Jewish children a great advantage, shown later in better school performance and greater power in resisting disease. In Hall's opinion this was not due to the surroundings, since Jews lived in quarters as dirty and run-down as their Gentile neighbors. Rather, "they had clean food and they freely used oil, fish and eggs. This," the editors of *JAMA* reported, "Dr. Hall regarded as the great secret of their health."[104]

What should we make of the strategy of translation and equivalence in the context of the first half of the twentieth century, in Europe and America? What did it mean at the time to want to make Judaism and eugenics compatible, to want to convince the world that Judaism, too, celebrated only the "healthy" and the "normal"; not only that "motherhood" was an integral aspect of Jewish tradition, but that the blind and deaf, the epileptic, the mentally ill and "defective," and all the others that the medical world had come to identify as inferior and dangerous to the well-being of the nation, had also been condemned to the margins or even worse by Judaism and the Jewish sages? What does it mean that the collective survival of the Jews was now the product of a Darwinian struggle for existence, evidence of Herbert Spencer's belief that persecution and persecution alone breeds strength and vitality? Notions of civilization and progress had shifted again, and the Jewish past and present would be reinterpreted accordingly. If the Jews "became white" over the course of the early twentieth century, then surely one way in which this occurred was that they became imbued with the spirit of racialism, eugenics, and colonialism. Not all of them were so imbued; but many, and many more than Jews and others after the end of World War II have acknowledged. And the fact that Jews were one of the main targets of this racialized worldview does not obviate the fact that, at certain points, they participated in it.

5

TB or Not TB, That Was a Jewish Question

Moses, *Kashrut*, and the Prevention of Tuberculosis

In March 1900, an individual identified only as "Medicus" wrote a letter to the *New York Times* about "the tuberculosis problem."[1] The very immediate and practical crisis of tuberculosis, "Medicus" suggested, could possibly be addressed and remedied through the ancient laws of Moses. It was now generally conceded, with the acceptance of the germ theory of disease, that tuberculosis was infectious and not hereditary. This meant that health officials and policy makers must begin to think not only or primarily about what to do with those who were already ill, but how to prevent the healthy from becoming sick.

"Medicus" devised an imaginary dialogue between an older, more traditional medical authority and a young, progressive voice. The former believes that treating TB means dealing with those already ill: those in an advanced state must be isolated, given whatever aid can be provided, and prevented from infecting others; those in the early stages of the disease should be treated and cured if possible. Then the progressive voice is heard. Why not try to prevent the disease? How? It is generally agreed that the cow and cow's milk are the origin of tuberculosis. "Keep your cattle in good shape, learn to recognize disease in them and consumption will cease." Where is the evidence for such claims? "Talmudic writings show that the wise men of Judea recognized the existence of tubercle in cattle and its consequent danger to human kind." "Medicus" then set out briefly the principles of *kashrut*, including the practice of inspecting meat and discarding anything that looks diseased or impure. Further evidence of the deterrent effects of the Jewish dietary laws lay in the statistics from Russia that showed that the Jews there, overwhelmingly still Orthodox, rarely died of the disease, while the death rates for non-Jews equaled and even exceeded those in the United States. "Medicus" ended on a practical, hortatory note: "If the State wants to save human life let it arrange to have every teacher in the land learn enough physiology to comprehend the wisdom of the sanitary and dietary laws of the Talmudists – let these views be imparted to the rising generation."

We can be fairly certain that "Medicus" was a medical professional, or at least someone self-identified as a medical authority. But was Medicus a Jew? Again, we might assume so (as we might assume with regard to Dr. Ratner in Chapter 4), given the celebration of the prophylactic and salubrious nature of Jewish dietary laws, and of the wisdom of the ancient rabbis. Yet, as we've seen, the ideas articulated by Medicus were as likely to be found among Christians as Jews. Medicus was hardly alone in his heartfelt belief that the scourge of tuberculosis might be stemmed if both Jews and non-Jews paid greater heed to "the wisdom of the sanitary and dietary laws of the Talmudists." In this chapter, a case study of sorts, I address the decades-long discussion within the medical community about Jews, Judaism, and tuberculosis, a discussion that both reflected and contributed to the broader interpretive tradition of the healthy Jew. Again, as in Chapter 4, on eugenics, I move here chiefly among three national contexts: Great Britain, the United States, and Germany. Without denying that national contexts matter, and that the same set of images and arguments meant different things in different places, the purpose here is less to highlight differences or discontinuities in these narratives along national lines than to point up the continuities; that is, to reconstruct and illuminate further the coherent interpretive tradition that is the subject of this book.

I.

Tuberculosis, Winslow Anderson, a medical authority, wrote in the *Journal of the American Medical Association (JAMA)* in 1894, is "the most dreadful scourge the human race has ever known."[2] He conveyed in dramatic terms the universal threat of infection, giving voice, like so many others, to the recent discovery of germs and their danger. Germs, he said, are in the air and in the soil. They are spread through dried sputum and dust, the two main vectors. Individuals are in danger at home and on the street, "from the air in the street cars, railway carriages, churches, theatres, the streets and public highways which are sure to contain the bacilli. . . . "[3]

Like "Medicus," Anderson reminded readers that tuberculosis was an infectious and not a hereditary disease, as had been commonly believed until newly proven otherwise by Robert Koch. This meant that physicians and the public had to be made aware of the ways in which the disease could be transmitted. Anderson called attention to the dangers of spitting. He also noted the well-established connection between cattle and consumption: cattle can become consumptive, and their meat "is capable of communicating tuberculosis by infecting the intestinal glands with the uncooked bacilli." More frequent than infection from meat was infection from milk; tuberculosis could be contracted from tainted milk and butter. While some studies estimated that at least one in three to five cows were infected with the tubercular germ, some placed the figure at 50 percent.[4] "The possibility of the transmission of tuberculosis from the lower animals to man has long been recognized," one physician at the University of Pennsylvania wrote in 1897. "The danger of contracting the disease through the consumption of the milk and meat of tuberculous cattle has been known to the scientific world for more than a hundred years."[5]

No vaccination against the disease had been discovered or produced, so even greater emphasis was placed on prevention.[6] This connection between tuberculosis and cattle, and more generally between disease and the quality of food, became a central element in the medicalized analyses of the Jewish dietary laws. The physician N. E. Aronstam, in a pamphlet on *Jewish Dietary Laws from a Scientific Standpoint* (1912), touted both the moral and health benefits of *kashrut*. After an extended polemic against those advocates of stunning who would condemn kosher slaughtering as inhumane, Aronstam celebrated the prophylactic ability of *kashrut* vis-à-vis tuberculosis, "the white plague of mankind," whose victims numbered in the thousands; "they constantly fall as a burnt offering, a holocaust upon the altar of death." One of the "potent sources of infection," Aronstam informed his readers, "is the *meat and milk of consumptive animals*."[7] Aronstam's pamphlet contained a rather detailed lesson in the methods of kosher slaughtering, its health benefits, and the correspondence of the ancient Mosaic code with today's scientific principles. "Every one is forced to admit that Moses – or be it, as modern research wants it, some other personality or group of codifiers – was a painstaking and thorough sanitarian." Finally, the laws of *kashrut* are linked with the quality of the Jews, the religious or moral nature of the biblical commandments are translated as scientific, and the example of the Jews used to rebuke contemporary state-sponsored health practices. All of these, as we shall see, were themes common to the literature on Jews and health:

> The longevity of the Jew may partly be explained by his faithful compliance with the doctrines of hygiene and the sanitary rules promulgated by the Bible. Our moral, mental, domestic, and social purity are but the reflection of the purity of our bodies. 'Clean ye shall be unto me,' is the command of the Bible, and 'clean ye shall be unto yourself,' is the dictum of science. Any animal that dies of disease is forbidden; meat kept for more than three days is rarely used by Jews. No such thing as indefinite or prolonged refrigeration or cold storage is permitted, so universally in vogue among Gentile packers and butchers. The meat that comes to the Jewish table is fresh, clean, wholesome, and free from pat[h]ogenic organisms, in short, it is 'kosher.' The '*shochet*' [ritual slaughterer] is indeed just as competent and efficient a meat inspector or veterinary as the government is capable of appointing. He is enabled by ritual inspection to recognize pathologic lesions in the entrails of the animal, and thus contributes no inconsiderable quota to the prevention of the disease and the maintenance of the health.

"The Bible," Aronstam concludes, "is the pioneer of the sanitary sciences of to-day."[8]

This sort of analysis was not limited to rabbis or Jewish physicians and scholars. It appeared in monographs and journal articles on tuberculosis, written by non-Jewish as well as Jewish authorities.[9] "The Jews have abnormally small proportions of deaths from consumption and pneumonia," wrote one American authority on race at the end of the nineteenth century. "This immunity can best be ascribed to the excellent system of meat inspection prescribed by the Mosaic laws."[10] Interpretations of *kashrut* and health were, in turn, part of a larger debate over Jews and tuberculosis, and Jews, Judaism, and health and race.

The relationship between Jews, Judaism and tuberculosis was a "question," but what sort of question? Jews, like everyone else, could and did contract tuberculosis. But were they at risk as Jews? If they were lucky enough to avoid the disease was this due to their Jewishness? The issue of Jews and TB raised much broader questions about race and environment, heredity and history, and the influence of Jewish dietary practices on the survival and health of Jewry.

In an 1856 tract on the comparative longevity of Jews and Christians, Eduard Glatter wrote of the Jews that "they possess the greatest immunity against malaria, convulsions, degeneration of the respiratory organs, a tendency to skin diseases, gastrointestinal ailments and hernias. And they suffer much less from TB than do other peoples."[11] Much the same opinion would be found seventy years later, in scholarly forums, both "Jewish" and general. Hans Ullmann, writing in the *Archiv für Rassen- und Gesellschafts-Biologie*, noted the low death rates of Jews from TB and attributed this to an immunity produced by natural selection; in this he was in agreement with Dr. H. Strauss, whose article on Jews and tuberculosis appeared in the *Zeitschrift für Demographie und Statistik der Juden.*[12] Hugo Hoppe listed tuberculosis as one of a number of infectious diseases from which Jews suffered far less than Christians, and from which Jews seemed to enjoy a relative immunity. "Indeed, there exists an astounding immunity amongst the Jews against tuberculosis!" And, Hoppe noted, this appears to be true despite vast differences in geography, national affiliation, and standards of living. Thus, Jews in Russia, England, Central Europe, the United States, and Tunisia all enjoyed lower rates of tuberculosis than the non-Jewish populations around them.[13] Leo Sofer, a Jewish racial scientist, referred to and quoted from an array of physicians and researchers who had written on Jews and disease; numerous studies demonstrated the resistance of Jews to TB. Even in Russia, where Jews on the whole lived in far worse conditions than did Christians, the statistics indicated that Jews enjoyed an advantage. Physicians in London observed the same thing; Cesare Lombroso, the famed Italian (and Jewish) social scientist, noted something similar for Italian Jewry.[14] Dr. Ludwig Silvagni, in an article on Jews and pathology in the Italian medical journal *Rivista Critica di Clinica Medica*, wrote that Jews are less subject to those harsh infectious diseases that decimate other populations: tuberculosis, pneumonia, typhus, and malaria.[15] There appeared to be something of a consensus, then, that the Jews suffered less from TB, and may even have enjoyed a relative immunity from it. This phenomenon, in turn, could be attributed in large part to the Jewish dietary laws, and particularly the laws governing the slaughter of meat. The Russian

Jewish anthropologist Samuel Weissenberg, writing in one of Germany's leading academic journals devoted to matters of race and hygiene, noted that "there is unanimity to the claim that Jews fall prey to this plague [tuberculosis] to a far less degree than the surrounding populations. And what is particularly noteworthy, as numerous clinicians have testified, is the far greater recovery rate among Jews." Weissenberg noted that this advantage on the part of the Jews was explained with reference to a number of factors, including moderate alcohol consumption, the Jewish culture of the family, and the laws of *kashrut* governing meat.[16] Finally, Jean Flamant, in his 1934 doctoral thesis for the Faculty of Medicine in Paris, summarized the data, which he described as "incontestable," and reached the same conclusion: the Jews are relatively immune to tuberculosis, along with syphilis and alcoholism.[17]

2.

In a letter to the *British Medical Journal*, dated April 6, 1889, Dr. C. R. Drysdale called attention to the latest alarming information on deaths from tuberculosis in France, Australia, England, and Scotland. These deaths had been linked to cattle. Drysdale then informed readers that Jews, it seemed, were relatively immune to tuberculosis, and that this could be explained by their dietary laws.

> My own experience of the Jews in the East End of London is that they very rarely indeed die of phthisis [an older term for tuberculosis], and they are, as all know, very particular about the kind of meat supplied to them for food. It seems to me that it is time that this question of the spread of tuberculosis in our large cities were thoroughly investigated, for it is deplorable to think that one disease should commit such terrible devastation on our race without using every means to prevent it.[18]

Drysdale made the point in order to stress the need for British officials to reform Britain's laws regulating slaughtering and inspection of cattle. I will take up the theme of the Jews as "models" for general reform in Chapter 6. Here, what is of interest is Drysdale's representation of Jews, and particularly poor, immigrant Jews living in London's East End, as suffering less from respiratory ailments than do the Christian population, and his explanation that this has to do with Jewish dietary practices.

Drysdale's intervention in the tuberculosis debate was first and foremost about the disease and the need of British officials to respond more vigorously. But the specific invocation of the Jews of the East End could not but remind readers of the ongoing debate over recently arrived Jewish immigrants from Eastern Europe, a debate occurring in Great Britain as well as in the major cities in continental Europe and the United States. As is well known, one key component of the anti-immigrant arsenal was the charge that immigrants were dirty and diseased, and so threatened the health of the nation.[19] Moreover, a debate over health and disease that included Jewish rituals of slaughter assumed a heightened import in 1889, one year after the Jack the Ripper killings in Whitechapel, a section of London's East End heavily populated with Eastern European Jewish immigrants. One of the earliest theories generated about the murderer portrayed him as a Jew who had employed the techniques of *shechitah* (kosher slaughtering) to kill more effectively. Thus, any intervention in the debate over Jews, health, and Jewish ritual slaughter would also, potentially, be an intervention into the contemporary politics of immigration.[20] And yet, it bears repeating that the intervention of medical authorities in public debates over "aliens" or immigrants was complex, and that medicine and science could lend its support to both pro-alienism and anti-alienism.[21] Moreover, as I've argued throughout this book, the narratives about Jews and health, including tuberculosis and *shechitah*, cannot be reduced to or sufficiently explained by reference to these contingent political events. Such events undoubtedly gave them force, but the narrative tradition preceded them.

Thus, Henry Behrend's influential articles on the subject of infectious disease, meat, and Jewish dietary laws first appeared in London's *Jewish Chronicle* in 1880 and 1881, before any concerted anti-immigration movement arose in Great Britain.[22]

Behrend's contribution may certainly have been motivated in part by an apologetic impulse – anti-Semitism certainly existed in Great Britain before the 1880s, and Jewish elites were already showing concern about the immigrants' ability to assimilate in the early 1880s. But Behrend, who studied medicine at University College Hospital in London and at the University of Manchester, and who in 1850 was elected to the Royal College of Surgeons of England, seemed motivated at least as much by a genuine enthusiasm about recent breakthrough discoveries in scientific and medical knowledge and a desire to spur British health officials to action on TB prevention as by a need to offer an apologia about Jews and Judaism.[23] The Jews, Behrend argued, are – or at least should be – of interest to everyone at present, given the widespread concern with communicable diseases such as tuberculosis, typhoid, and scarlet fever. These diseases are linked with the food supply, with cattle, milk, flesh and fluids; and the "relatively small death-rate of the Jewish, as compared with the general, population of Great Britain," has a clear lesson to teach the general society.[24]

In identifying tuberculosis as a communicable disease in 1880–1881, Behrend was actually adopting a position on the illness's etiology that was still under attack by most mainstream medical authorities. A few individual researchers had argued already in the 1850s and 1860s for the communicability of tuberculosis, and by the 1870s an increasing number of experiments involving the inoculation of animals with the tubercular bacillus produced a groundswell of support for the theory of communicability. Still, as Thomas Dormandy writes, "Respectable opinion still remained on the fence; in 1881, almost at the eleventh hour, Austin Flint and W. H. Welch, in the fifth edition of their magisterial textbook *The Principles and Practice of Medicine*, committed themselves to the statement that 'the doctrine of contagiousness of the disease . . . has its advocates but general belief supported by the weightiest of evidence is in its non-communicability.'"[25]

Behrend's 1880 article began with a discussion of the communicability of disease, the main contours of the new germ theory, and the clear connection between disease transmission and parasites found in cattle and pigs. Researchers had identified seven types of animal diseases that were believed to be transmissible to humans through the ingestion of tainted meat: cattle-plague, swine-typhoid, pleuro-pneumonia, foot and mouth disease, anthrocoid diseases, crysipelas, and tubercle. (While TB was usually linked with cattle, recent outbreaks of trichinosis in Britain in 1871 and 1877 made the subject of pigs also germane.) The main concern for Behrend, though, was tuberculosis. It was the most deadly of all the communicable diseases, "being accountable for at least one-fifth of the entire mortality of the country." The connection between the flesh and milk of diseased cattle and the contraction of TB by humans who ingest this material had only recently been demonstrated; but little doubt remained, he argued, that the malady could be produced in humans in this way. The only means of combating this, according to Behrend, was through ensuring that those in charge of the abattoirs were committed to a thorough inspection of meat and the destruction of diseased animals.

Into the early 1900s at least, a good deal of confusion reigned over the question of bovine and human tuberculosis. Could humans contract the disease from animals? What were the means of transmission?[26] Robert Koch, who had discovered the bacillus for tuberculosis, initially maintained that such transmission was indeed possible. Then, in 1901, he reversed his position and insisted "transmission of tuberculosis from cattle to humans was…negligible and possibly even non-existent."[27] But Koch's revised opinion met with stiff resistance, and many continued to believe that the disease could be transmitted from cattle to humans, through infected meat and milk.

Rabbi Hermann Gollancz certainly believed so. Medical science, he told his congregants in 1890, had now determined that the disease is transmissible from cattle to humans. Gollancz used this to remonstrate both the Jews and the British government. Jewish dietary laws recognized thousands of years ago the connection between health and the proper inspection of meat. England now needed to institute such a proper inspection process if it hoped to contain the TB epidemic. More mysterious than British official inaction, however, was the ignorance and neglect of Jews themselves in the face of a very real danger. Why, Gollancz asked, have Jews given up these dietary practices when just now British health officials are informing us that 80 percent of the cattle brought to the London market was tainted with the tubercular germ, and when we know that it has been adherence to *kashrut* that is largely responsible for the "pertinacity and persistence of the Hebrew people?" "Do men of science labor for nought? Or do we not take the trouble to read the latest results of scientific research? If Christians are beginning to marvel at the wisdom of the laws of the Bible, and are seriously thinking of adopting certain of them in Christian countries, should Jews show an utter disregard of these same laws, and treat them as obsolete ordinances?"[28]

Gollancz's certainty about the relationship between bovine and human tuberculosis did not mean that medical researchers and bacteriologists themselves had resolved the issue. Into the 1900s, the question remained unresolved. When Koch addressed the 1901 meeting of the International

Medical Congress in London, he left the question of bovine and human tuberculosis open, causing a panic in medical and administrative circles. He suggested that there was a possibility that humans could not in fact contract the illness from cattle. This led the British to form a Royal Commission to investigate the matter, and in 1904 they issued their findings: "The bovine strain of tuberculosis was readily transmitted from cow to man (and to other animals like pigs) both in milk and in meat."[29] Bovine and human tuberculosis are, in fact, particular strains of the disease; "bovine" does not refer to a type of TB that can only affect cattle. The bovine strain of the bacillus could affect humans, and the human strain could affect animals. Usually, pulmonary tuberculosis was produced by the human strain; intestinal tuberculosis, as well as tuberculosis of the bones and joints, often by the bovine strain.[30]

The Royal Commission's findings did not go unnoted by defenders of the Jewish dietary laws. Solomon Steinthal, a German Jewish sanitation official, maintained in a 1907 work, *Die Hygiene in Bibel und Talmud*, that

> everyone knows that the tubercles in cattle [*Perlsucht des Rindviehs*] and tuberculosis in humans is the same disease. Only recently, a scientific commission in London has made its research conclusions known, showing that the flesh of cattle can be a source of transmission of TB to humans. How much illness, how much suffering, how much misery have the Jews been spared because of adherence to *shechitah* and *bedikah*! [the ritual inspection of the animal's organs].[31]

The purported Jewish immunity from TB was one reason for such celebratory remarks about *kashrut*, focused on *shechitah*. Tuberculosis was undoubtedly a dreadful disease, a major scourge, and anything that offered some hope of its prevention or cure was going to be embraced at least by some people. And at a time, not unlike our own, when alternative forms of medicine and healing were extremely popular, and diet was of course the focus of so much of this alternative approach, an interest in *kashrut* does not seem all that strange. At the same time, as already noted, an apologetic argument that insisted on the positive effects of Jewish slaughtering must also be read within the context of the political or ideological debates produced in both Germany and Great Britain about *shechitah*. Linking the observance of *kashrut* with the prevention of tuberculosis would go a long way in deflecting the charges brought against kosher slaughtering methods not only by anti-Semites, but by anti-vivisectionists and animal rights advocates.

3.

Detailed discussions of Jewish slaughtering methods and the purported health benefits of *kashrut* were not confined to specialized books and journals. Readers of popular magazines were also offered specifics. In 1907, for example, Solomon Solis-Cohen told readers of the *Saturday Evening Post* about "the health laws of the Jews." In great detail, Solis-Cohen set forth the rules about the method of slaughter, the need to remove the blood through salting and washing, and the inspection of the lungs and other organs. It is worth noting at this juncture that the idea of blood as a prime transmitter of infectious illness and the consumption of blood as a thing to be avoided were in no way universal. In fact, into the twentieth century in some parts of Europe, for instance, people continued a long-standing tradition of eating and drinking blood – animal and human – for medicinal purposes.[32] Recall that Hermann Strack, with whom we dealt in Chapter 3, rooted his rebuttal of the charge of Jewish ritual murder in the copious evidence of peasant (Christian) consumption of blood. In the late eighteenth century, and well into the nineteenth, the Jews were often taken to task precisely for removing the blood from their meat. Thus, the French revolutionary, the Abbé Grégoire, in his famous tract on the physical and moral regeneration of the Jews, noted the ill-effects of the koshering process: "it is certain, that from a fear of eating blood, the Jews squeeze it almost entirely from their meat, and by these means deprive it of much of its nutritive juice."[33] Nothing had changed in the practice of *kashrut* over the hundred years between the Abbé's opinion and that of Behrend, Drysdale, and Solis-Cohen, among many others. The change had occurred in a more general knowledge and awareness of how diseases are transmitted, and the specific concern over tuberculosis and its communication from bovines to humans.

Inspection (Solis-Cohen introduced the readers of the *Saturday Evening Post* to the Hebrew term *bedikah*) would determine if any organ contains parasites, or if it "has at any time been affected with tuberculosis. True, the word 'tuberculosis' is not used, and as the bacillus of tuberculosis was not discovered by Koch until 1882, the rabbis of the Talmud were as ignorant as the rest of the world concerning it." Thus, Solis-Cohen was unwilling to equate the scientific and medical knowledge of the rabbis with modern-day research. However, if we look at the rules the rabbis set forth about the minute inspection of meat, it is clear that they were "guided by a large knowledge. We cannot better their tests today except with the microscope and the bacterial culture – methods obviously inapplicable to routine meat inspection."[34] And for Solis-Cohen, *kashrut* had "an enormous influence in preserving their [the Jews'] vitality under adverse conditions and in giving them a relative immunity from certain forms of disease – in especial from tuberculosis and from infection from animal parasites."[35]

Henry Behrend was of the same mind:

> I am myself decidedly of the opinion that the care bestowed upon the examination of meat for the use of the Jewish community is an important factor in the longevity of the race, which is at present attracting so much attention; and in its comparative immunity from Scrofula and Tubercle, to which Dr. Gibbon, the Medical officer of health for [the English town of] Holborn, has so markedly alluded in his last report. Naturally such cases do not produce an immediate effect, but their transmission through innumerable generations must eventually bring about a decided result, and exercise a considerable influence in building up the mental and physical toughness of the Jewish people, which has been so long an object of wonder. . . .[36]

A full year later, in 1881, Behrend published the second part of his article on the communicability of disease. Research carried out by German and French scientists, he was happy to report, confirmed even more forcefully what he had told his readers the year before. This new research validated "in a most singular manner, the wisdom of the sanitary laws laid down ages ago for the guidance of the Hebrew people."[37] And British officials were now finally paying attention to the question of the nation's meat supply. Behrend cited a number of articles and speeches by British health officials about the high rate of tainted meat used as food, including an article by Dr. Carpenter, in the *British Medical Journal* (October 7, 1879), who claimed that an inspector of the Metropolitan Meat Market "declared upon oath that 80 per cent of the meat sent to the London market had tubercular disease, and that to exclude it from the market would be to leave London without its meat supply. Is it then to be wondered at that our Medical Officers of Health should call attention to the comparative freedom from scrofulous and tuberculous affections enjoyed by the Jewish race?" Behrend then commented: "I would only point out how interesting it is, from a purely scientific standpoint, to notice the complete accordance of these latest investigations with the Mosaic prohibition of blood, 'as being the life,' and with the restrictions of the Talmudical dietary laws."[38]

If works on Judaism and Jews, health and disease served to better acquaint readers – professional and lay, Jewish and non-Jewish – with aspects of Jewish law and ritual, it is worth noting that such works also served, at least potentially, to provide readers with a working knowledge of medical and scientific matters. Thus, articles such as Behrend's, which contained a fair amount of technical information on the nature of diseases and the modes of their transmission, and which appeared in Jewish newspapers or popular magazines, constituted a form of general learning or instruction for Jewish readers. This was certainly not the only, or even the main, purpose of such articles. But popular articles on Jews, Judaism, and hygiene could serve as a sort of remedial instruction on contemporary medical and scientific findings. Behrend, for instance, told his readers that he was taking the opportunity to instruct them, in non-technical language, about the most recent developments in knowledge about disease transmission. In his 1881 article in the *Jewish Chronicle* he discussed, albeit briefly, definitions of bacteria, germ theory, Listerism, and the discoveries of Louis Pasteur.

A far more detailed account of such discoveries appeared in Behrend's much longer 1889 article in *The Nineteenth Century*.[39] In this case, of course, the intended audience would have been much vaster, and not confined to a predominantly Jewish reading public. Readers unfamiliar with Jewish dietary laws and practices would have an opportunity to learn about these (from a sympathetic perspective), while at the same time perhaps learning something about recent trends in tuberculosis research and treatment. The article dealt with tuberculosis ("the most deadly of all the maladies which afflict humanity"), and its transmission through impure meat. Behrend briefly described Koch's discovery that the tubercular bacillus was responsible for the disease in a healthy animal, and noted that his (Behrend's) two previous pieces had been published before the announcement of Koch's discovery in 1882. This article, then, was another update on the research about TB and its transmission. More particularly, Behrend was interested in the issue of the transmission of the disease from tainted animals to humans through alimentation.

The subject of meat contamination and tuberculosis, according to Behrend, had generated widespread concern during the 1880s. The Congress of Tuberculosis, held in Paris in July 1888, identified the issue as of special concern; so, too, in the Anglophone world. Health officials in the U.S. and Australia reported that a significant percentage of the meat available was diseased, and vowed to focus on the problem.[40] Throughout his narrative, Behrend invoked the Jews as counter-examples to the general population. The latter seemed rather apathetic about the high rates of TB and the consumption of tainted meat.[41] Many of the health officials he quoted also invoked the Jews and their laws of slaughtering, the statistics that showed that kosher inspection succeeded in catching tainted meat, and that as a result the number of Jewish deaths from infection was far lower than was the number in the general population. Dr. Klein, of the Brown Institution, told the _Glasgow Herald_ (May 27, 1889) that tuberculosis in man and cattle was the same disease, communicable by ingestion and distributed by the circulation of the blood: "Dr. Klein remarks that it is singular that, centuries ago, the Jewish Church seemed more alive to the dangerous _rôle_ that the meat of animals plays in affecting man than our rulers appear to be at this day, notwithstanding scientific discoveries and exact experimental evidence."[42]

Behrend presented the arguments of the French authority Noël Guéneau de Mussy, whom we've encountered before: the vitality of the Jewish race can be explained, in part, by "the selection of their food supply." Here, again, we find Guéneau de Mussy's argument that Moses' ultimate aim in his law code was hygienic – the assurance of the "regular evolution and normal functions of individual organisms, and the preservation and amelioration of races" – and that he understood all the fundamental principles of modern pathology and bacteriology.[43] More particularly, Moses excluded all animals especially prone to parasites; he understood that germs or spores of infection circulate in the blood, and so he commanded that all blood be thoroughly drained from animals destined for human consumption. And the Talmud builds on Moses' insights, and goes much further in regulating food.[44]

The image of Jews and Judaism offered here is one of health, vitality, hygiene linked with religion, and all these serving as a possible model in one way or another for the general society. Just as significant, it was not only ancient Israelites who benefited from these hygienic measures:

> These ordinances are to this day observed by Israelites faithful to the law, and duly appointed officers visit the slaughter-houses to superintend their execution. The chief rabbi of France says that sometimes as many as twenty-six out of thirty cattle are rejected on account of pleural adhesions. What an extraordinary prescience![45]

There is no reason to read statements such as these or the others reproduced here as anything other than what they purport to be: celebrations and appreciations of the hygienic quality of Judaism and of the concomitant health of the Jewish people, qualities that were in danger of being ignored in the face of anti-Jewish rhetoric.

Guéneau de Mussy and Behrend both advanced the notion that the Jews – identified as a race – enjoyed a relative immunity to tuberculosis, that this immunity was due in large part to their adherence to the laws of *kashrut*, and that this immunity in turn ensured them greater vitality and longevity. According to Behrend, the Jews' "comparative immunity from the tubercular diathesis has been recognized by all physicians whose special experience entitles them to express an opinion, and is the more remarkable when the adverse conditions under which the vast majority live are taken into consideration." British medical officials testified to the lower rates of tuberculosis among even the poorest Jews – for instance, those in Whitechapel – in Great Britain. Behrend insisted that he was not arguing for a mono-causal relation between *kashrut*, tuberculosis prevention, and the overall greater biological vitality of what he called "the Jewish race." No one factor, he wrote, could produce "constant and invariable biological results; all that I claim for that under consideration [*kashrut*] is that it is an important factor, and that operating during a countless series of generations, and acquiring increased force by constant hereditary transmission, it exercises an important influence in building up the physical toughness, and thereby the mental acuteness, so markedly characteristic of the Jewish race."[46]

Both Behrend and Guéneau de Mussy were invoked by numerous others who also insisted that the Jews enjoyed a comparative immunity from tuberculosis, and explained this with reference to the dietary laws. Marcus Adler, writing in the *Asiatic Quarterly Review*, provided a detailed account of rabbinical rules of meat inspection, and informed readers that in this regard the Talmud displays "a profound knowledge of physiognomy. An animal, the lungs of which are in any way affected by tubercules, has always been by Jews considered unfit for food." Then, referring to the research of Behrend (and Drysdale), Adler added: "it is only quite recently that the danger of eating the flesh of cattle suffering from pleuro-pneumonia has been generally admitted."[47] Proof of *kashrut*'s positive impact on the health of Jews, he said, could be found in the statistics compiled and published by insurance companies and by empirical evidence accumulated by physicians. "My own experience, which extends over thirty years, agrees with that of numerous physicians, and I can confidently assert that Jews are remarkably free from scrofulous and tubercular complaints."[48]

In a number of articles on Jews and tuberculosis, and Jews and disease in general, the American Jewish physician and anthropologist Maurice Fishberg made a detailed case for the relative immunity of Jews from TB, and cited Behrend's research in support of his own.[49] Tuberculosis usually struck those who lived in overcrowded, urban areas, who worked in particular occupations such as tailoring that exposed them to dust and other causal agents, and who, as a result, suffered greater mental and physical anxieties. One might expect, therefore, that immigrant Jews in New York, Philadelphia, Chicago, and other major cities would suffer in large numbers from the disease. Moreover, Fishberg noted, the Jews' physical appearance – short stature, flat or concave chests – would certainly lead one to assume this. Their living conditions, occupations, marriage patterns (consanguineous marriages), all would seem to point to Jews as prime candidates for tuberculosis. It was remarkable, then, that almost all leading medical authorities, from around the world, testified to the fact that Jews suffered less from TB than other groups. Fishberg cited the findings of physicians from Great Britain, Australia, North Africa, and the United States.[50]

How might this relative immunity be explained? Fishberg summarized competing explanations of earlier authorities, including Behrend's argument for the significance of *kashrut*.[51] "Of all these causes, the most plausible is the careful selection of the carcasses in Jewish slaughter houses. It has been repeatedly shown that meat from tuberculous cattle is infective to susceptible animals, and the meat inspection practiced by Jews surely has its effect in lessening the number of the tuberculous."[52] Fishberg did make a point of adding that other important factors – in particular the infrequency among them of both syphilis and alcoholism, and the frequency with which Jews tended to consult physicians, even for the mildest of ailments – contributed to the Jews' partial immunity.

In some cases, medical authorities could endorse the notion of a Jewish immunity to tuberculosis even as they challenged the notion of a Jewish immunity to other serious illnesses. Thus, in a note titled "Jewish Immunity to Cancer Denied," *JAMA* disseminated the idea of the relative immunity of Jews to tuberculosis. The note referred to B. W. Richardson's denial of the assertion that "the Jewish race" enjoys "an almost, if not total, immunity ... from cancerous affections." At the same time, Richardson did agree that Jews suffer less from TB than do Christians.[53] In addition to the widespread notion that the Jews suffered less from TB, this brief piece also alerts us to the fact that the idea that the Jews were immune to cancer was circulating in the late nineteenth century, and some felt the need to rebut the notion.[54] The debate over Jews and cancer yielded an interesting parallel to Fishberg's analysis on Jews and tuberculosis. In 1906 Hiram Vineberg published an article on the low incidence of cervical cancer in Jewish women. Vineberg was a gynecologist at Mt. Sinai Hospital in New York City. Over a decade and a half, he had seen close to twenty thousand patients, most of them from the immigrant Jewish population, and among these had encountered only nine cases of cervical cancer. "What especially interested this perceptive physician," Leonard Glick has written, "was that nearly all his patients exhibited the social and economic characteristics then thought to be associated with the disease: poor, prolific, overworked, and malnourished."[55] Vineberg asked himself the same question that Fishberg and others had asked about the Jews and TB: one would expect to find higher rates of the disease precisely among this very population, given the environmental factors; and yet the opposite proved true. How to account for this anomaly? Vineberg believed that it might have to do with laws promulgated in the Mosaic and talmudic codes concerned with marital sexual relations, the laws of *niddah*.[56]

4.

By the first decades of the twentieth century, then, the notion that Jews enjoyed some immunity, even if only partial, to certain diseases, tuberculosis among them, was clearly part of the medical discourse produced about Jews and disease. A 1925 German language article on the Jews and tuberculosis reproduced Fishberg's argument about the ghetto and the Darwinian selection process, and then claimed that "Fishberg's hypothesis has enjoyed especially wide dissemination, and is generally taken today as the explanation for the low level of tuberculosis among Jews."[57] Yet this claim was also being challenged. In a 1917 summary of recent findings on "the health status of the Jews," the Berlin sanitation official and Jewish community leader Louis Maretzki wondered about the widespread claims for a Jewish immunity to tuberculosis and other infectious diseases.[58] Citing a recently published dissertation on Jews and pulmonary tuberculosis, Maretzki noted that the author had concluded that Jews indeed do demonstrate a high proclivity to the disease, yet they rarely die of it and recover more easily from it than do non-Jews.[59] A bit later on in his essay, Maretzki referred to the large number of authorities who had produced statistical studies showing that Jews are less prone to tuberculosis than are non-Jews. At a minimum, the scholarship was at odds and Jewish immunity appeared open to serious question. Maretzki, though, was adamant about one thing: whatever resistance to infectious illness Jews might enjoy, this was not due to any "racial particularity" (*Rasseneigentümlichkeit*) on their part. Rather, if the Jews have been relatively healthy in the past, and if this continued into the present, the reasons were to be found in differential social, environmental, and historical conditions. One must look at hygienic rituals and practices, patterns of occupation and class, relative abstention from alcohol, and – here Maretzki invoked Fishberg – the centuries-long process of natural selection that took place in the ghettoes. In the end, though, Maretzki remained ambivalent and uncertain about what sorts of conclusions might be drawn about Jews and tuberculosis. "The rigid observance of the dietary laws hinders the passing on of the TB germs through the flesh. However, this is questionable, since TB is most widespread in Russia and Galicia, where ritual laws are still maintained."[60] Neither Jews nor non-Jews, Maretzki insisted, should invoke the purported immunity of the Jews from tuberculosis to assert an essential, racial difference between Jews and others. The Jews are distinct, but they are not qualitatively different. ("*Andersartig, aber nicht anderswertig sind die Juden.*")[61]

In the United States, as the number of Eastern European immigrants grew, as their living and working conditions, and the health problems resulting from these conditions, became the object of increased interest, health experts and others grew skeptical of a purported Jewish immunity. "No subject of medicine received more attention in the last 20 years than tuberculosis, its etiology and means of prevention," one medical authority, writing in *JAMA*, remarked. Theodore Sachs was a physician at the Maternal Jewish Hospital for Consumptives in Chicago. In a 1904 article on "Tuberculosis in the Jewish District of Chicago," Sachs challenged what he identified as the dominant notion among medical professionals and the public about Jews and TB.[62] He disabused readers about any racial immunity Jews might possess to the disease, stressing the environmental factors; and he raised the issue of class differences explicitly. Tuberculosis was fairly rare among the well-off, but quite common among the lower, poorer classes.

Sachs' understanding reflected a general change in the understanding of the disease that had occurred since the 1880s and Koch's discovery of the tubercle bacillus. Consumption, as the disease was known before 1882, was believed to be an inherited illness that struck indiscriminately, regardless of class or background. Tuberculosis, as the disease came to be called after Koch's discovery, was an infectious disease that, by the beginning of the twentieth century, came increasingly to be seen as a disease of the industrial, urban working classes and the poor.[63] Based on his own observations and research, Sachs concluded that tuberculosis was very prevalent among the poor Jews of Chicago, and that this was due to unsanitary conditions of homes and factories. "The so-called immunity of Jews from tuberculosis is greatly overestimated," he concluded.[64] A year later *JAMA* also challenged the idea of any sort of racial immunity on the part of Jews. The editors granted that "the Jews of western Europe have, relatively, little tuberculosis." But this was "not due to any true race immunity, as shown by the prevalence of the disease among the less favored members of this race in Poland, Russia, and in the ghettos of our own large cities."[65]

It is generally assumed that by the 1910s opinion had shifted and the notion of Jewish immunity to tuberculosis was overthrown for a more realistic position. Indeed, Maurice Fishberg, arguably the leading authority on Jews and TB, appeared to reverse himself in a 1908 address delivered to the Sixth International Congress on Tuberculosis in Washington, D.C.[66] Fishberg noted that while for the past half century or more it had been commonly believed that Jews enjoyed an immunity to the disease, now it was recognized that there were large numbers of Jewish tubercular patients. But statistics still seemed to indicate that Jews died at a much lower rate from tuberculosis than non-Jews. He presented his earlier findings on comparative mortality rates among immigrant populations in New York City, and added that similar conclusions could be drawn about the Jews throughout Europe and North Africa. In general, the mortality rate from tuberculosis for Christians was four to five times higher than for Jews; studies from Tunisia showed similar results when Jews were compared with Muslims.

Fishberg again called attention to the fact that Jews were overwhelmingly city dwellers, that they worked indoors, at particular occupations (above all, tailoring), and that their physical status was highly compromised (their flat or concave chests were especially notable). Each of these conditions was conducive to tuberculosis; taken together, one would certainly expect to find Jews dying at far higher rates from TB than was the case. He addressed the possible explanations. Racial immunity was dismissed, since the Jews were not a race, or at least not a pure race, and in any case all the evidence pointed to the fact that "tuberculosis displays no racial preference."[67] Fishberg also dismissed inbreeding, or endogamy, as the primary cause in the lower rates of tuberculosis among Jews. Albert Reibmayr, in monographs published in German in the late 1890s, had argued "Jews may abandon all their habits and customs, and so long as they abstain from intermarriage with non-Jews, their immunities to contagious diseases, including tuberculosis, will not be lost."[68] Fishberg rejected this argument as well, based on statistics from Berlin and Vienna on Jewish rates of intermarriage. The rate of intermarriage between Jews and Christians in Berlin in 1905 was close to 44 percent. We know, Fishberg wrote, "that certain racial immunities, like those of the negro against malaria and yellow fever, are impaired in the mulatto." So intermarriage between the races can lower or eliminate a group's resistance to certain diseases. We would then expect to find higher rates of tuberculosis among the Jews in Berlin, given their high rates of inter-marriage. Yet, that was not the case. Jews died from the disease at a far lower rate than did Christians. Moreover, mortality rates from tuberculosis among Jews in communities such as Vienna and Cracow, where the intermarriage rate was either quite low or non-existent, were far higher than in Berlin. More generally, the rates in Western Europe, England and the United States were lower than in Eastern Europe, even though Jewish communities in Eastern Europe experienced almost no intermarriage. This disparity also eliminated adherence to the Jewish dietary laws as a possible factor. The Jews of Eastern Europe continued to keep strictly to these laws, while Jews in Western Europe and America were abandoning them in greater numbers.[69]

"The incidence of tuberculosis among Jews depends more on their economic and social environment than on racial or ritual affinities." The poor suffer more, the better-off, less. Finally, Fishberg added the element of the Darwinian process of natural selection, a theme encountered in Chapter 4. Those most at risk for contracting tuberculosis are the rural dwellers that move into the cities; they possess no built-up resistance to the disease.

> It is this class of rural dwellers, not adapted to indoor city life, that is lacking among the Jews, who have for two thousand years lived exclusively in cities, and during Medieval ages [*sic*] were confined to the worst parts of cites, the Ghettoes.... Under such conditions, those Jews who were predisposed to tuberculosis succumbed, while many of those who survived left a progeny refractory to the disease. The same process is to-day going on with most other inhabitants of large cities. The Jews have only the advantage of having passed through a process of infection during past centuries. Hence their lower mortality to-day from tuberculosis.[70]

As we saw in Chapter 4, Arthur Ruppin reproduced Fishberg's argument regarding urbanism and natural selection, and the lower rates of tuberculosis among Jews. Yet unlike Fishberg, Ruppin accepted the idea that a relative Jewish immunity to TB could be explained by race as well as history and environment. His racial argument can be found in his two-volume *Die Soziologie der Juden* (1930), composed during the years that he headed up the Department of Sociology at the Hebrew University in

Jerusalem. Ruppin offered statistics from Europe and the United States to show that Jews suffer half as often from TB as do Christians. He granted that external factors, such as income levels and standards of living, impacted rates of TB. But were external factors alone responsible? Other factors may be at work. Ruppin reproduced data from Warsaw, from the year 1927: Out of every 100 deaths, TB was the cause in 19.9 of the cases for Christians, 10.6 of Jews. It was doubtful, Ruppin argued, that income levels and living conditions were better in Poland for Jews than for Christians. Moreover, one could not point to occupational differences, for TB attacked Jews from all professions. "A greater defense capability against disease based on race cannot be rejected as an explanation." There is reason to believe that Jews possess a racial immunity to TB not enjoyed by Christians. This was even more extraordinary given "the Jew's small chests. Here is an example of a phenotype (the external appearance of an individual), which is poorer than the genotype (procreative worth). The weak looking Jew can give birth to a healthy child." Thus, the Jew is different from others, those whose phenotype is better than their genotype (for example, on account of the persistent engagement in sport, which improves the body; yet these same people give birth to sickly children).[71] Other scholars argued that while Jews had historically demonstrated a notably lower rate of infection from tuberculosis, this had changed because of World War I. One authority, writing in 1925, concluded that "on account of the privation and upheaval brought by the War (especially for the Jews of Eastern Europe), a fatal reversal took place [in the numbers of Jews suffering from tuberculosis] and this terrible scourge will take innumerable victims among the Jews for decades to come."[72]

Nonetheless, the idea of a special immunity on the part of the Jews to tuberculosis retained its force, and not only among Jewish physicians and writers. In a lengthy article on immunity to TB, Edward Baldwin repeatedly singled out the Jews as the one group "within the White race" that enjoyed a heightened resistance to the disease. Baldwin was the assistant director of the Saranac Laboratory at the famous Saranac Lake sanitorium in New York. In his article, published in the *American Journal of the Medical Sciences* in 1915, Baldwin referred to Fishberg's authoritative studies, and endorsed the idea that a combination of genetics and history explained the Jews' present-day resistance to the illness. "All uncivilized races long removed from infection are very susceptible, but the white races, especially the European Jews, have acquired a certain degree of immunity by inheritance and almost universal infection."[73] It is at this very time, as Baldwin is identifying the Jews as the epitome of civilization in racial terms, that nativists such as Edward Ross and Madison Grant are inveighing against dirty, uncivilized Polish Jews and working for immigration restriction. The two contrary visions of what the Jews represented circulated at the same time; that the nativists and restrictionists had their way nearly a decade later does not mean that the era as a whole was "anti-Semitic" or that one outcome was inevitable.

5.

The idea of a Jewish immunity to TB, explicable with reference to genetics, history, and/or observance of the Mosaic laws, was in no way limited to academic medical journals and textbooks. It made its way repeatedly into the national newspapers, and so circulated beyond the limited circle of elite physicians. We began with a letter to *The New York Times* at the turn of the twentieth century from "Medicus" about the medical wisdom of Moses and the prophylactic value of Jewish law. The *Times* published numerous articles and letters along these lines over the decades, as did other national newspapers such as the *Washington Post*. "Five thousand years before Koch gave to the world the results of his researches in bacteriology," the *Post* told its readers, "the Mosaic law pointed out the danger to man from tuberculosis in cattle, but did not forbid infected poultry as food. It was only a few years ago that German specialists discovered that fowl tuberculosis was harmless to man."[74]

In late 1908 both the *New York Times* and the *Washington Post* published articles on Jewish immunity to tuberculosis.[75] Both included a brief summary of Maurice Fishberg's argument about Jewish history and natural selection. Two thousand years of city dwelling have produced an inborn resistance to the disease. The Jew "has paid the price for urbanization already for several hundred years." This bio-historical experience of the Jews was contrasted to that of the Italians. According to Dr. Antonio Stella, Italians suffer and die from tuberculosis in very high numbers in the United States. They do not come to America with the disease; they contract it once they are in the country. Italians come from largely rural areas, without a history of either urban dwelling or the disease, and so they do not carry with them a resistance. In America, they settle in cities, in highly congested areas, and so die in very high numbers. Indeed, the numbers themselves hardly reflect the true scope of the tragedy, since many Italians who fall ill in the United States travel back to Italy to live our their lives and die. Italy, in turn, had developed a problem with tuberculosis because emigrants were returning from America and spreading the disease among the native population.

Jews and Italians were again linked in a discussion of resistance to tuberculosis in a series of articles on the power of garlic to prevent and heal the disease. In June 1916, the *Washington Post* picked up a story from the *Houston Post* on "garlic as a medicine."[76] Numerous medical authorities, including the *Lancet* in Great Britain, had recently called attention to "the success of the garlic treatment" in treating TB. After the appearance of the long article in the *Lancet*, Dr. Leo Summers, identified as an eminent New York physician, publicly claimed "that garlic is responsible for the relative immunity of Jews and Italians to tuberculosis, an immunity that has been so marked as to excite the wonder of the medical world."[77] Italians, the *Post* writes, consume garlic "almost as freely as we consume onions."[78] Italian physicians apply infusions and poultices of garlic as a treatment for TB, and Italian mothers "give their children garlic syrup at the first indication of a cold." Like the Jews, the Italians here are racially and culturally different in America, but difference does not necessarily mean inferiority. The *Post*'s "we" (Italians consume garlic "almost as freely as we consume onions") suggests a group of readers, most likely middle- and upper-class "Anglo-Saxons," made up of something less than the full population of the United States at the time. Simultaneously, these readers are invited to see Italians and Italian customs as healthy, at least with regard to the threat of tuberculosis. The article then cites Fishberg: "Dr. Maurice Fishberg in discussing the prevalence of tuberculosis among Jews of New York said: 'The Jews always have been garlic-eating people and almost immune from tuberculosis, but when they come to America they cease to eat garlic and become susceptible to the disease.'" Here then, it seems, is a shift or reversal on Fishberg's part. Now it is culture or custom rather than history that explains the Jews' resistance; despite the natural selection process, Jews seem to be susceptible to the disease in America after all, and this because they have ceased to eat garlic.[79]

6.

By 1940, Emil Bogen, the Director of Laboratories and Research at Olive View Sanatorium in California, could write in *Medical Leaves* that the evidence on Jews and tuberculosis appeared contradictory. But "the supposition that the Jewish dietary customs, the rejection of unclean meat, the meticulous care in food preparation, the ritual hand-washing before meals and other hygienic measures might lessen the frequency of ingestion tuberculosis, is now of only historic interest."[80] Still, even Bogen felt it necessary to add that Jews do seem to possess a greater resistance to the disease than their non-Jewish neighbors. Just why this was so, though, remained somewhat of a mystery. Bogen rejected not only explanations rooted in religious ritual or culture, but also those based on racial or inherited resistance, due either to Lamarckian or Darwinian mechanisms. Rather, he favored a more prosaic cultural explanation, one that participated in another set of popular stereotypes given credence by medicine. Jewish health could be explained in part by Jewish hypochondria. Jews, more than most other groups, were not only "more hygienic," but more likely to take quick advantage of medical care.[81] In Bogen's terms, Jews are more neurotic and given over to hypochondria when it comes to TB, complaining and taking a cure even before any physical symptoms appear. This almost neurotic concern with health probably contributes to early detection and cure.

> Perhaps, the apparent resistance to tuberculosis among the Jews depends not upon some mysterious genetic or acquired constitutional cellular or humoral, immunological mechanism, but rather on the behavior both of the individual and community with regard to the disease. The provision of generous facilities for the care of tuberculosis by their co-religionists, and the readiness of individual Jews to seek medical care and follow medical advice may be already reaping their reward in the lessened toll from this disease.[82]

Thus, even if the Jew is neurotic, it is ultimately in the service of better health.

Nonetheless, the notion of a Jewish immunity to tuberculosis persisted into the post-World War II period. Writing on "Tuberculosis Among Jews" in the *American Review of Tuberculosis* in January 1953, the Jerusalem-based physician Joseph Rakower noted that "the high resistance" of Ashkenazi, Sephardi and Middle Eastern ("Oriental") Jews to tuberculosis "is an old and a well-known problem which has received considerable attention. These groups were always cited as an example of a highly immune ethnic group in contradistinction to the marked susceptibility of the non-white races. This well-known fact was confirmed once again by the first published tuberculosis mortality rate in Israel in 1949." The newly formed State of Israel had one of the lowest tuberculosis rates in the world.[83] The only exception to this pattern appears to have been the Jews of Yemen, and Rakower's article is an investigation into this anomaly. Rakower concluded that the high rate of tuberculosis among Yemenite Jews was the product of emigration, of their move from an agricultural, rural setting "where tuberculosis was almost unknown," to an urban setting "where tuberculosis was endemic." Fishberg, recall, had argued that Jews were resistant to TB in part because they had dwelled for hundreds of years in cities, and that this experience had acted to immunize them against the ravages of the disease. It was the largely peasant populations, like the Italians, who were devastated when they moved from rural to urban environments. Echoing Fishberg and others, Rakower argued that

> due to the process of natural selection, the Ashkenazi, Sephardi, and Oriental Jews, who were for centuries exposed to tuberculosis in urban communities, acquired a greater degree of resistance to this infection. Yemenite Jews, i.e., the section of Jews who lived under desert conditions such as are found in Yemen far from the rest of the people, are now paying the same price as any other group would pay which had been free from previous contact with the tubercule bacillus.[84]

7.

What impact, if any, did the elite medical analysis of Jews and tuberculosis have on the way Jews actually lived? In other words, what was the connection between discourse and material or social reality? Despite or regardless of any notion of an immunity to the disease, Jews of course did get tuberculosis. And this meant that by the first decades of the twentieth century, a host of institutions had either been created *de novo* to deal with Jewish tubercular patients or had expanded their missions to include disease prevention and cure. In the United States, for example, the Educational Alliance, the Workmen's Circle, Jewish hospitals – chief among them Montefiore, but also Mt. Sinai and others, and sanitoria, the best known the two competing institutions in Denver, Colorado – all now made care for Jewish tubercular patients a priority.[85] At the same time, as late as 1925 complaints could still be heard that the organized Jewish communities were not devoting enough attention and money to the prevention, rather than treatment, of the disease.[86] In any case, it would be difficult to imagine that the mass of Jews – like their non-Jewish counterparts – were unaware or unconcerned by the threat of the illness. Daniel Bender has shown just how conscious Jewish labor-ers themselves were of disease, and in particular tuberculosis, and how they understood the relationship between their working and living con-ditions as impoverished immigrants and the effect of this on their bod-ies. "Jewish workers viewed work as an inevitable confrontation with weakness and disease, and this image represented an important part of how Jewish workers articulated their common experiences as garment workers." Jewish workers "used images of disease and enfeeblement to describe workplace conflict; questions of health and curing workers' bod-ies lay at the heart of their organizing."[87] However, this understanding of the relationship between work in a factory or sweatshop and the con-traction of tuberculosis did not necessarily translate into an immediate or full understanding of bacteria and the transmission of disease. Nancy Tomes notes that at the outset of the twentieth century the heightened awareness of germs remained limited for the most part to the upper and middle classes. By the second decade of the twentieth century, "the epi-demiological havoc wrought by tuberculosis and other communicable diseases had become much more class and race specific. From the late 1800s onward, the ailments that the gospel of germs sought to prevent increasingly became identified with the poor and sanitarily disadvan-taged." Tuberculosis, for instance, ceased to be a "house disease" that potentially ravaged anyone unlucky enough to contract it, and became, as Tomes writes, a "tenement house disease."[88] Jewish workers and the Jewish poor, like the working classes and the poor in general, now had to be instructed in the basics of bacteriology and disease prevention. Popular medical texts, many written in Yiddish, and aimed at the Jewish working classes, conveyed a basic knowledge of biology and physiology, of dis-eases and how to prevent or treat them. Such books and pamphlets were merely the Yiddish versions of more mainstream or general health guides directed at a lay audience. Seeking to calm and reassure an increasingly worried public, bacteriologists and physicians began in the late 1800s to publish popular works that described "'what bacteria do' and what precautions health-conscious citizens should adopt."[89]

Paradoxically, it was the material written in the so-called parochial language of the Jews – Yiddish – that spoke to the Jewish masses in a universal way about health and disease, preventive care and treatment.[90] The content belied the form. "There is no race or class of humans who are exempt from potentially contracting tuberculosis," Dr. A. Sztylman told his readers in *Layb un Leben*. "Only newborns show no reaction to Koch's tuberculin bacillus. Once we reach the age of twenty, every human seems at risk."[91] There is no hint here of a Jewish immunity to tuberculosis or any other illness. If there was an agenda in these Yiddish works, aside from the obvious and practical one of attempting to ensure the reader's well-being, it was decidedly not a Jewish apologetics. Thus, a Yiddish work titled *Reinlichkeit un Gezunt (Cleanliness and Health)*, published in Vilna in 1901, began with the assertion that while in the past Jews were known as the purest or cleanest of people, with an abiding adherence to laws of hygiene, today the opposite held true. Cleanliness is ignored, considered "a Gentile attribute." Rather than Moses, the author invoked the Romans, who long ago gave us the motto *mens sano in corpore sano*.[92] The author, a Dr. Jevnin, proceeded to inform his readers about the nature of infectious disease, and the central role played by the microbe. "Every infectious disease has its microbes, and they multiply in filth (*shmutz*)." Therefore, everything must be clean – clean air, clean dwelling, clean body, clean clothing, clean bed and bedding. "Open up the gates!" he implored. "Open the doors and the windows, let some fresh air in. Let the sun shine in your shuttered rooms. Don't fear the fresh air, or a bit of cold. Take my word for it, I'm a doctor!"[93] He made a special point of discussing tuberculosis, and the need to keep one's living space free of dust. Only once, when discussing the benefits of clean water, did Jevnin mention a Jewish ritual or practice. "The old *minhag* [custom] of *Erev Shabbat* [Friday night], of going to the bath is a very good tradition. If you can't bathe at home, at least you can bathe in a public bath."[94] However, any hint of the sort of reinterpretation of the Mosaic or talmudic laws along the lines that we have been concerned with is absent. The concern in these advice books lay elsewhere.

A more likely impulse to these practical works than a Jewish apologetics was the advancement of a socialist or reformist perspective, one that included a more or less explicit attack on a capitalist system that placed owner's profits far above workers' health. This was most evident, of course, in the writings produced by doctors and popular medical writers associated with the Workmen's Circle (*Arbeter Ring*) and other Jewish socialist organizations.[95] For example, in a long, three-part article on "medicine from a social standpoint," Dr. A. Kaspe offered a basic lecture on the nature of capitalism, and he made his point about the sacrifice of the health of the workers to the wealth of the owners through a discussion of tuberculosis.[96] His is a wonderful example of a work aimed at the Yiddish reading public that sought to educate Jews about the nature of the illness, the discovery of germs (with accounts of Pasteur and Koch, but also the details of the French researcher Villemin's experiments in the 1860s with injecting live tubercles into hares and rabbits in order to establish the infectious nature of the illness), and current thinking about prevention and cure.[97] Kaspe included a protracted discussion of the relationship between human and animal tuberculosis, instructing his readers that one could contract the disease by either breathing infected air or consuming tainted milk or meat. But nowhere did he mention Moses and the rabbis, or the hygienic value of Jewish law – though, admittedly, a celebration of traditional Jewish religious practice, even if reinterpreted as scientific, would be unexpected from a Jewish socialist.

There were, to be sure, works in Yiddish that spoke of "Jewish diseases," but in the main, only in passing and only to dismiss the very category. "Is it true that there are particular Jewish diseases?" Benjamin Dubovsky asked in his work of popular medical advice, *Gezunt un Leben*. Certainly not. "This is pure fantasy (*bloyz an aynraydnish*)."[98] Works in Yiddish on health were intended as practical instructional or educational texts, not academic treatises. If information on the history of medicine did appear, it was more likely to follow the dominant narratives than reimagine Moses and the rabbis at the center of the story. When L. V. Zwisohn, a New York physician, asked "*Vos is higiene?*" (What is hygiene?) in his 1904 work on how to prevent and treat tuberculosis, he mentioned Hippocrates and his teacher Herodicus, who Zwisohn credited with introducing the notion of physical exercise as a means of improving health.[99] Moses, the rabbis, Maimonides – they are nowhere to be found. And when he discussed the various measures poor Jews ought to take to prevent the disease, he listed all the common pieces of advice found in such works at the time: fresh air, exercise, diligence in washing and disinfecting one's house, clothes, and linen. He even warned his readers about the dangers of kissing household pets, for dogs, cats and birds could also transmit tuberculosis to humans. And he warned about the dangers of impure foods and liquids. But there was no mention of *kashrut*, or the benefits that might come from adhering to the Jewish dietary laws.

Popular tracts in Yiddish were "Jewish" insofar as they were written in a language that is generally identified as "Jewish" and were aimed presumably at a Jewish audience. But they did not concern themselves with issues such as biblical and talmudic medicine, the Jewish contribution to health and medicine, or even the historical or contemporary differences between Jews and non-Jews when it came to matters of health and disease. When such discussions appear in Yiddish, it is in the pages of the *YIVO Bleter*, the journal of the Yiddish Institute for Scientific Research, or in monographs aimed at a more limited and elite audience.[100]

If ordinary Jewish workers, or those writing for them, did not necessarily take seriously the discourse on Moses and hygiene, then who did? Jewish elites like Fishberg, but also non-Jewish elites, Christian physicians and authors, who offered up Jewish law (together with historical experience) not only as the most likely explanation for Jewish survival and vitality, but as a possible means by which Gentile societies could meet present and future challenges to their individual and collective health.[101] As Chapter 6 demonstrates, the notion that Jews had proven relatively immune to tuberculosis, along with a host of other illnesses, served as a powerful impulse to the belief that the Jews and Judaism provided a model for Christians when it came to matters of health and hygiene.

6

"Then What Advantage Does the Jew Have?"

Judaism as a Model for Christian Health

I.

"In the Greeks alone we find the ideal of what we should like to be," Wilhelm von Humboldt wrote in his essay *Über das Studium des Altertums und des Greicheschen inbesondere* (1793).[1] By the late eighteenth century at the latest, ancient Greece, for better or worse, was regarded by many as the ideal and model for European culture.[2] At the same time, as is well known, there were others who insisted that the worship of all things ancient and Greek was misplaced, that modernity was superior to the ancient past, and that modern Europeans would do well to reject the idealization of the ancients. Progress, in the view of the moderns, was linear, and for the most part those who lived now were better off than their ancestors. Were these the only two models offered an educated public interested in the relationship between the ancient and the modern, and the questions of knowledge, well-being, and progress?

As I've tried to show in this book, over the course of the nineteenth century an intellectual tradition developed that reinterpreted the Mosaic and rabbinic law codes as medical hygiene codes. Physicians, rabbis, professional and popular medical writers, and others working within this interpretive paradigm demonstrated the efficacy of the laws by pointing to the historical and contemporary vitality of the Jews, their longer individual life spans, their purported immunity from certain diseases, and their 3,000- year-long survival as a distinct race or *Volk*. The Jews owed their vitality and health ultimately to the Mosaic and rabbinic codes. Why, many Christians asked, could not this Jewish health and vitality become a model for government and society in general? If Christians adhered to those Jewish religious proscriptions that were now shown to be of hygienic value, could they not also expect to decrease disease and suffering?[3]

The period between the Renaissance and Enlightenment had witnessed the publication of numerous works by Christian Hebraists on the ancient Hebrew "republic" or "commonwealth," studies intended not only as scholarly investigations into Jewish political and social customs but, as one seventeenth-century writer put it in dedicating his work to the magistrates of Holland and West Frisia, as an "example" to be imitated.[4] The idea of the Jews as a model or example for Christians, then, precedes by centuries the interpretive tradition of the Mosaic law as a hygienic code to be followed by individual Christians and implemented by Christian policy makers and administrators. However, the discursive link between Jewish law and health was a radical departure from and at least an implicit repudiation of Enlightenment and Reform Jewish perspectives. Perhaps even more startling, though, is this discourse's repudiation of Christian theology and the Christological understanding of history, startling because, as I hope I've demonstrated, so many of the contributors to this reinterpretation of Judaism and the Jews were Christians. Max Grunwald, a Viennese Jewish scholar, opened his introduction to the 1911 collection *Die Hygiene der Juden*, by noting how many non-Jewish experts had testified to the wisdom of the ancient Jewish hygiene laws and regretted that Christians had neglected them until recently. The Scottish minister and theologian Alexander Rattray, for instance, had explained this as a product of the long-standing belief among Christians that the laws of the Old Testament were obsolete and therefore could be discarded and forgotten. It was only with the emergence of modern biblical criticism that Christians rediscovered the import of the Pentateuch's laws.[5]

Granted, there is no sure way to determine the levels of "religiosity" for many of these Christian writers. Nonetheless, it is not far-fetched to assume that these men, having grown up and been educated in cultures that were still deeply Christian, would at least carry with them some residual notion of traditional Christian belief. In any case, the interpretive tradition they helped produce departed, at least implicitly, from this traditional Christian theology about the Jews and Judaism. Jewish law does not, as St. Paul would have it, signify corruption, sin, and death.

Jesus' dictum, in the Gospel of Matthew, that it is "not that which goes into the mouth that defiles a man, but what comes out of a mouth that defiles a man" (Matthew 15: 11), this had to assume a different meaning in the light of tuberculosis, and the accepted idea of the transmission of the disease through meat and milk. When it is widely acknowledged that circumcision prevents cancer, among a host of other maladies, what answer does one then give to Paul's question to the Roman community, "What is the profit of circumcision?" (Romans 3: 1). When the Jewish laws were heralded as necessary and healthy, where did that leave the theological repudiation of these Jewish practices? Once Jewish law is medicalized (and therefore at some level de-theologized), once it is reframed positively as a prodigious set of hygienic rules, then the traditional Christian understanding is overturned.

"Then what advantage does the Jew have?" Paul asked in Romans 3: 1. According to the Christian physicians and medical authorities writing in the nineteenth and twentieth centuries, "much in every way! Because first of all, they were entrusted with the oracles of God" (Romans 3: 2). And Christian authorities insisted that the laws, as hygienic rules, could benefit Christians as much as they had benefited Jews. Of course, this did not mean a repudiation of the fundamental theology of salvation through faith. But if Christians would not be saved spiritually by the laws, they could be saved physically, through a greater resistance to tuberculosis, cancer, and a whole host of lesser ailments.

2.

If thou wilt diligently hearken to the voice of the Lord thy God, and wilt do that which is right in his sight, and wilt give ear to his commandments, and keep all his statutes, I will put none of these diseases upon thee, which I have brought upon the Egyptians: for I am the Lord that healeth thee. (Exodus, 15: 26; Deuteronymy 7: 15)

The Lord your God shall bless thy bread and thy water; and I will take sickness away from the midst of thee. (Exodus 23: 25)

The Reverend Charles Richson invoked these verses towards the beginning of a sermon he delivered in the cathedral in Manchester, England, on Sunday morning, April 30, 1854. The sermon's title, "The Observances

of the Sanitary Laws, Divinely Appointed, in the Old Testament Scriptures, Sufficient to Ward off Preventable Diseases from Christians as well
as Israelites," was indeed the main thrust of the Reverend's argument.
Like the ancient Israelites, Richson told his congregants, we have suffered the scourge of disease and pestilence: cholera in 1832 and 1849;
scarcity in 1847, which became famine in Ireland; fever, and the destruction of war at present in the Crimea. How important it is, then, "that we
endeavor to ascertain, for our practical guidance in seeking to obtain the
like advantages for ourselves [of preventing disease], what are the statutes
and commandments of Divine institution that related to *the avoidance
of bodily affliction, and the maintenance of physical health.*"[6]

An expanded version of the sermon was published in 1854, with notes
by John Sutherland, a physician who sat on the General Board of Health
in London. When we read Richson's sermon together with Sutherland's
notes, it is possible to see even more clearly both the process of the medicalization of religious discourse and the way in which Christian authorities, speaking in the name of Christianity and Science, could advocate
for the adoption of Jewish laws.

Everything that is unclean is to be abhorred, Richson tells his listeners. The Bible celebrates a land "rich in farinaceous and other vegetable
productions, and abundant in the supply of purest water"; it warns us
"the deterioration of race, by the intermarriages of close kindred, was to
be strictly avoided"; it instructs us repeatedly to respect the distinction
between clean and unclean food. In an extended footnote, the physician
Sutherland suggests that a prohibition against the breeding and eating
of pork would go a long way toward advancing the cause of health. He
contextualizes the definition of clean and unclean food, granting that
in particular climates certain nations and races become ill from certain
foods. True, pork does negatively affect those who in the main live in a
warm climate. But Sutherland focuses on the dangers involved in breeding pork, which are universal. Thus, "a simple enactment prohibiting
the use of swine's flesh as an article of food, if it could be carried out,
would put an end to a great cause of disease and degradation in our large
cities and towns, even if it were at the same time admitted that pork was
perfectly wholesome food." Sutherland connects the raising and keeping
of pigs in English villages and towns with cholera, fever, higher mortality
rates in general, as well as moral degradation that comes as a result of

people living in darkness and filth. He then invokes Moses, and suggests that Britain itself would be better off following his basic dietary precepts:

> The Hebrew legislator provided against the degradation which might have arisen among his people from the rearing of certain animals, by pronouncing them unclean, and prohibiting their use as food. If we had the same opportunity of observation in regard to all the prohibited animals as we have in regard to swine, we should doubtless obtain similar proofs of the wisdom of the prohibition.[7]

Richson mentions the Jews for the first time explicitly in his discussion of alcohol. Moderation, he advises, is the rule. In his footnote, Sutherland moves into the present, arguing that all empirical evidence shows that drunkenness compounds the effects of epidemic diseases, cholera especially. The suggestion here is that the British would be well advised to follow the Jews in this regard also, as they are renowned for their moderation in drink and for their health.

Richson proceeds to discuss clothing, and the dangers of dirty clothes. Mosaic law paid great attention to clothing, and its inspection as a signal of diseases such as leprosy. Again, Sutherland insists that the English present falls short of the ancient Jewish past. The "washing and burning of foul apparel and household linen is a common precaution in the present day against epidemic diseases, but as usual it is done *after* the disease has appeared, and not *before*, as was the case under the Jewish law."[8]

Sutherland's comments on Richson's text make the social and practical point explicit, translating the religious into the medical and weighing the British present against the Jewish past, finding the former wanting. Ancient Jewish law understood the connection between refuse and infectious disease, and commanded that all refuse, animal and human, be destroyed by fire immediately. Unfortunately, according to Sutherland, "our present practice is directly the reverse of that commanded by the Jewish lawgiver." In Great Britain, any man may not only retain refuse, but may turn it into a product for profit. Boiled bones, catgut, artificial manure, animal oils, anything "whereby he can make money" is countenanced. Until "our sanitary police" act as the Jewish legislator did, and ensure the swift removal of all sorts of refuse, "it can never be said that proper attention is paid to the health and habits of our working population." Modern science and experience are now catching up with the ancient wisdom and law regarding human refuse and disease, and validating these ancient insights. Modern science, after centuries of barbaric practices in Europe, has discovered "that the Hebrew practice is the only one consistent with a proper regard to public health and public decency."[9]

While it is perhaps not surprising that Sutherland, the physician, medicalized religious rules, Richson too subsumed the religious and the ritual within the sanitary. It was necessary, he argued, for the divine rules of health to be cast as religious ceremonials so that they would more likely be observed. But the principles upon which this code was founded were "the physical nature and constitution of man." The Divine laws contained in the Bible were sanitary regulations not only in their effect but also in their intent.[10] Richson, of course, felt obliged to address himself to the obvious question: are these sanitary regulations contained in the Old Testament binding upon Christians as well as Jews? His answer was yes, and he invoked modern science to defend this argument. Science was at that time demonstrating that the observance of Mosaic law "is absolutely indispensable to the maintenance of physical health, and that they [the laws] are now, as formerly, the only conditional preservatives against pestilence and disease." According to Richson, "it is one of the especial duties of a minister of Christ to insist on the religious obligation of the sanitary laws. But be the opinion what it may on the religious aspect of this question, no one, except the most ignorant person, doubt the expediency, particularly at the present time, of giving serious attention to sanitary regulations."[11] In the end, Richson also invoked the contemporary Jewish condition to reinforce his claims about the sanitary laws. He implored his congregation to read the Old Testament and contemplate the disparity between those who keep the Mosaic laws and the contemporary condition of Christians.

The comparison is important; both because it will lead you to consider how far we may reasonably expect the Divine blessing upon our own proceedings; and also because it will help you to appreciate a recorded fact that during the visitation of cholera in 1848–49, the Jews in London, many of whom are of the very lowest class, 'suffered much less from the disease of cholera than the other classes of the community; probably not more than thirteen deaths occurring out of a population of 20,000;' and 'this comparative immunity,' after an official investigation, could be accounted for, only by their partial observance of the Mosaic Institutions.[12]

Sutherland expanded on Richson's point about the functional aspect of the sanitary rules being cast in religious and ritualistic terms. He also linked the Jews' own condition to their laws, arguing that historically

> Jewish people escaped pestilence during the whole period of their national existence.... Even till this present day they suffer less, in proportion to their numbers, than any other race, except in certain special cases where the governments under which they live flagrantly neglect their duty. A large volume might be written to show that the fundamental principles of all sanitary legislation and practice, whether national, domestic, or personal, are contained in the Old Testament.

Sutherland proceeded to repeat his point that contemporary life in towns and cities throughout the country testify to the disease, misery, and death that result from "the neglect of the Old Testament sanitary principles."[13]

3.

The contribution of Jews to medicine, then, lay in the first place in the past, in Moses having given his own people, and then, through Christianity, the world, this health code. But the Jews still had a contribution to make in the present and future. As John Sutherland's gloss on Richson's sermon indicates, health authorities saw in the Mosaic code a very real and practical guide to contemporary health issues. They took an enormous interest in questions of Jewish group survival, immunity from certain diseases, and the connection between purported Jewish health and allegiance to the Mosaic code. In turn, if a causal connection between Jewish health and survival could be linked with their historical observance of Jewish law, then should not the observance of Jewish rituals in some form or other be instituted for all civilized countries?

To be sure, not every invocation of the Hebrew Bible by a Christian physician can or should be taken as a philosemitic gesture, or as evidence of an acceptance of Jews as a model for Christians. The Mosaic code was, of course, also part of the Christian scriptural tradition, and Christian intellectuals could invoke the Old Testament entirely as Christians, without a nod to Jews or Judaism. Thus, for instance, when

G. S. Franklin, a physician from Ohio, spoke in 1886 about "Purification and Sanitation by Fire," and opened his essay by citing eight passages from the book of Leviticus, he did so as a believing Christian and as a medical authority. The sanitary practices contained in the law of Moses demonstrated, he argued, the happy confluence of religion and science, and justified a Christian's faith. It is "gratifying to the believer when the progress of science brings us to a more exact comprehension and belief in doctrines and practices taught and enjoined by the inspired lawgiver over 3,000 years ago."[14] Moses, Franklin made clear, was equal to or ahead of modern science in his understanding of purification by fire. So, he already directed that nitrogenous waste be destroyed quickly, and outside of the camp. He commanded that this be done no later than the third day, and we now knew, said Franklin, that "infection becomes powerful by the third day." In the end, Franklin implicitly suggested that contemporary modes of sanitation fall short of those of the ancient Hebrews. He offered an extensive list of dangers posed by germs and by the failure to destroy with fire everyone and everything that had been infected; he then asked when the day would come when intelligent and efficient boards of health would turn their full attention to "this great sanitary problem."[15]

Franklin never mentioned Judaism or the Jews, and there is no reason to assume that in invoking Moses he meant to do anything other than celebrate ancient wisdom in light of modern science and lend support to his recommendations for contemporary sanitary measures by juxtaposing them with biblical proscriptions. Yet, for many other Christian authorities, the ancient Hebrew past and the Jewish present were merged, and Jews and Judaism had a contribution to make in terms of the future health of all nations. The American physician Edward T. Williams insisted that the Jews had something to teach the Christian world about sexual health. Williams' 1882 article, "Moses as a Sanitarian," is yet another example of translation and equivalence. "So far as we know," Williams stated at the outset, "Moses was the creator of preventative medicine, an idea thought to be peculiarly modern."[16] Among other topics Williams explored, he took up briefly one that, as we have seen, concerned a large number of writers on Jews and health in the two centuries under discussion here: the health benefits of circumcision. These were benefits that accrued first of all to Jews, yet also, potentially, to Christians.

Circumcision, Williams argues, bestows clear hygienic benefits upon its practitioners. It helps, for instance, to prevent syphilis and other such diseases; and "it is known that Jews rarely have syphilis...."[17] In addition,

> the removal of the foreskin is acknowledged to be useful as a preventative of masturbation. It not only renders the act itself more difficult, but by diminishing the sensibility of the part and favoring the removal of irritating secretions diminishes also the propensity to the act. It is certain that this vice is a prolific cause of nervous diseases and even of insanity among Christian nations.... The habit itself when fully formed, and a species of paralysis resulting from it, have in numerous instances been cured by circumcision. Hence one of the strongest arguments in its favor.

Circumcision prevents phymosis (the inability of the foreskin to retract), and the retention of sebaceous secretion, and thus helps to prevent balantitis, the inflammation of the glans of the penis. "Lastly, it probably promotes continence by diminishing the pruriency [sic] of the sexual appetite."[18]

Williams then offered up his more general conclusion, in which he cast the Jews as a much-needed model for Christian civilization:

> The remarkable exemption of the Jews from insanity and nervous diseases, even their general good health and longevity, may in no small degree be attributable to these causes [circumcision and the curbing of the sexual appetite]. At any rate it is a fact that the Jews are the healthiest race in existence. They have produced the greatest men, and contributed more to the advancement of civilization than any nation known to history. However degenerate, morally speaking, some of their modern descendents may be, they certainly have not degenerated physically, a sufficient answer to the often repeated assertion that civilization tends to physical weakness, for the Jews have been longer civilized than any other highly civilized people. May we not then venture the inference that the rite of Abraham, or Moses, has had its share, in the production of these wonderful results, and that it might perhaps be profitably imitated by other nations?[19]

A number of points are worth noting about this passage. Williams was a Christian, and his celebration of Jewish health and civilization illustrates the fact that the "healthy Jew" was a figure not only of the Jewish, but also of the Christian, imagination. Of course, the Jews in Williams'

narrative here are not absolutely healthy; the modern Jew has degenerated morally. In this regard, as well, Williams was articulating, albeit
in a vague and undeveloped way, a wider notion that became a crucial
part of the scientific discourse about Jews in the late nineteenth and early
twentieth centuries. The Jews of the past, those who kept their religious
laws and maintained themselves in a traditional, orthodox community,
were healthy; those Jews who were modern, who surrendered their commitment to Orthodoxy for secularism, were diseased. Williams, writing
in the early 1880s, offers only a partial version of what would become, in
the writings of both Jews and non-Jews, a full-blown theory of contemporary Jewish abnormality and illness. Many later writers would extend
the image of Jewish disease to the physical and mental, which Williams
did not do. It is worth noting that Williams, contrary to the prevailing
view at the time, insisted that the Jews are exempt from insanity and nervous disorders. For Williams, modern Jews are only morally degenerate;
they remain physically and mentally healthy, "the healthiest race in existence," and a model for Christians in this regard.

In many cases the notion that Christians would do well to take up circumcision or another Jewish ritual for health reasons can only be inferred
from what Christian authorities wrote. Thus, in an 1876 article in the
Lancet, Dr. Gibbon, from Holborn, argued that because of circumcision
the "Hebrew race" enjoyed an immunity from syphilis and scrofula. In
response, Dr. Edgar Sheppard insisted that the absence of such diseases
among the Jews was not due to circumcision, but to the fact that the
Jews "were more moral and religious than Christians"; they "carry their
religion more into the details of their daily life."[20] Gibbon and Sheppard
disagreed on the reasons for the immunity Jews seemed to enjoy, but
they agreed on the fact that the Jews possessed such immunity. And both
seemed to suggest, if only implicitly, that Christians might benefit from
following the Jews.

Often, though, Christian medical authorities were quite explicit about
the advisability of following the Jews. Jonathan Hutchinson, medical
historians agree, was one of the most influential advocates of universal
circumcision in the nineteenth century.[21] Hutchinson was a surgeon at
the Metropolitan Free Hospital in London, and a tireless promoter of circumcision as a prophylactic against venereal disease and other maladies.
He fervently urged its universal adoption. Working from statistics he

collected during a single year (1854) on Jewish and non-Jewish patients suffering from venereal disease, Hutchinson concluded that "the circumcised Jew is . . . very much less liable to contract syphilis than an uncircumcised person." This was a fact that had been, he wrote, "long entertained by many surgeons of experience."[22] Circumcision, for Hutchinson, was a matter of both covenant and health. It was "probable that circumcision was by Divine command made obligatory upon the Jews, not solely as a religious ordinance, but also with a view to the protection of health. . . . One is led to ask, witnessing the frightful ravages of syphilis in the present day, whether it might not be worthwhile for Christians also to adopt the practice."[23]

Over forty years later, S. M. I. Henry, in her popular work *Confidential Talks on Home and Child Life*, noted that circumcision was "still in existence among the Jews, and as some special forms of venereal disease become more and more manifest among other nations . . . the Jews [go] almost entirely free." The "old rite," she suggests, has "a value for both boys and girls as a cleansing and preventative process."[24] We should not necessarily conclude from passages such as this that Christians in Victorian Britain had ceased to see Jews as different, as non-Christians and probably not quite British. It may very well be that Henry harbored an extreme unease about the Jews in her midst. Her advocacy, and the advocacy of other non-Jewish writers, of Jewish rituals as hygienically sound did not necessarily translate into tolerance, let alone fondness, for actual Jews. But, nonetheless, we are faced with an image of Jews and Judaism as healthy, and as a model of hygienic and moral practice for Christians that challenges to some degree our understanding of how the Jewish body was imagined in the late nineteenth and early twentieth centuries.

The advocacy of circumcision did tend to translate into a developing notion of a healthy and hygienic Jewish body. Hutchinson, for instance, published in 1890 a "Plea for Circumcision," in which he wrote of "the superior cleanliness of the Hebrew penis."[25] Scholars have argued that the circumcised penis had by the nineteenth century become a metonym for the Jew, and that the evaluation was almost always negative. The circumcised penis was both cause and sign of Jewish sexual lust, exclusion and segregation, and an unhealthy sense of superiority.[26] If so, then in the texts we are discussing here, we can see a counter-discourse developing around the circumcised penis and the Jew.

Circumcision, however, was just one of the ancient Mosaic rituals that Gentile physicians recommended for adoption by states and citizens. As we saw in Chapter 5, numerous medical authorities touted *kashrut* as key to a preventive program against tuberculosis. It was noted that Jews seemed historically resistant to the disease, and governments and populations were urged strongly to consider adhering to Jewish dietary restrictions. Thus, in August 1912, the *New York Times* delivered the findings of J. A. Lindsay, a professor of medicine in London, on "How Races Differ in Disease Immunity."[27] Professor Lindsay, the *Times* reported, "discusses the advantages the Jew is generally believed to enjoy." Lindsay's evaluation of the Jews was mixed. They seemed to suffer less from a host of illnesses, including alcoholism, venereal diseases, skin diseases including leprosy, and many epidemic diseases. On the other hand, "the Jew suffers more than the average from diabetes, hemorrhoids, nervous diseases in general, especially blindness and color blindness, the deaf and dumb defect, and insanity...." Lindsay also discussed the common belief that Jews suffer less or have proven resistant to tuberculosis. He listed the familiar arguments for this, but in the end rejected the idea of Jewish immunity.

For this reason, Lindsay did not advocate that Britain or any other country take up the Jewish dietary laws. Nonetheless, he did report that in Greece, physicians had started a campaign to have the Greek populace follow *kashrut* laws to prevent tuberculosis. "The alleged infrequence of tuberculosis among Jews as a result of the care they exercise in their choice of meat for food has resulted in a campaign in Greece for the adoption there of the ancient Jewish ritual slaughter of cattle and the providing of kosher meats throughout the kingdom." At an anti-tuberculosis congress in Wala, Greece, the chief physician of Larisa, on the Aegean coast, Dr. Erepidas, "read a paper to prove that tuberculosis is less frequently met with among Jews than among other peoples." Erepidas attributed this to the *kashrut* laws governing the slaughter and preparation of meats. "He concluded that these laws are a protection against tuberculosis, and he proposed that the congress adopt a resolution urging the Government to introduce the Jewish mode of slaughtering cattle into all slaughter houses of Greece. The resolution of Dr. Erepidas was adopted, and all Greek newspapers are now discussing the interesting proposal."[28]

Two years earlier the *Washington Post* had published a story with the headline "People of Britain Urged to Follow Jews by Physician."[29] Dr. Allison, "prominent physician and authority on nutrition," urged Britons to follow the Jewish dietary practices. According to the article, Allison claimed that as a race, the Hebrews were "practically immune from consumption." The Jewish people, he maintained, through the centuries of oppression had survived because it was the best fed race on earth. Jewish mothers were greatly to be commended for bringing up their children on fatty foods." Already by the last quarter of the nineteenth century, Victorians such as Ernest Hart and Alexander Davidson were juxtaposing Jewish health with the squalor and disease of urban industrial spaces, and holding up the Jews' advanced notions of hygiene as a model for general society. Hart, writing in *Sanitary Record*, compared the Mosaic hygiene laws to the contemporary public health acts, and admitted that Britain lagged behind the ancient Hebrew code. The Jews were clean, industrious, sober, focused on family, and demonstrated immunity to numerous ailments, particularly to what he labeled "filth diseases": cholera, typhoid, typhus, and other infectious plagues. Jewish children, he added, "have no hereditary syphilis and scarcely any scrofula. Their greater tenacity of life is therefore due not only to better maternal care and nursing, but to the inheritance of a better physical constitution than the Christian child."[30] Even when, by the 1890s, this problem of 'filth diseases' in urban areas was being addressed, the Jews could still be celebrated in other contexts. For instance, during the Boer War, the poor performance of the British soldiers called up fears about the physical condition of recruits and national decline and degeneration. According to Robert Darby, "the Committee on Physical Deterioration (1904) was particularly interested in how Jewish parents looked after their children, and many of the witnesses confirmed that they were better nourished, stronger, and healthier than their Christian neighbors, and that Jewish parents were thriftier, more abstemious, and generally better housekeepers. In their chastity, sobriety, industriousness, cleanliness, and family feeling, the Jews had become model Victorians."[31]

Clearly, part of the attraction of the medicalization of Jewish religious texts, for both Jews and non-Jews, was the way in which contemporary political and social policies and practices could be critiqued vis-à-vis these ancient texts. Ernest Hart's criticisms of Britain's approach to urban poverty and disease are one example of this. Or take the American physician Edward T. Williams' talk on Moses as a sanitarian, delivered before the Norfolk Medical Society in 1881, and published in the *Boston Medical and Surgical Journal* the following year.[32] Among other things, Williams spoke of discharges from male and female genital organs, and the regime mandated by Moses for the treatment of someone so afflicted. The individual affected was designated "unclean," isolated from the community, and mandated to abstain from sexual relations and even touching others. Then Williams castigated contemporary policy makers:

> It is easy to see that these rules if faithfully carried out would be an efficient preventative of gonorrhoea. Yet we, in our enlightened age and country, dare not legislate on the subject of venereal disease, blindly refusing the protection of the law not only to the guilty victims of illicit pleasure, but to great numbers of innocent men, women, and children, who have to suffer and often to die for the faults of others. Leaving wholly out of view the humane aspect of the question, the mere pecuniary loss to the State from such defective legislation is incalculable.[33]

Even if the healthy Jew served only a functional purpose in such texts, the image and idea were disseminated, and constituted part of a larger discourse that could break free of its intended purpose.

Oftentimes, the Jews were represented as a barometer or bell-weather of the future. The signs, however, were usually negative. "The Jew," according to Anatole Leroy-Beaulieu, in his oft-quoted work *Israël chez les Nations*,

> is the most nervous, and, in so far, the most modern of men. He is by the very nature of his diseases the forerunner, as it were, of his contemporaries, preceding them on that perilous path upon which society is urged by the excesses of its intellectual and emotional life, and by the increasing spur of competition. The noisy army of psychopathics and neuropathics is gaining so many recruits among us that it will not take the Christians long to catch up with the Jews in this respect. Here, again, there are no ethnic forces in operation.[34]

However, in the case of celebrations of Mosaic law, Jews were represented as a possible positive model for the future. If societies plagued by tuberculosis were to adhere more closely to the laws of kosher ritual slaughter, then the death rates from the century's greatest scourge would presumably be lowered; if circumcision could be universalized as a medical practice, then all sorts of pathologies from masturbation to insanity and certain types of cancer could be prevented or cured.

In his recent study of the history of circumcision, Leonard Glick presents a number of examples of Gentile physicians who advocated that Christians follow the Jews. A. U. Williams, an Arkansas physician, wrote in 1889 in a Chicago medical journal, "I would follow in the footsteps of Moses and circumcise all male children." J. Henry C. Simes, a prominent Philadelphia urologist, argued one year later that there was no doubt about the "hygienic advantages" of circumcision, "and that the first and great teacher of hygienic medicine, Moses, certainly had this view in his mind when he gave forth the order, that all male children of Israel must be circumcised." Simes wondered why more Christians had not yet taken up this ritual, and highly recommended that they do so. A New Orleans physician recommended circumcision for Christians because, in Glick's words, "anyone familiar with the healthy state of 'the Jewish type' knew the benefits of the practice."[35]

As Glick and others have recently pointed out, by the late nineteenth century, Gentile physicians in Anglophone countries were increasingly vocal in urging circumcision as a universal practice. This was no longer understood as a religious ritual, but rather as a medical procedure believed to prevent or cure a wide array of maladies. And, remarkably, circumcision did become an almost universal practice in Great Britain, Canada, the United States, and other English-speaking countries during the twentieth century.

Why, then, did the dietary laws not take hold among non-Jews in the same way? *Kashrut*, too, as we've seen, came to be medicalized in the late nineteenth century and linked, as a preventive measure, with the most devastating disease of the time, tuberculosis. By the 1940s an antitubercular vaccine was being successfully tested, and within a short while the disease could be controlled if not cured. Very quickly, tuberculosis went from being a fatal to a manageable illness. Nonetheless, that still leaves more than half a century during which TB threatened the lives of millions of people, and *kashrut* could have been taken up and universalized in a way similar to circumcision. Yet this was not done.

The universalization of circumcision and the failure of *kashrut* in this regard is even more striking when we recall the quite different natures of the two ritual practices. While there was and is an ongoing debate about these issues within the general medical community (and now among Jews), circumcision for many was seen as painful and highly stress-inducing for the infant and for the parents and relatives who had to watch. The surgery itself came with risks such as infection and mutilation that while fairly rare, were nonetheless present. And the removal of the foreskin was permanent.

Kashrut, on the other hand, was none of these things, seemingly far more benign to imagine and carry out. Yet, non-Jews did not adopt *kashrut* in appreciable numbers, while circumcision became standard practice, at least in the English-speaking world.[36] The reason for this may lie with the divergent natures of the two practices and the different demands they place on individuals. Circumcision is a one-time thing; *kashrut* makes demands on a daily basis. As an obstetrician at Johns Hopkins once put it, "One nice thing about circumcision is that when it is done it is finished. The foreskin never grows back."[37] Circumcision is also a private, intimate matter; if it has any ongoing physical and emotional effects – one of the standard claims, reaching back centuries, is that circumcision reduces sexual pleasure and performance – this is going to affect only the individual man and his partner. *Kashrut*, on the other hand, is a public matter, affecting as it does choices of food and therefore family, friends, community. It also literally costs in terms of time and money; kosher meat must be purchased from a reliable kosher butcher, and is usually more expensive than non-kosher meat.

While most Jews over the past century have ceased to practice some or even most of the proscribed religious commandments, the vast majority still circumcise their sons. This, according to scholars, is a product of a combination of religious or communal and health imperatives (even if there is enormous debate within the medical establishment over the genuine health benefits of the practice). While overall circumcision rates have been dropping over the past decades, nonetheless Gentiles in Anglophone countries at some point did indeed follow a Jewish model, if only in the case of circumcision. Yet in other cases, and *kashrut* especially, non-Jewish health officials and physicians were strong advocates of extending this practice of following the Jews. What does this tell us, if anything, about the shifting mentality of Christians vis-à-vis Jews and Judaism?

4.

Even if *kashrut* was not taken up by large numbers of Gentiles, it is nonetheless significant that such a course was advocated, and that this occurred not at the fringes, but among some of those with access to the most important medical and popular outlets at the time. The discourse on "the healthy Jew" was a direct engagement with the interpretative tradition that had marginalized or eliminated Judaism and Jewry's role in the progress of "civilization," that is, of Europe and America. It was also an engagement with Christianity, at least implicitly, and with the theology of supercession: the principle that with the coming of Jesus, and the Jews' rejection of his messiahship, the love and grace of God had passed from the old Israel (the Jews) to the new Israel (the Church). What is worth noting here is that the body of literature with which this study deals offered up the notion, at least implicitly, that when it comes to matters of health and disease, of purity and impurity, of the life and death of individuals, nations and races, Christianity as such was at best an afterthought. This was the case whether the writer was Jewish or Christian. Once science replaced theology in framing the terms of the debate, and the Mosaic laws became not a matter first and foremost of the soul but of the body – an individual and collective body understood in terms of its materiality, not as metaphor – then the supercession of the synagogue by the church ceased to really matter. If the Mosaic and rabbinic laws were hygienic rules and regulations that worked in the past, then Jesus' career as a healer may or may not provide further evidence for the efficacy of these laws; Christ, though, can no longer matter in the same way when these laws are discussed. And, indeed, the Christian physicians and scientists we encounter here paid far less attention to their New Testament than they did to their Old, representing the former, when they did invoke it, as an appendage, in terms of a continuity of healing traditions. They might invoke "the Lord Jesus Christ" now and again, but this reads as rather formulaic; the New Testament adds nothing substantial or new with regard to health and healing to what is found in the Hebrew Bible.

Moreover, as I've attempted to show throughout this book, the Christian physicians and medical writers more often than not made no effort to distinguish in any meaningful way ancient Hebrews from contemporary

Jews, or biblical from post-biblical Judaism. That is, they did not participate in the older intellectual tradition of a Christianity-infused interpretation of Jewish history, in which the Jews and Judaism remain alive and vital until the appearance of Jesus and Christianity. The medicalized reinterpretation of Jews, Judaism, and Jewish history posited continuity between the biblical and post-biblical eras, and the interpretive tradition analyzed here framed the entirety of Jewish history in terms of health and hygiene.

7

Conclusion

I.

Where does this discourse about Jews, Judaism, health and medicine fall within the longer trajectory of modern Jewish history? Did the narratives of "the healthy Jew" that appeared in the nineteenth and early twentieth centuries signal a growing confidence among German, French, American and British Jews, or a residual unease, a continuing need to demonstrate the "natural" relationship of Judaism to a progressive modernity, to civilization, and to those societies in which Jews resided? The latter seems more likely given the explicit apologetic impulse to so much of the scholarship. But perhaps, too, we might discern some of the former, some confidence or assertiveness in the dissemination of these stories of Jewish contribution. Consider the assertion discussed in Chapter 6 about the way in which Jewish ritual could and should serve as a model for societies in general. Gentiles made such a suggestion, but so, too, did Jews. Such an assertion is an implicit critique of current practices, a suggestion that what health officials are currently doing is insufficient and even dangerous. It is also, perhaps even more impudently for many, an implicit suggestion that Christianity erred in dismissing the Mosaic laws as unnecessary or irrelevant. Taken as a whole, the literature produced by Jews and non-Jews on the nexus of Torah, Talmud, and health suggests a continuing relevance of Jewish law that runs counter to Christian and European philosophical notions of supercession, and the more prosaic dismissal of the continuing relevance of Jewish religious observance. That Christians produced narratives about the healthy Jews, and that these appeared not only in scholarly monographs but also in prestigious medical journals, newspapers, and popular forums reveals something significant about Christian and Jewish relations over the past two centuries, something that in the post-Holocaust era might too easily be overlooked. While the image of the "dirty Jew" was undoubtedly powerful and widely disseminated, it was not the only image of Jewry out there. That Jews produced such texts certainly needs to be understood within the context of Jewish apologia; but perhaps we might also see aspects of this interpretive tradition as a sign of comfort and confidence as well.

At the same time, the texts produced about "the healthy Jew," written by Jews and Christians, and published in Jewish and general forums, reveal something about the complex relationship between religion, medicine, and science in the modern world. Granted, these were not revolutionary texts that transformed disciplines or produced a shift in interpretive paradigms. Yet, many of them did appear in mainstream medical and academic journals, even if they failed to have much of an impact on the grand narrative of the history of modern medicine or science. Nonetheless, these texts do tell us something important about the story some physicians and medical researchers once told about their own profession. The place of ancient Jewish laws and rituals at times moved from periphery (or invisibility) to center; Moses, Judaism, and the Jews exerted an influence on the modern medical imagination that opened up the possibility of a reconceptualization of the history of medicine and science. This, it seems, did not occur in any significant way. However, the literature on "the healthy Jew" illuminates a negotiation between religion and science that is not one-directional, that does not comport with a simplistic notion of secularization or the irrelevance of older forms of knowledge. Thus, it offers a more complex picture both of the recent past of Jewish and Christian intellectual exchange, and of the narrative of medical historiography.

2.

In the end, did the nineteenth- and twentieth-century medical writers discussed in this book believe that Moses was indeed a sanitarian, an ancient Pasteur or Koch? Or was this a collective literary strategy whose end was social and practical rather than historiographical or theological? We have at least to be open to the very great possibility that this large group of physicians and medical writers, as well as religious figures of course, believed not only in the historical existence of Moses, but also that he understood at some level the scientific and medical principles and concepts ascribed to him. Those who contributed to this interpretive tradition certainly wrote as if they believed it. They read and interpreted the biblical narratives in a hyper-literalist way, diagnosing the illnesses and medical conditions of biblical figures such as Abraham and Sarah; translating descriptions of ancient ailments into modern terminology; historicizing the Bible even as they collapsed time and made historical difference all but vanish through the strategy of equivalence.

It would be easy, intellectually, to distance ourselves epistemologically from these physicians, rabbis, ministers, and popular writers, to believe that a chasm exists between what they were capable of believing about Jews, race, medicine and health, and what we today know and believe. And yet, many of the questions and issues raised by researchers fifty or one hundred years ago are still with us, matters of legitimate or normative and unresolved scientific inquiry. True, the notion of Moses and the ancient rabbis as forerunners of modern hygiene officials is less likely to appear in medical journals, though the remarkable knowledge of the rabbis as well as of medieval figures such as Maimonides in matters related to genetics/eugenics is still celebrated.[1] Yet, what of the health value of specific ritual practices such as *kashrut* or circumcision? If there has been no recent campaign among physicians celebrating the health benefits of a kosher diet, nonetheless the idea that "kosher" translates into healthy and pure retains its power at the popular level.[2] The debate over the health benefits of circumcision is still very much alive, among both medical authorities and the interested public. Moreover, the issue is often presented in much the same terms as it was a century ago.[3]

The boundaries between normative and peripheral, legitimate and illegitimate are oftentimes fluid. As the historian of medicine James Harvey Young remarked about the relationship between folk medicine, patent medicine, and orthodox medicine, they are all open-ended, evolving systems, "each containing at any given time some therapeutic practices centuries old and others only recently acquired, while in all three systems hitherto viable practices become obsolescent and then die out from lack of usage."[4] Without leveling the differences between various types of medical and scientific bodies of knowledge and practice to the point of silliness, it is nonetheless possible to acknowledge the contingency of medical and scientific knowledge, and to grant that an understanding of the relationship of religion and medicine, of normative to unconventional knowledge is as often cyclical as it is linear.

Certainly, there are still books being published on the topic of Judaism, health, and medicine that trace the profound engagement of Jews with health back to the Bible and then forward into the present.[5] The biblical *cohanim*, David M. Feldman has written, were "custodians of public health, wardens in charge of the social hygiene regulations that feature prominently in Leviticus and elsewhere. And if a health factor is discerned in the dietary laws and rules of sexual relations, then a large proportion of the 613 biblical commandments can be said to be hygienic *in intent.*"[6] Moses was not an epidemiologist, as many in the nineteenth century believed.[7] Nonetheless, he was deeply interested in matters of health and hygiene. Moreover, it is not merely that Moses' laws had hygienic effects; rather, *kashrut* and other laws regulating bodily purity were motivated by sanitary considerations. Even the eugenic impulse to Jewish law makes an appearance, and without declamatory remarks. Feldman's work appeared in the mid-1980s; other recent accounts of Judaism and medicine include similar claims.[8] Unsurprisingly, popular books on Judaism and health emanating from Orthodox circles celebrate the prophylactic effects of an observant life. Yet, they too sometimes feel it necessary to support their claims with reference to medical science. "Studies have established," one such guide informs its readers, "that there is a lesser incidence of heart attacks among Torah-observant Jews than there is among the general population. The *International Journal of Cardiology* explains this phenomenon: 'It is possible that the strong belief in a Supreme Being and the role of prayer may in themselves be protective.'"[9]

There continue to exist questions about certain diseases to which Jews are believed susceptible, and the role of genetics and natural selection in relation to particular "Jewish diseases" or "Jewish traits." If these questions vanished or went underground for half a century, this was for political reasons: Nazism and the Holocaust made asking questions that touched on Jewish identity and race, genetics, and predisposition to disease extremely difficult and dangerous. But this did not mean that science had arrived at any definitive answer to such questions. Consider the recent intense interest in the "discovery" of the Y-chromosome in those claiming to be *cohanim*, or descendents of the priestly caste in ancient Judea, who trace their origins back to Aaron, Moses' brother. It is unclear (at least to me) just what is gained by possession of this "truth" about one's ancestry, but the discovery has generated enormous excitement among those involved. There are, then, Jews out there searching for the genetic key to their own history and identity, even as others invoke the Jewish tradition to try to curb some of this enthusiasm for "the genetic self."[10] It does seem, at any rate, that this is one way for the notion of a "Jewish race" in some form or another to sneak back into mainstream science, more than half a century after the Holocaust. Have historians, sociologists, or anthropologists established a period of time that must pass before ideas that have become tainted or illegitimate are permitted to reappear as acceptable and valid? Is it half a century in the case of a Jewish race? Are the Jews in the United States comfortable and secure enough now that such a notion can gain some traction without the debilitating fear that it will produce another Nazi Germany?

The discovery of a genetic link between today's Cohens and the ancient *cohanim* is an example of the power of the myth of continuity, of a legitimacy and perhaps even a superiority (in relation to what, though?) that is derived from a link with thousands of years ago. It is also testimony to the continuing need for the "truth" that science alone appears to offer. The mere assertion of such a continuity in the language of faith or tradition would, of course, be less than noteworthy. But science, through DNA testing, has now established the scientific basis of the myth of the *cohanim*. So, again, is it religion or science that is elevated in this negotiation, or more likely, both? Finally, we have here a latter-day example of the sort of biblical literalism married to science that constituted one of the main modes of interpretation dealt with in this book. The entire intellectual and cultural exercise of discovering a priestly line through DNA depends on taking the biblical account of Aaron and his descendents at face value. Moreover, if, as we saw in Chapter 4 on Darwinism and eugenics, Jewish thinkers in the past sought to demonstrate a symbiosis between the contemporary scientific breakthroughs of the day and Judaism, many Jews today are seeking the same. The content of that science has, of course, changed in important ways; few Jews today would tout the racial hygienic elements in ancient Jewish law, for instance. But the impulse to identify the elective affinities between Judaism and science, including medicine, is still a powerful one.

Nor are discussions of Jewish identity and difference rooted in genetics and natural selection a thing of the past. Are Jews more intelligent than other groups, and is this advantage a product of a Darwinian process of selection? In an interview published in 1982, the Yiddish writer Isaac Bashevis Singer sought an explanation for why the Jew is an intellectual, or at least why every Jew is a potential intellectual: "Perhaps because Judaism was persecuted, sooner or later the ignorant, the anti-intellectual, had no reason to stay. They left. Who stayed with the Jews? Generation after generation of believers, scholars, and because they did not intermarry, we have a great reservoir of intelligence among the Jews."[11] Now Singer was in many ways mischievous, and he may have been playing here with his interlocutor. Yet there is just as good a chance that he meant what he was saying, picking up consciously or not an idea that, as we have seen, circulated widely earlier in the century. Jewish intelligence is the product in large part of a Darwinian-like winnowing out process of the less intelligent Jews.

This notion of a naturally selected "Jewish intelligence" has recently reappeared in scholarly debate over how to account for so-called Jewish diseases. Are the genetic diseases commonly associated with Ashkenazi Jews – Tay-Sachs, Gaucher disease, Niemann-Pick disease, and mucolipidosis Type IV – a result of random chance, genetic drift, or are they part of a selection process that conveys to Jews a "hidden advantage"? Questions about a purported "Jewish intelligence" and "Jewish diseases" (and the connections between these two phenomena) remain open questions, debated by scientists in specialized academic journals and widely reported by the press, framed as one component of a larger discussion over genetics and race.[12] For our purposes, the conclusions reached recently by three geneticists at the University of Utah are the most illuminating. In their article "Natural History of Ashkenazi Intelligence," Gregory Cochran, Jason Hardy and Henry Harpending argue that Ashkenazi Jews possess higher IQs on average, and that this translates into greater economic success (since IQs are reliable predictors of economic and social success): "Ashkenazi Jews have the highest average IQ of any ethnic group for which there are reliable data. . . . During the twentieth century, they made up about 3 percent of the U.S. population but won 27 percent of the U.S.

Nobel science prizes and 25 percent of the ACM Turing awards. They account for more than half of world chess champions."[13] This advantage in intelligence, they argue, is genetic, developed through natural selection in Europe during the Middle Ages (800–1600). This selection process for the single trait of intelligence, however, also had a deleterious effect, what the researchers call the "cost of selection": it produced the genetic diseases Tay-Sachs and Gaucher's.[14]

What were the precise mechanisms in this selection process? Cohran and his colleagues focus on the economic and social role of the middleman played by Jews in medieval Europe: In "pre-Diaspora times, the Jews did not occupy an unusual ecological niche nor did they yet exhibit unusual cognitive traits." It is only when they settle in significant enough numbers in Europe that a particular social and occupational pattern develops, one that is due to a unique set of factors: high literacy rates, strong discouragement of intermarriage, and a high level of stability in social arrangements. Prosperity and survival of the group depended on success as merchants and middlemen. "Jews who were particularly good at these jobs increased reproductive success."[15] Selection pressures led to a favouring of traits that reproduced the talents needed to survive and thrive, which in turn produced "high status and wealth." Among the causal factors of Jewish intelligence the authors also list "winnowing through persecution" – "only the smartest Jews survived persecution" – though why this should have been so, they admit, is not clear. They also raise the argument about sexual selection by the wealthy for talmudic scholars, or more likely selection for excellence and intelligence in general. (They do grant that far more historical demographic information would be needed to test this hypothesis.)

At the most abstract or broadest level, what is still functioning here is the ontological status of essential difference. This difference is maintained even in America, where levels of "assimilation" – however that is defined and whatever its effects – are said to be highest. Even here, the Jews are different; or, it must be emphasized, Ashkenazi Jews, for the authors are quick to point out that non-Ashekenazi Jews demonstrate no evidence of abnormally high IQ scores. Thus, it was the particular historical-genetic development within Central and Eastern Europe that determined both higher Jewish intelligence and greater risk for a group of hereditary disorders. Different IQ levels, different "ability distribution: great success in mathematics and literature, and more typical results in representational painting, sculpture, and architecture," different diseases, and so on. The politics of this difference, as Steven Pinker points out, are ambiguous. Certainly, as he writes, an explanation of Jewish superiority that hinges on IQ is better than one built on the theory of a worldwide conspiracy of Jewish elders. Nonetheless, the essential difference remains. So, too, the more specific references to Jewish health and disease, and to the Darwinian selection process, whose mechanisms included not only occupational patterns but also what Pinker calls "the weirdest example of sexual selection in the living world: [the idea] that for generations in the *shtetl*, the brightest yeshiva boy was betrothed to the daughter of the richest man, thereby favoring the genes, if such genes there are, for Talmudic pilpul."[16]

Pinker refers to this notion as a "folk theory." But in doing so he ignores the history of the idea itself, and he distances us from those "weird" notions that Jews and non-Jews believed about Jews in the past. In calling attention to the continuities over time in the discussions by educated elites about Jewish traits, identity, health and disease, I neither wish to validate the earlier narratives about the healthy or diseased Jew by linking them with contemporary, up-to-date scientific inquiry, nor suggest that contemporary scientific inquiry into such matters is somehow less than legitimate because we can identify such continuities. My point here is only that these questions are unresolved. What is the epistemological status of the truth-claims made about Jews and health, about Judaism and medicine?

Pinker, for instance, questions some of the hypotheses offered by the geneticists in Utah to explain Jewish intelligence, but he does not question the reality of Jewish success or its link with IQ and selection. "Jewish achievement is obvious; only the explanation is unclear," he writes. Despite the discomfort caused by such discussions and debates, "reality is what refuses to go away when you do not believe in it, and progress in neuroscience and genomics has made these politically comforting shibboleths (such as the non-existence of intelligence and the non-existence of race) untenable."[17] If these questions remain unresolved for many geneticists, then do they not remain unresolved for the rest of us as well, except at the level of myth, faith, or politics? Moreover, and this follows from the previous question, epistemologically and culturally we cannot easily distance ourselves from a not-so-distant past in which ideas such as the existence of a Jewish race, specific and identifiable Jewish diseases or immunity from diseases, and Jewish culture, religion, and history as crucial factors in the process of natural selection and the survival of the "Jewish people" were discussed and debated by physicians, scientists and educated lay people.

Jewish genetic identity over thousands of years; Jewish diseases passed on hereditarily; a Jewish advantage intellectually, passed on genetically, that explains the statistical overrepresentation of Jews in the arts and sciences – these are all images and ideas that are circulating again. Such examples offer us further evidence of the larger point: epistemologically and culturally the investment in such arguments and debates encountered in this book has not vanished. Again, what is the epistemic status of such knowledge? Did Singer believe what he was saying? On what grounds might we evaluate the beliefs and ideas of medical and religious authorities of a century or more ago when the relationship between religion, science, and medicine remains so highly contentious?

Notes

Introduction

1. James E. Reeves, "The Eminent Domain of Sanitary Science, and the Usefulness of State Boards of Health in Guarding the Public Welfare," 612.
2. Yosef Tennovim, "Review of *Torat ha-Hygienia* by Dr. A. Goldenstein," 59.
3. My purpose in this book is decidedly not to reconstruct the actual conditions of health and disease in the Bible and Talmud, or the level of medical knowledge of the rabbis or Jewish physicians in the Middle Ages. Among the many works devoted to this, see the comprehensive work of Julius Preuss, *Biblisch-talmudische Medizin; Beiträge zur Geschichte der Heilkunde und der Kultur überhaupt* (Berlin: 1911). The work was translated into English by Fred Rosner under the title *Julius Preuss' Biblical and Talmudic Medicine* (New York: Sanhedrin Press, 1978). Nor is my purpose to make sense of purity rules and rituals within their own contexts. Mary Douglas offered the seminal interpretation of biblical purity laws from an anthropological perspective. See her *Purity and Danger: An Analysis of Concepts of Pollution and Taboo*. Finally, this is not an attempt to write a comprehensive history of Jews and medicine; numerous works exist on this subject. Most recently, John Efron, *Medicine and the German Jews: A History*. See as well Nora Goldenbogen (ed.), *Hygiene und Judentum*; Nora Goldenbogen (ed.), *Medizinische Wissenschaften und Judentum*; Robin Judd, "German Jewish Rituals, Bodies, and Citizenship"; David Ruderman, *Jewish Thought and Scientific Discovery in Early Modern Europe*; Joseph Shatzmiller, *Jews, Medicine, and Medieval Society*. For a more popular and celebratory history of the subject, see Frank Heynick, *Jews and Medicine: An Epic Saga*. And the extraordinary corpus of Harry Friedenwald remains immensely valuable. See, among many works, *The Jews and Medicine: Essays*.
4. I have cited in the following chapters some works in Italian, though only those summarized in languages that I know. I do not have direct access to the Italian literature, but there is every indication that the Italian sources are far more extensive than I suggest in this study. I have not looked at literature produced in Russian or Polish, since I do not read these languages. Nor have I looked at the books and articles published in Ladino and Spanish. The extent of the

interpretive tradition I explore here could, therefore, be far more extensive than my work suggests.

5. The literature is substantial. Authoritative works include Henry Friedlander, *The Origins of Nazi Genocide: From Euthanasia to the Final Solution*; Robert Proctor, *Racial Hygiene: Medicine Under the Nazis*; Benno Müller-Hill, *Murderous Science*. See also Klaus Hödl, *Die Pathologisierung des jüdischen Körpers: Antisemitismus, Geschlecht, und Medizin im Fin de Siècle*.

6. See especially Sander Gilman, *The Jew's Body*, and *The Case of Sigmund Freud: Medicine and Identity at the Fin de Siècle*. See also John Efron, *Defenders of the Race: Jewish Doctors and Race Science in Fin de Siècle Europe*; Mitchell B. Hart, *Social Science and the Politics of Modern Jewish Identity*; Mark H. Gelber, *Melancholy Pride: Nation, Race, and Gender in the German Literature of Cultural Zionism*; Joachim Doron, "Rassenbewusstein und Naturwissenschaftliches Denken im Deutschen Zionismus während der Wilhelminischen Ära." See also, most recently, the essays devoted to Jews and race in *Jewish History* 19, 2005. Michael Stanislawski has analyzed the impact of Social Darwinian thinking on select Jewish thinkers in connection with the emerging conceptualization of Zionism in *Zionism and the Fin de Siècle: Cosmopolitanism and Nationalism from Nordau to Jabotinsky*.

7. And even those, such as Dohm, who conceived of an original Mosaic religion that had degenerated, did not associate the law with that original spiritual purity. My argument throughout this book is that in contrast to Enlightenment thinkers and then nineteenth-century, mainly Protestant, biblical critics, who saw Judaism as degenerate precisely because of its legalism, nineteenth- and twentieth-century Christian and Jewish medical authorities sought to recover this very legalism and reinterpret it as the source of vitality and health. On Dohm's view, see James Pasto, "Islam's 'Strange Secret Sharer': Orientalism, Judaism, and the Jewish Question."

8. Jan Assmann, *Moses the Egyptian: The Memory of Egypt in Western Monotheism*, 7–9.

9. Adam Sutcliffe, *Judaism and Enlightenment*. See also Arthur Herztberg, *The French Enlightenment and the Jews*.

10. I take the phrase from Sutcliffe, *Judaism and Enlightenment*, 211 and passim.

11. See Sutcliffe's discussion, ibid.,191f.

12. Efron, *Medicine and the German Jews*, 65.

13. John Murray Cuddihy, *The Ordeal of Civility: Freud, Marx, Levi-Strauss, and the Jewish Struggle with Modernity*. For recent discussions of the history of the idea of civilization and its import, see Jean Starobinski, "The Word *Civilization*"; Bruce Mazlish, *Civilization and Its Contents*.

14. Medical texts written in Hebrew are *sui generis*, intended for an elite yet highly circumscribed audience, Jews educated in and still engaged with Hebrew-speaking Jewish culture.

15. On this see Derek Penslar, *Shylock's Children: Economics and Jewish Identity in Modern Europe*; Hart, *Social Science*, especially chapter 7.

16. J. Hoberman, *Bridge of Light: Yiddish Film Between Two Worlds*, 68.

17. At times, in reaction against philhellenism, Egypt and the Orient also functioned in this way. See Suzanne Marchand, "Philhellinism and the *Furor Orientalis*."

18. Sven Lindquist, *"Exterminate All the Brutes": A Modern Odyssey into the Heart of Darkness.*

19. This is, by no means, an argument that has disappeared. In his 2005 book on the history of the Jews in Eastern Europe, the Austrian-born British writer Paul Kriwaczek notes that although it is now largely forgotten, the Yiddish-speaking Jews were "one of Europe's nations.... What is more, their contribution to central and eastern Europe's economic, social and intellectual development was utterly disproportionate to their numbers. The Yiddish people [i.e., the Jews] must be counted among the founder nations of Europe. (Please take note Ireland, Spain, Italy and Poland, who have pressed for 'the Christian roots of the continent' to be proclaimed in the constitution of the European Union)." Paul Kriwaczek, *Yiddish Civilization: The Rise and Fall of a Forgotten Nation,* 3.

20. Persecution, in the form of marginality, is also at the heart of the explanation of the overrepresentation in the twentieth century of the Jews in the sciences, including medicine. See Shulamit Volkov's influential article, "Juden als wissenschaftliche 'Mandarine' im Kaiserreich und in der Weimarer Republik; neue Überlegungen zu sozialen Ursachen des Erfolgs jüdischer Naturwissenschaftler."

21. Gil Anidjar, *Semites: Race, Religion, Literature.*

22. On the notion of the "ancient Jewish commonwealth" and its role in early modern debates over republicanism, and the place of the Jews in European society, see Lea Campos Boraleva, "Classical Foundational Myths of European Republicanism: The Jewish Commonwealth"; Kalman Neuman, "Political Hebraism and the Early Modern 'Respublica Hebraeorum': On Defining the Field."

23. I take the phrase from Ivan Davidson Kalmar and Derek J. Penslar, "Orientalism and the Jews: An Introduction," xviii.

24. Ibid., xxviii.

25. Thus, to offer just one example, in a summary of the 1889 International Congress of Dermatology and Syphilography, held in Paris in connection with the Universal International Exposition, the *Medical News* could report enthusiastically on papers delivered covering a myriad of syphilis-related maladies: "syphilis of the nose to syphilis of the vagina; from syphilis of the child to the same disease in the aged, including both Turk, Jew, and infidel. There were a number of important papers on lepra, lupus, sarcoma, epithelioma, and tuberculosis." Lanterne, "Correspondence." The "Turk, Jew, and infidel" was an old clichéd phrase, but it could still easily be invoked in conjunction with the most dreaded illnesses of the late nineteenth century, and used to unite Jews and Muslims as different and diseased. On the identity of Jews and Arabs in the European imagination see Gil Anidjar, *The Jew, the Arab: A History of the Enemy.*

26. Edward Said writes about the "process of conversion" as central to the Orientalist project, as crucial to the nexus of discourse and power: "Yet the Orientalist makes it his work to be always converting the Orient from something into something else; he does this for himself, for the sake of his culture, in some cases for what he believes is the sake of the Oriental." The strategy of translation that I explore in this book can be understood as one instance of this wider process of

conversion, though of course crucial differences or developments emerge when the subject and object of discourse (in this case, the Jew) begin to merge; fundamental issues of discourse and power, "us" and "them," need to be addressed in a different way. Edward Said, *Orientalism*, 67.

27. The relationship between science and religion I explore in this book is different from the issue of the causal connection between the values of Christianity and the rise of modern science. I am not arguing that the debate about Judaism and health was some sort of parallel to the debate over Puritanism and its role in the emergence of modern science in seventeenth-century England; I have not encountered anyone who sought to connect Judaism to modern science in a causal way. On the debate over Christianity and science see the introductory essay by David Lindberg and Ronald Numbers in Lindberg and Numbers (eds.), *God and Nature: Historical Essays on the Encounter Between Christianity and Science*.

28. John Hedley Brooke, *Science and Religion: Some Historical Perspectives*, 5. See also Edward B. Davis, "Fundamentalism and Folk Science Between the Wars"; Lindberg and Numbers (eds.), *God and Nature*, especially the introduction; David C. Lindberg and Ronald L. Numbers, "Beyond War and Peace: A Reappraisal of the Encounter Between Christianity and Science"; and Christine Rosen, *Preaching Eugenics: Religious Leaders and the American Eugenics Movement*, 8–9 and passim.

29. This is less true for scholarship on the premodern period. And Christine Rosen, in *Preaching Eugenics*, does include a chapter on American rabbis and eugenics.

30. Ludmilla Jordanova, *Sexual Visions: Images of Gender in Science and Medicine Between the Eighteenth and Twentieth Centuries*, 74.

31. For an extended and highly suggestive analysis of the categories "religion" and "secularization," and the role such categorical distinctions have played in European (Christian) politics and culture over the past two centuries, see Anidjar, *Semites*.

32. Nancy Tomes, *The Gospel of Germs: Men, Women, and the Microbe in American Life*.

33. Aleida Assmann, "Translation as Transformation," 21.

34. On this counter-history of Moses and the Exodus story, see Amos Funkenstein, *Perceptions of Jewish History*, 36–40.

35. For other images of Moses during this period see Richard I. Cohen, "Urban Visibility and Biblical Visions: Jewish Culture in Western and Central Europe in the Modern Age."

36. Charles Weiss, "Medicine in the Bible," 286–9; emphasis in the original.

37. Israel Zangwill, "The Jewish Race," 274.

38. I am of course hardly the first to come to this conclusion. On the relationship between texts and contexts see Dominick LaCapra, *Rethinking Intellectual History: Texts, Contexts, Language*, 116f. David Biale has also made the point recently in the preface to his *Cultures of the Jews*, xxvi.

39. For a recent challenge to this interpretive tradition, however, see Jeffrey Herf, *The Jewish Enemy: Nazi Propaganda During World War II and the Holocaust*.

40. Alan Levenson, *Between Philosemitism and Antisemitism: Defenses of Jews and Judaism in Germany, 1871–1932*, xii.

41. Caroline Bynum, "Why All the Fuss About the Body? A Medievalist's Perspective."
42. Howard Eilberg-Schwartz, "Introduction: People of the Body"; Daniel Boyarin, "Tricksters, Martyrs, and Collaborators: Diaspora and the Gendered Politics of Resistance"; Daniel Boyarin, *Unheroic Conduct: The Rise of Heterosexuality and the Invention of the Jewish Man*; Daniel Boyarin, *Carnal Israel: Reading Sex in Talmudic Culture.* For the deep tensions in Boyarin's early work, see Naomi Seidman, "Carnal Knowledge: Sex and the Body in Jewish Studies," 130f.
43. Sander Gilman, *Franz Kafka, the Jewish Patient*, 21.
44. For only one example of the influence of Gilman's notion of the Jewish body and a restatement of the argument, see Paul Root Wolpe, "Bioethics, the Genome, and the Jewish Body."
45. Seidman, "Carnal Knowledge," 118–19. On the impact of body studies on Jewish studies, see in addition Charlotte Fonrobert, "On Carnal Israel and the Consequences: Talmudic Studies since Foucault."
46. Gilman, *The Jew's Body*, 38. As David Luft remarked, "One could only wonder what this could mean or how one could test it empirically." David Luft, review of *The Jew's Body*, 573.
47. Gilman, *The Jew's Body*, 59.
48. Ibid., 60.
49. Gilman, *Franz Kafka*, 12.
50. Laura Engelstein, in her review of *The Jew's Body*, asked "What has led him to select just those sources on which he relies and not others?" (759).
51. Naomi Seidman has noted the irony in this recent turn to the body in Jewish Studies in terms of apologia. The earlier spiritualization of Judaism has been repudiated as apologetic; yet, is the re-embodiment of the Jews, she asks, not also apologetic, aimed at a largely Christian audience that now embraces sex and the body?
52. For insightful discussions of these larger issues see Kenneth Gergen, *The Saturated Self: Dilemmas of Identity in Contemporary Life*; Paul Root Wolpe, "If I Am Only My Genes, What Am I? Genetic Essentialism and a Jewish Response."
53. For other such strategies, and in particular those taken up by theologians, see Richard Cohen, "Urban Visibility and Biblical Visions." While I touch on the intersections between the medicalized hermeneutics of Jewish texts and developments within the world of theology and biblical criticism, a full treatment of the latter is beyond the scope of this book.

1. "'Tis a Little People, But It Has Done Great Things"

1. For an introduction to the historiography on Jews and medicine, and its relation to modern Jewish historiography in general, see Robert Jütte, "Die jüdische Medizingeschichtsschreibung im 19. Jahrhundert und die Wissenschaft des Judentums."
2. Moritz Steinschneider, "Schriften über Medicin in Bibel und Talmud und über jüdische Aerzte."

3. Ibid., 434. Steinschneider was not the only Jewish authority at the time to reject this mode of interpretation. In his work on Jewish racial traits, the Anglo-Jewish scholar Joseph Jacobs rejected the notion that the rabbis were the "anticipators of Koch and Pasteur" and the argument that Jewish religious laws were efficacious in preventing disease. See Jacobs, "On the Racial Characteristics of Modern Jews," *Studies in Jewish Statistics*, footnote 1, viii. Years later, the Russian Jewish anthropologist Samuel Weissenberg rejected this sort of ahistorical interpretation in terms similar to Steinschneider's. "We might believe that Moses saw God; but he did not see trichinae." Weissenberg argued that the real reasons for the commandments were still unclear; nonetheless, their positive effects on the Jews biologically had to be acknowledged. See Samuel Weissenberg, "Zur Sozialbiologie und Sozialhygiene der Juden," 409. On Jacobs and Weissenberg in general, see John Efron, *Defenders of the Race: Jewish Doctors and Race Science in Fin-de-Siècle Europe*.

4. Hans Golsar (ed.), *Hygiene und Judentum: Eine Sammelschrift*, 7.

5. Ernest Renan, *Etudes d'histoire religieuse*, 88, quoted in Gil Anidjar, *Semites: Race, Religion, Literature*. On Renan and the context of his ideas of race, see Michael Marrus, *The Politics of Assimilation: The French Jewish Community at the Time of the Dreyfus Affair*, 10–27.

6. Joseph Jacobs, *Jewish Contributions to Civilization: An Estimate*, 18.

7. Ibid., 41.

8. Ibid., 42.

9. Ibid., 153.

10. Ibid., 202.

11. For examples of this "minority" response to dominant narratives, see the essays collected in Sandra Harding (ed.), *The 'Racial' Economy of Science*.

12. For a comparative analysis of this type of literature, and the difficulties posed to its conceptualization and production, see Sander Gilman and Nancy Leys Stepan, "Appropriating the Idioms of Science: The Rejection of Scientific Racism."

13. Yaakov Shavit, *Athens in Jerusalem: Classical Antiquity and Hellenism in the Making of the Modern Jew*, 65.

14. Ibid., 70.

15. Ibid., 71. Aristotle's conversion appears in footnote 50.

16. Marc Brochard, *L'Hygiène Publique chez les Juifs, son importance, et sa signification dans l'histoire générale de la civilisation*, quoting from 7.

17. On modern Jewry and the question of "civilization" see John Murray Cuddihy, *The Ordeal of Civility: Freud, Marx, Levi-Strauss, and the Jewish Struggle with Modernity*; Jean Starobinski, "The Word *Civilization*"; Bruce Mazlish, *Civilization and Its Contents*.

18. Suzanne Marchand, *Down From Olympus: Archaeology and Philhellenism in Germany 1750–1970*; Frank M. Turner, *The Greek Heritage in Victorian Britain*; Frank M. Turner, "Why the Greeks and Not the Romans in Victorian Britain." On the United States see Carl Diehl, *Americans and German Scholarship, 1770–1870*.

19. Turner, *The Greek Heritage in Victorian Britain*, 8–9.

20. Ibid., 1.
21. Marchand, *Down From Olympus*, 20–1. According to Marchand (21, note 62), "In his university lectures, Wolf frequently depreciated the Jews as 'the nation that the Greeks described as having invented nothing at all.'"
22. Turner, *The Greek Heritage*, 169. On Victorian Britain see as well Gregory Claeys, "The 'Survival of the Fittest' and the Origins of Social Darwinism," especially p. 238f., and the literature cited therein. Claeys notes the "racial polarity between so-called Anglo-Saxons, Britons, Greeks, and Romans supposedly derived from a common Aryan ancestry" and non-"White" or Anglo races that took hold in the 1880s.
23. Suzanne Marchand, "Philhellenism and the *Furor Orientalis*," quoting from 335. George Mosse, in his history of racism in Europe, demonstrated the crucial role of aesthetics, and in particular the ideal of classical Greek beauty, in the making of modern racism. Mosse, *Toward the Final Solution: A History of European Racism.*
24. See Edgar Feuchtwanger, "'Jew Feelings' and Realpolitik: Disraeli and the Making of Foreign and Imperial Policy"; Anthony S. Wohl, "'Dizzi-Ben-Dizzi': Disraeli as Alien"; David Feldman, *Englishmen and Jews: Social Relations and Political Culture, 1840–1914*, ch. 4.
25. In Emmanuel Eze (ed.), *Race and the Enlightenment: A Reader*, 106.
26. Martin Bernal, *Black Athena: The Afroasiatic Roots of Classical Civilization*, 33. Bernal's work on the relationship between ancient Egypt and Greece, and his bid to replace what he believes to be the racist and hyper-nationalist "Aryan" model of scholarship with a revised "Ancient model" have certainly produced controversy. Whatever one thinks of Bernal's arguments about the reality of the ancient world, the first volume of *Black Athena* is without doubt the most exhaustive recent treatment of the politics of scholarship about Egypt, Greece, and the question of the origins and development of Western civilization. However, Suzanne Marchand, in *Down From Olympus*, does offer a brilliant and extensive analysis of philhellenism in Germany, and in the process a corrective to Bernal. As she insists in a number of places, the German engagement with the ancient world was the product of a host of forces, only one of which was the development of racism.
27. Bernal, *Black Athena*, 118 and passim.
28. See Mary Lefkowitz and Guy Maclean Rogers (eds), *Black Athena Revisited*.
29. Quoted in Alan Levenson, *Between Philosemitism and Antisemitism: Defenses of Jews and Judaism in Germany, 1871–1932*, 72–3.
30. L. Wallerstein, "Behind the Pioneer Role of Jews in Medicine: The Traditional 'Jewish Doctor' Explained," quoting from 249. The argument remains integral to narratives about Jews and medicine. See, for instance, David M. Feldman, *Health and Medicine in the Jewish Tradition*, ch. 5, in which the role of the Jews as "translators and transmitters of Greek medicine to Europe" is stressed.
31. Jacobs, *Jewish Contributions to Civilization*, 142. Jacobs distinguished between at least two types of translation activities: terminal and junctures. A translation into Hebrew was terminal, since it did not then easily pass into the larger European culture. Juncture, taken from railroad terminology, signifies the

translation from the Latin, since this would allow many "trains" to pass in different directions. This sort of translation facilitiated multiple movements and new avenues.

32. Max Neuburger, "Jewish Physicians at the Beginning of Modern Times," 145. On Neuburger, see Solomon Kagan, "Professor Max Neuburger: A Biography and Bibliography." Neuburger was born in Vienna in 1868, the child of German Jewish parents from Munich and Hamburg.

33. Isak Munz, *Die jüdischen Aerzte im Mittelalter*, 3.

34. Ibid., 107.

35. Wallerstein, "Behind the Pioneer Role of Jews in Medicine," 249.

36. Max Thorek, "The Jew in Medicine."

37. Neuburger's article on Jewish physicians was translated and published in a shortlived American Jewish journal, *Medical Leaves*. The editors sent out a letter that accompanied complimentary issues of the first volume of the journal in 1937. It informed those who received it that the journal's publication was tied directly to what was going on in Europe. "Can we, the 15,000 Jewish Physicians of America thus remain aloof during this hour of destiny in the life of our people? Is it not our imperative duty to rally our moral and economic support to those who are fighting heroically so that we may survive?" Letter, found in volume 1, 1937 of *Medical Leaves*, in the Jewish American Historical Society Archives, Center for Jewish History, New York City.

38. J. K. Walker, "On the State of the Medical Art Among the Jews, as Recorded in the Bible," quoting from 169.

39. Ibid., 173.

40. Brochard, *L'hygiène publique chez les Juifs*, 18.

41. Lawrence Irwell, "Talmudic and Jewish Medicine," 471.

42. Irwell provided no source for this quotation.

43. Irwell, "Talmudic and Jewish Medicine," 474.

44. Ibid., 474. Irwell incorrectly listed the publication date as 1802. On Cabanis see Georges Canguilhem, "P. J. G. Cabanis."

45. Max Danzis, "The Jew in Medicine from Biblical to Modern Times." The article originated as a public lecture, given at the Men's Club of Temple B'nei Abraham in Newark, New Jersey. References here are to the reprinted version by the American Jewish Historical Society. Danzis was born in Russia in 1874, and came to the United States in 1889. He graduated from the University and Bellevue Hospital Medical College in 1899. On his biography, see Solomon Kagan, *Jewish Contributions to Medicine in America*, 391.

46. Danzis, "The Jew in Medicine from Biblical to Modern Times," 5–8.

47. Heinrich Haeser, *Lehrbuch der Geschichte der Medicin und der epidemischen Krankheiten*, 59. Haeser's work went through a number of editions. It appeared first in 1845 under the title *Lehrbuch der Geschichte der Medicin und der Volkskrankheiten*; it then appeared as a revised work under the title *Lehrbuch der Geschichte der Medicin und der epidemischen Krankheiten* (1853–65), and in a second edition between 1875 and 1882.

48. Alfred Nossig, *Die Sozialhygiene der Juden und des altorientalischen Volkerkreises*, 66.

49. Ibid., 67.

50. Haeser, *Lehrbuch*, 60.
51. Ibid., 60–1.
52. These were David Carcassone, *Essai historique sur la médecine des Hebreux anciens et modernes*; Isidore Breug, Diss. De medicis illustribus Judaeorum qui inter Arabes vixerunt; Eliakim Carmoly, *Histoire des médecins juifs, anciens et modernes*. Haeser did remark that Carmoly's work was "unreliable": *Lehrbuch*, 548.
53. Haeser, *Lehrbuch*, 551.
54. Hasdai ibn Shaprut serves as an example of the "elevated place and influence occupied by Jews in the transplantation of Oriental knowledge to Spain...." Haeser, *Lehrbuch*, 551–2.
55. Ibid., 554.
56. Ibid., 554.
57. Quoted in Percival Wood, *Moses: The Founder of Preventive Medicine*, 18.
58. Ibid., 18–19.
59. Rudolf Virchow "Morgagni and Anatomical Thought," quoted in Arturo Castiglione, "The Contribution of the Jews to Medicine," 194. In a postscript at the end of the essay, Harry Savitz (M.D.) identifies Castiglione as an Italian Jew, professor of medical history at Padua and then at Yale. Castiglione died in 1953.
60. Castiglione, "The Contribution of the Jews to Medicine," 195; Moritz Steinschneider, *Die hebräischen Übersetzungen des Mittelalters und die Juden als Dolmetscher*.
61. Heinrich Rosin, *Die Juden in der Medizin*, 2.
62. Ibid., 3.
63. Jules Askenasi, *Contribution des Juifs á la Fondation des Écoles de Médecine en France au Moyen-Age*, 8.
64. Ibid., 11–12.
65. Charles Singer, quoted in Wallerstein, "Behind the Pioneer Role of Jews in Medicine," 250. Singer's essay was part of a collection of essays about Jews and civilization, written by eminent Jewish and Gentile Britons, and published under the title *The Legacy of Israel* (Oxford: Clarendon Press, 1927).
66. Yehuda Katznelson, *Ha-Talmud ve-Chochmat ha-Refuah*, 7–8, emphasis in original. Katznelson emphasized "most of their pronouncements" because he wanted to make clear that "most, but not all" rabbinic pronouncements were in agreement with what modern science has discovered. There are clearly places, he wrote, where the Talmud's take on pathology fails to comport with modern research (8).
67. The literature on these general developments is of course extensive. For general introductions to developing notions of hygiene, see George Rosen, *A History of Public Health*; Dorothy Porter, *Health, Civilization, and the State: A History of Public Health from Ancient to Modern Times*, especially her chapter on Victorian Britain; Judith Leavitt and Ronald Numbers, "Sickness and Health: An Overview"; Suellen Hoy, *Chasing Dirt: The American Pursuit of Cleanliness*; Paul Weindling, *Health, Race and German Politics Between National Unification and Nazism, 1870–1945*.
68. Thurman B. Rice, *Racial Hygiene: A Practical Discussion of Eugenics and Race Culture*, 14.

69. C. H. von Klein, *Jewish Hygiene and Diet, the Talmud and Various Other Jewish Writings Heretofore Untranslated*, 20–1. Reprinted from the *Journal of the American Medical Association* (1884). Von Klein's New York Times obituary (Dec. 13, 1913) identified him as a widely known authority on "the medical lore of the ancients." In 1883–1884, von Klein lived in Hamilton, Ohio, where he maintained his office as a practicing physician. My thanks to the Butler County Historical Society for this biographical information.

70. Ibid., 8–9.

71. The work was published originally as a long article in Westermann's *Jahrbuch der Illustrierten Deutschen Monatshefte* 41 (1876–1877), and then reprinted numerous times as a short monograph. It was quickly translated into French, Hebrew, Russian, and Italian, and appeared in English as *The Importance of the Jews for the Preservation and Revival of Learning during the Middle Ages*, published in the United States in 1883 and Great Britain in 1911.

72. Schleiden, *The Importance of the Jews*, 42–3.

73. Ibid., 47.

74. Ulrich Charpa, "Matthias Jakob Schleiden (1804–1881): The History of Jewish Interest in Science and the Methodology of Microscopic Biology." Schleiden, as Charpa notes, is best known as one of the pioneers in general cell theory.

75. Ibid., 221–2.

76. Ibid., 222.

77. Ibid., 230. Nor was Schleiden alone in this belief. Schleiden's teacher, Jacob Friedrich Fries, who was himself antagonistic to Jews, produced other students who shared Schleiden's idea: the botanist Heinrich Friedrich Link and the physicist Heinrich Wilhelm Dove. See 231, footnote 49.

78. Ibid., 238–9.

79. Ibid., 229.

80. Hermann Gollancz, "Preface," 5.

81. Maurice Kleimenhagen, "Introduction," 7. In his brief introduction to the Hebrew translation (*Mifalot ha-Yehudim: Le'kiyum ha-Chochmat ve-ha-Madayim b'Yamay ha-Baynayim ve-Harchbatam*), Arieh Gordon also made explicit reference to Schleiden as a "Christian believer," and contrasted his wisdom and courage in giving "honor to Israel" to the wickedness of the anti-Semites and those who supported them. The French edition, translated and published under the auspices of the Alliance Israélite Universelle, did not contain an introduction.

82. Schleiden, *The Importance of the Jews*, 53–4.

83. Ibid., 55.

84. Ibid., 56.

2. Moses the Microbiologist

1. *Die Sozialhygiene der Juden und des altorientalischen Völkerkreises (SJaV)*. This was a *"Separat-Abdruck"* of a somewhat longer work, *Einführung in das Studium der Sozialen Hygiene* (Stuttgart: Deutsche Verlags-Anstalt, 1894), which Nossig published in the same year.

2. See "Alfred Nossig," Walther Killy and Rudolf Vierhaus (eds), *Dictionary of German Biography*, vol. 7, 468.

3. Nossig, "Einleitung," in *SJaV*, 1–4.

4. Throughout the work, Nossig used the terms *Volk. Stamm.* and *Rasse* interchangeably. The term *Rasse* was widely used by both Jews and non-Jews to describe the Jews into the twentieth century; in some, but not all, cases it indicated a belief in biological differences between Jews and others. But the term "Jewish Race" also often appeared in the writings of those who clearly understood the Jews as a product of historical and cultural, rather than biological, forces.

5. A similar definition was offered thirty years earlier by Marc Borchard in his work on the significance of hygiene for the Jews. See Borchard, *L'Hygiène Publique chez les Juifs, son importance, et sa signification dans l'histoire générale de la civilisation*, 5–6. And see as well the definition of social hygiene and "the hygiene of the Jews" by O. Neustätter, in his introduction to Max Grunwald (ed.), *Die Hygiene der Juden*, v–vi. For the definition of social hygiene within the context of a discussion of ancient and contemporary Jewry, see Samuel Weissenberg, "Zur Sozialbiologie und Sozialhygiene der Juden."

6. Nossig, *SJaV*, 3. Nossig intended to expand the definition of social hygiene to include all aspects of communal, as well as much of individual, life. On his contribution to the redefinition of social hygiene in Germany, see Rudolf Thissen, "Die Sozialhygiene als selbstständige Wissenschaft und ihre Terminologie."

7. Nossig, *SJaV*, 1.

8. Ibid., 24, 25, 28, 37.

9. On the political and socioeconomic contexts of public health in the nineteenth century and the professionalization of medicine, see George Rosen, *A History of Public Health*, chs 6 and 7; Roy Porter, *The Greatest Benefit to Mankind: A Medical History of Humanity*, chs 11–13 and 20. On Germany, see also Paul Weindling, *Health, Race and German Politics Between National Unification and Nazism, 1870–1945*; Donald Light, Stephen Liebfried, and Florian Tennstedt, "Social Medicine vs. Professional Dominance: The German Experience"; Alfons Labisch, "Doctors, Workers, and the Scientific Cosmology of the Industrial World: The Social Construction of 'Health' and the 'Homo Hygienicus'"; Michael Kater, "Professionalization and Socialization of Physicians in Wilhelmine and Weimar Germany"; Ute Frevert, "Professional Medicine and the Working Classes in Imperial Germany"; and Claudia Huerkamp, "The Making of the Modern Medical Profession, 1800–1914: Prussian Doctors in the Nineteenth Century."

10. See Nossig, *SJaV*, 67–68, 93.

11. On Nossig and Zionism see Shmuel Almog, "Alfred Nossig: A Reappraisal"; Ezra Mendelsohn, "From Assimilation to Zionism in Lvov: The Case of Alfred Nossig"; and N. M. Gelber, *Toldot Ha-Tenuah Ha-Tzionit Be-Galizia 1875–1918*, vol. 1, 84–7.

12. Mitchell Hart, "Moses the Microbiologist: Judaism and Social Hygiene in the Work of Alfred Nossig."

13. Nossig, *SJaV*, 67–8.

14. Ibid., 52.

15. See Ismar Schorsch, *From Text to Context: The Turn to History in Modern Judaism*; David Sorkin, *The Transformation of German Jewry, 1780–1840*; Michael Meyer, *The Origins of the Modern Jew*.
16. Nossig, *SJaV*, 1–4. Nossig subsequently equates social hygiene with morality and attributes this insight to Moses. Mosaic law addresses itself to the very principle of the interconnection between moral and physical health. Moses understood that "just as the soul and body are one in Man, so too morality is hygiene and hygiene is morality.... So he could promise health, long-life, and many descendants to those who followed the law, and he would declare that the sins of the father are passed on to the fourth generation, and this also in a physical sense" (34).
17. On the importance of social hygiene culturally and politically in Germany at this time see Michael Hau, *The Cult of Health and Beauty in Germany: A Social History, 1890–1930*.
18. Nossig, *SJaV*, 35, 70–3.
19. Ibid., 94–5, 96, 112.
20. Ibid., 56, 59, 82–3.
21. Ibid., 57–8.
22. Ibid., 139–40. On the image of the Jew as unfit for military service, and the political implications of this, see Sander Gilman, *The Jew's Body*, particularly Ch. 2, "The Jewish Foot."
23. Nossig, *SJaV*, 45.
24. John M. G. Barclay, "Manipulating Moses: Exodus 2.10–15 in Egyptian Judaism and the New Testament," 32. Artapanus's insertion of Moses into the center of Egyptian history must of course be understood within the context of Ptolemaic Jewish apologetics and politics. According to Barclay, Artapanus was clearly responding to the denigration of Moses and the Jews found in Manetho and elsewhere, but he was also, as a proud assimilated Egyptian Jew, celebrating the syncretism or integration of Jewish and Egyptian culture. "Artapanus has managed to use Exodus 2.10–15 to produce a faultless Moses, as fully integrated into Egyptian life and culture as Artapanus himself." Barclay, 34.
25. Barclay, "Manipulating Moses," 35–6.
26. Ton Hilhorst, "'And Moses Was Instructed in all the Wisdom of the Egyptians' (Acts 7:22)."
27. On this, see Barclay, "Manipulating Moses"; M. Dibelius, *Studies in the Acts of the Apostles*; John. J. Kilgallen, *Stephen Speech: A Literary and Redactional Study of Acts 7*; J. C. O'Neill, *The Theology of Acts in its Historical Setting*.
28. John G. Gager, "Moses the Magician: Hero of an Ancient Counter-Culture?" See also John G. Gager, *Moses in Graeco-Roman Paganism*.
29. Philo does write at one point that Moses' words of consolation to the Hebrew slaves were "like a good physician, he [Moses] thought to relieve the sickness of their plight, terrible as it was" (*Life of Moses*, Book I, 42). But this, of course, is hardly making Moses into a physician.
30. Hilhorst, "'And Moses Was Instructed in all the Wisdom of the Egyptians'", 158. See also Rob Kugler, "Hearing the Story of Moses in Ptolemaic Egypt: Artapanus Accommodates the Tradition."

31. Jan Assman, *Moses the Egyptian: The Memory of Egypt in Western Mono-theism*, 33–6. For Funkenstein's notion of counter-history, which Assman rejects, see his *Perceptions of Jewish History*, 36f.

32. Jan Assman, *Moses the Egyptian*, 34–6.

33. L. Wallerstein, "Behind the Pioneer Role of Jews in Medicine: The Traditional 'Jewish Doctor' Explained," 246.

34. Arnold J. Band, "The Moses Complex in Modern Jewish Literature," 306.

35. In each case, Band argues, we can see not only a particular version of Moses, but also an individual who believed himself to be the latter-day incarnation of Moses.

36. Nossig, *SJaV*, 35.

37. Ibid., 35–6.

38. Ibid., 39–40.

39. Ibid., 46–7.

40. Ibid., 84. Nossig's remarks here were part of a larger debate in Germany and elsewhere over *shechitah*. Jewish ritual slaughter had long been linked in popular and scholarly forums with ritual murder. In the nineteenth century *shechitah* was attacked not only by anti-Semites, but also now by animal rights activists, anti-vivesectionists and others who claimed that it violated universal norms of humaneness. Defenders of *shechitah* made the claim that it was the most humane way to slaughter animals. As we shall see in Chapter 5, *shechitah* was also defended as a means of preventing tuberculosis. On the debates over *shechitah* see Robin Judd, "Jewish Political Behavior and the 'Schächtfrage', 1880–1914"; Robin Judd, "The Politics of Beef: Animal Advocacy and the Kosher Butchering Debates in Germany"; John Efron, *Medicine and the German Jews: A History*, Ch. 6.

41. Nossig, *SJaV*, 85–7.

42. Ibid., 86. Nossig then quotes Anatole Leroy-Beaulieu, whose work, *Israël chez les nations* (Paris: Calmann Lévy, third edition, 1893), played a significant role in nineteenth- and early twentieth-century Jewish apologetics. Leroy-Beaulieu also pointed to the advanced state of Jewish medical knowledge and suggested that Christians follow talmudic slaughtering practices in order to lessen illness (Nossig, *SJaV*, 86–7).

43. See, among the many accounts of nineteenth-century discoveries, John Waller, *The Discovery of the Germ*; Roy Porter, *The Greatest Benefit to Mankind*, ch. 14; Weindling, *Health, Race, and German Politics*, 159; and Bruno Latour, *The Pasteurization of France*, ch. 1.

44. Weindling stresses this connection between bacteriology and state support and interests, arguing that the institutionalization of bacteriological research and practice marked a decisive turn away from the liberal social medicine of Rudolf Virchow and Max von Pettenkoffer toward a science with clear authoritarian overtones.

45. Weindling, *Health, Race, and German Politics*, 170. Elsewhere in his book, Weindling makes the same point about the general reaction to germ theory: "The spectacular advances in bacteriology during the 1880s and 90s greatly enhanced the public prestige of laboratory science. There was widespread adulation of

Koch: Thousands of handkerchiefs on which his face was embroidered were sold" (167).

46. Alex Bein, "Der jüdische Parasit: Bemerkungen zur Semantik der Judenfrage," 127. Bein makes clear the continuity between the appropriation of natural scientific ideas and methods by the social or human sciences and the biologization of the discourse on Jews and Judaism. See also James M. Glass, "Against the Indifference Hypothesis: The Holocaust and the Enthusiasts for Murder."

47. Studies on racial hygiene have stressed that conceptualizing social and political issues in biological and medical terms was in no way limited to the extreme Right. Social Darwinism, eugenics, and social biology were equally popular and legitimate as scientific disciplines and as tools of social reform among socialists, feminists, and liberals, as well as conservatives. See Gregory Claeys, "The 'Survival of the Fittest' and the Origins of Social Darwinism"; Robert Proctor, *Racial Hygiene: Medicine Under the Nazis*; Weindling, *Health, Race, and German Politics*, 6–7; and Sheila Faith-Weiss, "The Race Hygiene Movement in Germany."

48. Cited in Bein, "Die jüdische Parasit," 128–9.

49. Bein, "Die jüdische Parasit," 129, 131.

50. See Ismar Schorsch, *Jewish Reactions to German Antisemitism, 1870–1914*, 103–16; Hillel Kieval, "Representation and Knowledge in Medieval and Modern Accounts of Jewish Ritual Murder."

51. Hermann Strack, *Das Blut im Glauben und Aberglauben der Menschheit* (München: Beck, 1900). Published in English as *The Jew and Human Sacrifice: Human Blood and Jewish Ritual*. On Strack and his research on Judaism in general, see Ralf Golling and Peter von der Osten-Sacken (eds), *Hermann L. Strack und das Institutum Judaicum in Berlin*. Golling discusses Strack's *The Jew and Human Sacrifice* within the context of contemporary theological and political debates on pages 39–50. On Strack more generally, as a German Christian scholar of the Talmud and as a philosemite (with an admittedly ambivalent relationship to Judaism), see Christian Wiese, *Challenging Colonial Discourse: Jewish Studies and Protestant Theology in Wilhelmine Germany*, 136–58.

52. For the general background to this see Johannes T. Gross, *Ritualmordbeschuldigungen gegen Juden im deutschen Kaiserreich, 1871–1914*; George L. Mosse, *Toward the Final Solution: A History of European Racism*, ch. 9.

53. For a more recent demonstration of the centrality of blood for European culture, including the use of blood for ritual and medicinal purposes, see the exhaustive survey by Uli Linke, *Blood and Nation: The European Aesthetics of Race*. See also David Katz, "Shylock's Gender: Jewish Male Menstruation in Early Modern England"; Piero Camporesi, *The Juice of Life: The Symbolic and Magic Significance of Blood*.

54. The link between *shechitah* and ritual murder advanced in an 1892 pamphlet by Rohling was taken up and disseminated by politicians and the press in Austria and Germany. In 1891–92, a Jewish butcher was the object of suspicion when a young boy's corpse was found in Xanten, in the Rhine province, "and it was declared in wide circles that undoubtedly a Jewish ritual murder had been perpetrated for the sake of obtaining blood, and people soon talked about a Jewish butcher's cut [*Schächterschnitt*]" (Strack, *The Jew and Human Sacrifice*,

215–18). Strack cites numerous other examples of this imaginative link between ritual murder, ritual slaughter, and circumcision. In addition, see Robin Judd, "Circumcision and Modern Jewish Life: A German Case Study, 1843–1914"; Helmut Walser Smith, *The Butcher's Tale: Murder and Anti-Semitism in a German Town*; William Jordan, "Problems of the Meat Market of Béziers 1240–47: A Question of Antisemitism."

55. Nossig, *SJaV*, 74–5.

56. For prime examples, see Heinrich Haeser, *Lehrbuch der Geschichte der Medicin und der epidemischen Krankheiten*, vol. 1; August Hirsch, *Geschichte der medizinsche Wissenschaft in Deutschland*.

57. See Steven Aschheim, *Brothers and Strangers: The East European Jews in German and German-Jewish Consciousness, 1800–1923*; Steven Aschheim, "The East European Jew and German Jewish Identity," especially 5–7; Trude Maurer, *Ostjuden in Deutschland 1918–1933*, 12–16; Trude Maurer, "The East European Jew in the Weimar Press: Stereotype and Attempted Rebuttal"; Jehuda Reinharz, "East European Jews in the *Weltanschauung* of German Zionists, 1882–1914"; Jack Wertheimer, *Unwelcome Strangers: East European Jews in Imperial Germany*. On the link between the immigrant Jew and dirt and disease in the social scientific and medical literature in Great Britain, see Colin Holmes, *Antisemitism in British Society 1876–1939*, ch. 3.

58. Aschheim, "The East European Jew and German-Jewish Identity," 5–7.

59. On the theme of orientalizing the Jews see the essays in Ivan Davidson Kalmar and Derek J. Penslar (eds), *Orientalism and the Jews*. There was also a tradition, reaching back into the seventeenth century, that orientalized the Jews by situating them in China. On this, see Zhou Xun, "The 'Kaifeng Jew' Hoax: Constructing the 'Chinese Jew.'"

60. On this romanticization of the Orient among Jews, see Paul Mendes-Flohr, "Fin-de-Siècle Orientalism, the Ostjuden and the Aesthetics of Jewish Self-Affirmation." The engagement with "the East" or "Orient" was surely not limited to Jews, let alone to Jewish nationalists. In the last quarter of the nineteenth century, German scholars, politicians, and entrepreneurs "discovered" the Orient anew, a passion born of a combination of political and cultural imperialism, scholarly competition and debate, and greed. On this, see Suzanne Marchand, *Down From Olympus: Archaeology and Philhellenism in Germany, 1750–1970*, 188–227.

61. The best example of this sort of work is Felix Theilhaber's *Der Untergang der deutschen Juden*. At one point, in his discussion of the centrality of sexual and racial hygiene for the survival of the Jews as a people, Theilhaber cites Nossig's book, calling it the standard work on the subject of Jews and social hygiene (17–18).

62. On the middle class sensibility of the *Wissenschaft* movement and its impact on the interpretation of Jewish history, see David Biale, *Gershom Scholem: Kabbalah and Counter-History*.

63. The general literature on this subject is enormous. For example, see Daniel Pick, *Faces of Degeneration: A European Disorder, c. 1848–1918*; Mark Adams (ed.), *The Wellborn Science: Eugenics in Germany, France, Brazil, and Russia*. For Germany, see Weindling, *Health, Race, and German Politics*, ch. 3.

64. On the moral purity campaign in Germany see John C. Fout, "Sexual Politics in Wilhelmine Germany: The Male Gender Crisis, Moral Purity, and Homophobia."

65. See, for example, Ratner, "Die perverse Geschlechtsempfindung in der jüdischen Lehre. Sexual-hygienische Skizze," who began his discussion of Jewish hygiene with reference to §175, and Judaism's accord with Germany's decency laws.

66. Nossig, *SJaV*, 53–5.

67. Maimonides, *The Guide for the Perplexed*, III, 49, 69. It is worth noting that at least as far back as Philo of Alexandria, it was not only the Mosaic laws that put a healthy damper on sexual desire. Moses himself was represented as the model for such healthy repression. Philo tells us that when it came to the "pleasures that have their seat below," Moses evinced little interest: "Save for the begetting of children, they [sexual desires] passed altogether even out of his memory." *Life of Moses*, Book I: 28–9. On Maimonides and circumcision, see Elizabeth Wyner Mark, "Crossing the Gender Divide: Public Ceremonies, Private Parts, Mixed Feelings," xix.

68. Nossig, *SJaV*, 52.

69. On the medical debates over circumcision, see Leonard Glick, *Marked in Your Flesh: Circumcision from Ancient Judea to Modern America*; David L. Gollaher, *Circumcision: A History of the World's Most Controversial Surgery*.

70. For numerous examples of this climatic explanation of racial characteristics, see the selections in Emmanuel Chukwudi Eze (ed.), *Race and the Enlightenment*.

71. See Lloyd Gartner, "Anglo-Jewry and the Jewish International Traffic in Prostitution, 1885–1914."

72. His book on social hygiene, however, did resonate among Jewish and non-Jewish scholars. In 1908, H. L. Eisenstadt delivered a lecture on the need for a renaissance of Jewish social hygiene to the members of the Lehranstalt für die Wissenschaft des Judentums. Eisenstadt built explicitly on Nossig's work, pointing up the concern of the ancient Jewish law code with preventive care, infectious diseases, and sexual hygiene, and he called for the greater dissemination of hygienic knowledge to the Jewish masses. See "Mitteilungen." On Nossig's influence within the broader social hygiene literature, see Thissen, "Die Sozialhygiene als selbstständige Wissenschaft und ihre Terminologie."

73. Nossig's interest in the subject seemed to wane almost immediately. One year later, he published a critique of Spinoza, *Über die bestimmende Ursache des Philosophirens: Versuch einer praktischen Kritik der Lehre Spinoza* (Stuttgart: Deutsche Verlags-Anstalt, 1895); in 1901–2, he published a two-volume analysis of socialism and Judaism, *Revision des Socialismus* (Berlin: J. Edelheim, 1901) in which, interestingly, he attempted to prove that genuine socialism had its roots not in nineteenth-century European thought, but in the Mosaic laws and customs of the Bible. A selection from this work was published in the Zionist newspaper *Die Welt* as part of its ongoing debate over "the intellectual, physical, and economic uplifting of the Jews." Nossig offered his idea of Jewish socialism as a model for the future economy and society of Palestine (see his "Das social-wirtschaftliche Revisionssystem nach der altjüdischen Verfassung"). On the reception of his work on socialism, see Almog, "Alfred

Nossig," 7. Nossig did write a very brief, two-page piece on Jewish social hygiene for the 1930 collection *Hygiene und Judentum*, in which he discussed the connection between the Mosaic code, as a social hygiene system, and Jewish survival. Alfred Nossig, "Die jüdische Sozialhygiene als Erzieherin zur seelischen Vervollkommung."

3. Healthy Hebrews, Healthy Jews

1. Hermann Adler, "Sanitation and the Mosaic Law," 1340.
2. Ibid., 1340.
3. On the politics of *shechitah* in Great Britain, see Tony Kushner, "Stunning Intolerance: A Century of Opposition to Religious Slaughter."
4. Adler, "Sanitation and the Mosaic Law," 1341.
5. Percival Wood, *Moses: The Founder of Preventive Medicine.*
6. Madison C. Peters, *Justice to the Jew: The Story of What He Has Done for the World* (New York: F. T. Neely, [1899] 1910). Cited in Yuri Slezkine, *The Jewish Century*, 56.
7. *Washington Post*, "Mosaic Laws Sanitary."
8. Matthew Frye Jacobson, *Whiteness of a Different Color: European Immigrants and the Alchemy of Race.* For a full treatment on the subject of Jews and whiteness in America, see Eric Goldstein, *The Price of Whiteness: Jews, Race, and American Identity.*
9. Lothrop Stoddard, *Reforging America*, 256–7, quoted in Jacobson, *Whiteness of a Different Color*, 98.
10. Jacobson, *Whiteness of a Different Color*, 183.
11. Quoted in Christine Rosen, *Preaching Eugenics: Religious Leaders and the American Eugenics Movement*, 108.
12. J. K. Walker, "On the State of the Medical Art Among the Jews, as Recorded in the Bible," 165. Walker is identified as a medical doctor in Buddersfield. I have identified him as a Christian because in the text he refers to the Gospel of Mark and "the sayings of our Savior."
13. Ibid., 166.
14. Ibid., 166.
15. Ibid., 173.
16. John M. B. Harden, "Notes on the Medicine of Moses."
17. Solomon Kagan, "Talmudic Medicine," 164.
18. Ibid., 164–8.
19. Ibid., 164. On Katznelson, see the discussion in Chapter 1. For another example of this sort of attempt to degrade the Greeks and Romans and elevate the Jews, see Julius Magil, "Medicine and Physicians Among the Jews – From Bible, Talmud, and Ancient History."
20. Fielding H. Garrison, *An Introduction to the History of Medicine*, cited in Solomon Kagan, "Talmudic Medicine," 167.
21. Solomon Kagan, "Talmudic Medicine," 167.
22. Noël Guéneau de Mussy, "The Hygienic Laws of Moses." Originally published in *L'Union Médicale*, Jan. 4, 8, 15, 1885.

23. Ibid., 81.
24. Ibid., 82. Guéneau de Mussy was the best-known and most often invoked French authority on this subject. But he was not the first to be cited by American medical writers. In his 1859 article on the sanitary laws of the Hebrews, Mark Blumenthal quoted the French lawyer and writer Claude Emmanuel de Pastoret (*Moyse, considéré comme législateur et comme moraliste*, 528): "One of the most distinguishing traits in the character of Moses as a legislator and one in which he was the most imitated by those who, in after ages gave laws to the eastern world, was his constant attention to the health of the people." Mark Blumenthal, "The Sanitary and Dietetic Laws of the Hebrews, as Related to Medicine," 345.
25. Blumenthal, "The Sanitary and Dietetic Laws of the Hebrews," 84.
26. Ibid., 85.
27. Walker, "On the State of the Medical Art among the Jews," 164.
28. W. C. Bitting, "Address: Biblical Medicine," 370. Bitting is identified as a "reverend," not a physician.
29. Ibid., 373.
30. Ibid., 371.
31. Ibid., 386.
32. Ibid., 384. The exact same sentiment would be expressed by some Jewish physicians writing a decade or two later. See the discussion of Yiddish language health books in Chapter 5.
33. Max Danzis, "The Jew in Medicine from Biblical to Modern Times," 1. Reprinted by the American Jewish Historical Society. Originally given as a talk before the Men's Club of Temple B'nai Abraham of Newark, New Jersey.
34. Benjamin Lee Gordon, "Medicine Among the Ancient Hebrews," 219. Gordon was born in Neustadt, in Lithuania, and raised in an observant Jewish environment. He came to the United States in 1890 and attended medical school in Philadelphia. See his autobiography, *Between Two Worlds: The Memoirs of a Physician*.
35. Gordon, "Medicine Among the Ancient Hebrews," 220.
36. Ibid., 229.
37. Edward T. Williams, "Moses as a Sanitarian." Read before the Norfolk Medical Society, November 29, 1881. Quoting from 6.
38. David A. Stewart, "Diseases and History," 366.
39. James K. Hosmer, *The Jews: Ancient, Medieval, Modern*, 148–9.
40. Nuphtuli Herz Imber, "The Medical Science of the Talmud," 513–14; Lester Levyn, "Biostatistics of the Jewish Race: Pertaining Especially to Immunity and Susceptibility."
41. Blumenthal, "The Sanitary and Dietetic Laws of the Hebrews," 339. This originated as a paper read before the New York Medical Union, on Feb. 24, 1859.
42. Ibid., 340.
43. Maurice Fluegel, *Die mosaische Diät und Hygiene: Von physiologischen und ethischen Standpunkte*, 4–5. This was originally delivered as a lecture, on May 27, 1880, Temple B'nai Israel in Kalamazoo, Michigan. Fluegel cited other British physicians and health officials as authorities, who were contributors to the *Lancet* and to the *London Sanitary Record*.

44. Hermann Gollancz, *The Dietary Laws*, 4. This originated as a sermon delivered on October 18, 1890, at the Dalston Synagogue. There were also rabbis who invoked medicine and science to attack the continued adherence by Jews to the dietary laws. For example, the German reform rabbi Adolf Wiener blamed *kashrut* for a host of physical problems suffered by Jews, including skeletal weakness, intestinal diseases, scrophula, and hemorrhoids. See Wiener, *Die jüdische Speisegesetze nach ihren verschiedenen Gesichtspunkten zum ersten Male wissenschaftlich methodisch beleuchtet*, cited in Thomas Schlich, "The Word of God and the Word of Science: Nutrition Science and the Jewish Dietary Laws in Germany, 1820–1920," 111.

45. On the significance of the medicalization of the circumcision debate see Leonard Glick, *Marked in Your Flesh: Circumcision from Ancient Judea to Modern America*, chs 5 and 6.

46. See the discussion in Robin Judd, "Circumcision and Modern Jewish Life: A German Case Study, 1843–1914."

47. Todd Endelman, *The Jews of Georgian England, 1714–1830: Tradition and Change in a Liberal Society*, 142–9, for the earlier period. On the nineteenth-century rabbinate in America, see Hasia Diner, *A Time for Gathering: The Second Migration 1820–1880*; Jonathan Sarna, "The Evolution of the American Synagogue."

48. Thomas Schlich has pointed this out in his discussion of nutritional science and the reinterpretation of the laws of *kashrut*. See Schlich, "The Word of God and the Word of Science."

49. N. D. Stebbins, "Evidences of a General System of Medical Practice Being Taught by Scripture, and a Comparison of this System with Rational Medicine and Exclusive Homeopathy," 11.

50. See, for example, *Medical News*, "Summary of the Proceedings of the International Congress of Dermatology and Syphilography, Held in Paris in 1889." Also, Alan Kraut, *Goldberger's War: The Life and Work of a Public Health Crusader*. On the decline of leprosy as a focus of concern, see the comments in Henry E. Sigerist, "The Philosophy of Hygiene," particularly 323; Ernest Muir, "The Control of Leprosy"; Esmond R. Long, "The Decline of Tuberculosis with Special Reference to Its Generalized Form."

51. See Adam Sutcliffe, *Judaism and Enlightenment*; Jan Assman, *Moses the Egyptian: The Memory of Egypt in Western Monotheism*, 33–6; Amos Funkenstein, *Perceptions of Jewish History*, 36–40.

52. Stebbins, "Evidences of a General System of Medical Practice," 11–12.

53. Ibid., 16.

54. Wood, *Moses*, 70–1. We might, it is true, also see here a response and repudiation of an earlier intellectual tradition that cast priests and the priestly class as the bane of progress and culture. Significantly, this was linked explicitly to the ancient world, particularly Egypt and China. According to Martin Bernal (following Frank Manuel): "The Egyptians and Chinese were perceived as having been mathematicians, philosophers and metaphysicians. Unfortunately, in both civilizations these 'sciences' had been sapped by superstition and priestly dogmatism. Just as Bishop Warburton had tried to exculpate the priests on this issue out of 'clerical solidarity,' so intellectuals like Turgot and Condorcet were

delighted to have yet another stick with which to beat them, for here, as in the modern world, priests could largely be blamed for the decadence." Martin Bernal, *Black Athena: The Afroasiatic Roots of Classical Civilization*, 199.

55. Wayne Meeks, "Moses as God and King," 367.

56. On the factionalism within medicine and the process of professionalization in the American context see John S. Haller Jr., *American Medicine in Transition, 1840–1910*; Paul Starr, *The Social Transformation of American Medicine*. According to Starr, the "consolidation of professional authority" occurred during the years 1850–1930, just in those decades under discussion here.

57. On the history of alternative medicine in the Anglo-American context, see Mike Saks (ed.), *Alternative Medicine in Britain*; Norman Gevitz (ed.), *Other Healers: Unorthodox Medicine in America*. On Germany, see Robert Jütte, "The Historiography of Nonconventional Medicine in Germany: An Overview."

58. Ronald Numbers, "The Fall and Rise of the American Medical Profession."

59. Ibid., 227.

60. Harden, "Notes on the Medicine of Moses."

61. William Morrow Beach, "The Importance of Sanitation."

62. Ibid., 254.

63. This theme will be taken up in greater detail in Chapter 6.

64. Herman Bendell, "The Physician of Sacred History," 59.

65. Ibid., 59.

66. "It is only within recent years that the necessity has arisen to assign to hygiene a separate place among the sciences." J. Snowman, *Jewish Law and Sanitary Science*, 1.

67. Ibid., 2–3.

68. Ibid., 3.

69. Ibid., 4. Leviticus, for instance, is of scientific interest because it offers "remarkably early examples of the diagnosis and treatment of disease. The thirteenth chapter of Leviticus is quoted as a masterly piece of differential diagnosis, and the precautions to prevent infection remain to this day in principle unimproved."

70. Ibid., 15.

71. Ibid., 18.

72. The continuities and discontinuities of the narrative tradition of the healthy Jew into the present are discussed at greater length in Chapter 7.

73. Nancy Tomes, *The Gospel of Germs: Men, Women, and the Microbe in American Life*, 158.

74. Judith Walzer Leavitt and Ronald L. Numbers, "Sickness and Health: An Overview," 8.

75. See the discussion in Suellen Hoy, *Chasing Dirt: The American Pursuit of Cleanliness*, chs 2 and 3.

4. From Ghetto to Jungle

1. This was, for instance, the question with which Gobineau began his essay on human inequality. Accounting for the birth of civilizations, he believed, was

simple; but "the fall of civilizations is the most striking, and, at the same time, the most obscure of all the phenomena of history." Cited in Bruce Mazlish, *Civilization and Its Contents*, 59.

2. Moreover, in Weimar Germany Jews, too, were engaged in eugenic research and writing, and helped to fund institutes involved in eugenic research. See the discussion in Paul Weindling, *Health, Race, and German Politics Between National Unification and Nazism, 1870–1945*, 431–82; Robert Proctor, *Racial Hygiene: Medicine Under the Nazis*.

3. On the history of these efforts see Shai Cherry, "Three Twentieth-Century Jewish Responses to Evolutionary Theory"; Shai Cherry, "Creation, Evolution and Jewish Thought"; Marc Swetlitz, "American Jewish Responses to Darwin and Evolutionary Theory, 1860–1890"; Marc Swetlitz, "Responses of American Reform Rabbis to Evolutionary Theory, 1864–1888"; José Faur, "The Hebrew Species Concept and the Origin of Evolution: R. Benamozegh's Response to Darwin"; Lois C. Dubin, "Pe'er Ha'Adam of Vittorio Hayim Castiglioni: An Italian Chapter in the History of Jewish Response to Darwin"; Naomi Cohen, "The Challenges of Darwinism and Biblical Criticism to American Judaism." A number of the essays in Geoffrey Cantor and Marc Swetlitz (eds), *Jewish Tradition and the Challenge of Darwinism* (University of Chicago Press, 2006), are directly relevant to my discussion. I regret that the book appeared only after the completion of my manuscript and I was unable to integrate it into this chapter.

4. James Moore, "Deconstructing Darwinism: The Politics of Evolution in the 1860s," 359, cited in Ronald L. Numbers, *Darwinism Comes to America*, 49.

5. W. M. Feldman, "Ancient Jewish Eugenics."

6. Ibid., 28–9.

7. James Crichton-Browne, "Introduction," xxiii.

8. Ibid., xxiv–xxv. On Salaman and his Mendelian approach to the Jews see Todd Endelman, "Anglo-Jewish Scientists and the Science of Race"; Dan Stone, "Of Peas, Potatoes, and Jews: Redcliffe N. Salaman and the British Debate over Jewish Racial Origins."

9. Thurman B. Rice, *Racial Hygiene: A Practical Discussion of Eugenics and Race Culture*.

10. Ibid., 13.

11. Ibid., 13.

12. The literature on Darwinism, social Darwinism, and eugenics in the Anglo-American context is enormous. For a recent treatment see Mike Hawkins, *Social Darwinism in European and American Thought, 1860–1945*; Daniel Kevles, *In the Name of Eugenics: Genetics and the Uses of Human Heredity*. See also Numbers, *Darwinism Comes to America*. On the debate between religion and science in the wake of Darwin see Christine Rosen, *Preaching Eugenics: Religious Leaders and the American Eugenics Movement*; Edward J. Larson, *Summer for the Gods: The Scopes Trial and America's Continuing Debate over Science and Religion*.

13. Mark Blumenthal, "The Sanitary and Dietetic Laws of the Hebrews, as Related to Medicine," 341.

14. Max Reichler, *Jewish Eugenics and other Essays*.
15. Blumenthal, "The Sanitary and Dietetic Laws of the Hebrews," 340.
16. This does not mean that evolutionary language did not exist prior to Darwin's *Origin of Species*. Ideas about organic evolution had circulated before Darwin. Yet, it was not until after the publication of Darwin's work that the subject became a topic of intense public discussion and debate, and scientists felt comfortable enough voicing what still were highly heterodox views. Darwin, it should also be noted, did not introduce the phrase "struggle for existence" until the fifth edition (1872) of his book. See Gregory Claeys, "The 'Survival of the Fittest' and the Origins of Social Darwinism," 223, note 2. Nor do I want to suggest here that Blumenthal, as a doctor or scientist, would inevitably, after 1859, have adopted Darwinian language. The reception of Darwinian evolution among scientists in America and elsewhere was highly variegated. On this see Numbers, *Darwinism Comes to America*, ch. 1.
17. Darwinism and eugenics were not the only "languages" with which scholars and others had to work. As vital, perhaps, was the role of statistics (in the development of which Galton, the "founder of eugenics," played a significant part). Thus, at the outset of his book on Jewish disease and mortality, the Central European social scientist Hugo Hoppe noted the "extraordinary" or unique quality of Jewish survival. He then quoted Eduard Glatter (*Über die Lebens-Chancen der Israeliten gegenüber der christlichen Confessionen*), the former head of the Vienna Statistical Office, on the remarkable "tenacity of survival" of the Jews: "There is no analog in the history of nations to the [Jewish] condition." "For a long time," Hoppe continued, "it has been known that the Jews, in general, have possessed a far greater tenacity of life [*Lebenszähigkeit*] than the peoples amongst whom they reside. However, it is only with the modern science of statistics that we possess the numerical proof for this assertion." Hugo Hoppe, *Krankheiten und Sterblichkeit bei Juden und Nichtjuden*, 1.
18. By Jewish historiography here I mean not only works written by Jews about Jews, but any text that takes Jews as its object and utilizes the methods of historical analysis.
19. By no means, however, did the older theological or supernatural explanation of Jewish survival cease to function. For examples see Richard I. Cohen, "Urban Visibility and Biblical Visions: Jewish Culture in Western and Central Europe in the Modern Age," 47–8.
20. *Jewish Chronicle*, "Jews and Eugenics."
21. *Jewish Chronicle*, "Eugenics and the Jew. Interview for *The Jewish Chronicle* with Sir Francis Galton."
22. Reichler, *Jewish Eugenics*, 8–9.
23. Ibid., 7.
24. Ibid., 7.
25. I have been unable to identify Ratner any further. He does not appear in *Wer ist Wer?* for those years, or in any of the German biographical and bibliographical source works I was able to consult. The catalogue of the German National Library lists a 1914 medical dissertation from Basel by a Yitzak-Isaac Ratner ("Über die Bestimmung der Blutmenge: Vergleich der Behringschen mit der

Welckerschen Methode"). His 1909 article identifies him as a medical doctor, so he may have obtained his doctorate after completing medical school.

26. Ratner, "Die Psychotherapie und Volksmedizin bei den Juden"; Ratner, "Die perverse Geschlechtsempfindung in der jüdischen Lehre. Sexualhygienische Skizze"; Ratner, "Sociale und hygienische Fürsorge im altjüdischen Staate"; Ratner, "Die Gedächtnishygiene in den jüdischen Bräuchen sowie in der altjüdischen Literatur"; Ratner, "Die Geschlechtliche Hygiene in der altjüdischen Literatur"; Ratner, "Die Rassenhygiene, Familienforschung, Eugenik und einiges über die Vererbung geistiger Eigenschaften im altjüdischen Schriftum." This last article identifies Ratner as a Wiesbaden physician by origin who is now located in Cophenhagen.

27. Ratner, "Die Rassenhygiene," 249.

28. Ibid., 250.

29. Ibid., 250.

30. Ibid., 251–2.

31. W. M. Feldman, "Ancient Jewish Eugenics," 35.

32. Max Danzis, "The Jew in Medicine from Biblical to Modern Times," reprinted as a pamphlet by the American Jewish Historical Society, quoting 4.

33. Alfred Nossig, *Die Sozialhygiene der Juden und des altorientalischen Volkerkreises*, 57–8. On the impact of Darwinism on social and racial hygiene in Germany, see Weindling, *Health, Race, and German Politics*, ch. 1; and Günter Mann, "Rassenhygiene – Sozialdarwinismus."

34. W. M. Feldman, "Ancient Jewish Eugenics," 28–9.

35. Isidore Simon, "La Gynécologie, L'Obstétrique, L'Embryologie et la Puériculture dans la Bible et le Talmud," 26.

36. Arthur Ruppin, "Die sozialen Verhältnisse der Juden in Preussen und Deutschland," 380. One year later Ruppin elaborated on his understanding of Darwinian thought and its application to social policy in his prize-winning essay *Darwinismus und Sozialwissenschaft* (Jena: G. Fischer, 1903). He was unconcerned for the most part with Jews in this volume. On this work and its place in Ruppin's overall thinking see Derek Penslar, *Zionism and Technocracy*, 86–7; Yfaat Weiss, "Central European Ethnonationalism and Zionist Binationalism," 106–7.

37. Maurice Fishberg, "Rassenzüchtung der Juden," 80–4.

38. Ibid., 80–4.

39. Alfred Nossig, "Die Auserwähltheit der Juden im Lichte der Biologie," 2. Nossig's article was, it should be said, a direct response to an article by the non-Jewish authority Curt Michaelis ("Die jüdische Auserwahlungsidee und ihre biologische Bedeutung," *Zeitschrift für Demographie und Statistik der Juden* 1, 1905), who argued that the idea of chosenness had led to an unfortunate sense of racial pride among the Jews, and was the cause of the hostility and hatred directed at them by other peoples. Nossig's argument, then, was in part a response to what was widely seen as a piece of anti-Semitica (published in a Jewish journal), but, as I argue, its content cannot be reduced to that.

40. Max Levy, "Jewish People and the Laws of Evolution," 187.

41. Hyman Morrison, "A Biologic Interpretation of Jewish Survival," 98.

42. Ibid., 100–1.
43. Ibid., 98.
44. On the ghetto as an imagined site or space of degeneration, see Jürgen Heyde, "The 'Ghetto' as a Spatial and Historical Construction – Discourses of Emancipation in France, Germany, and Poland"; Alina Cala, "The Discourse of 'Ghettoization' – Non-Jews on Jews in 19th and 20th Century Poland"; Katrin Steffen, "Connotations of Exclusion – 'Ostjuden,' 'Ghettos,' and Other Markings."
45. Martin Engländer, *Die auffälend häufigen Krankheitserscheinungen der jüdischen Rasse*, 11.
46. Cesare Lombroso, *L'antisemitismo e le scienze moderne* (Torino: L. Roux e C., 1894). The work appeared immediately in German as *Der Antisemitismus und die Juden im Lichte der modernen Wissenschaft*, and I have used this translation here, quoting from 51–3.
47. On Sombart and his interpretation of Jews and capitalism, see Derek Penslar, *Shylock's Children: Economics and Jewish Identity in Modern Europe*, 164–5, and passim.
48. Arthur Ruppin, *Die Juden der Gegenwart*, p. 48. A version of this argument, has recently figured prominently in the thesis advanced by three researchers in genetics at the University of Utah that seeks to explain the purported higher intelligence of Ashkenazi Jews. See Gregory Cohran, Jason Hardy, and Henry Harpending, "Natural History of Ashkenazi Intelligence." And see the comments of Steven Pinker, "Groups and Genes: The Lessons of the Ashkenazim."
49. Leo Sofer, "Zur Biologie und Pathologie der jüdischen Rasse," 89.
50. Caleb Saleeby, *Parenthood and Race Culture: An Outline of Eugenics*, 297.
51. Ibid., 297.
52. Ibid., 317.
53. Lester Levyn, "Biostatistics of the Jewish Race: Pertaining Especially to Immunity and Susceptibility," 982.
54. Ibid., 982.
55. For the fullest treatment of this negative image of the Jewish body, see Sander Gilman, *The Jew's Body*.
56. Louis Wirth, *The Ghetto*.
57. Ibid., 24.
58. Ibid., 65–6.
59. Ibid., 66.
60. Israel Cohen, *Jewish Life in Modern Times*, 116. Cited in Wirth, *The Ghetto*, 66–7.
61. Ernst Mayr, *One Long Argument: Charles Darwin and the Genesis of Modern Evolutionary Thought*, 640.
62. "New Jews and Judaism," *American Hebrew*, 14 March, 1884, 66, cited in Swetlitz, "American Jewish Responses to Darwin and Evolutionary Theory," 227. Swetlitz makes the point that this sort of argument was part of a longer tradition of apologetics, by which traditional Jews sought to defend Jewish ritual by tying it with hygienic precepts.
63. Maurice Fishberg, "The Comparative Pathology of the Jews," 580.
64. Maurice Fishberg, "Tuberculosis Among the Jews," 1080–1.

65. Matthew Frye Jacobson, *Whiteness of a Different Color: European Immigrants and the Alchemy of Race.*

66. On Jews and the textile industry, including a discussion of tuberculosis, see Daniel Bender, *Sweated Work, Weak Bodies: Anti-Sweatshop Campaigns and Languages of Labor.*

67. Fishberg, "Tuberculosis Among the Jews," 1081.

68. Maurice Fishberg, *The Jews: A Study in Race and Environment.*

69. Arthur Ruppin, *Die Soziologie der Juden*, vol. 1, 268.

70. Hoppe, *Krankheiten und Sterblichkeit bei Juden und Nichtjuden*, 18–19.

71. Heinrich Graetz, "Historic Parallels in Jewish History," 4–5. Emphasis in original.

72. "Der auf- und Niedergang im Völkerleben, sowie die Wechselfälle im Leben des jüdischen Volkes brachten nämlich seit der grausigen Bertreibung der Juden aus Spanien und Portugal und der unmenschlichen Verfolgung der marranen einigen Scharfbeobachtenden Juden die Überzeugung bei, daß nicht der Zufall in der Geschichte walte, sondern daß sie eine höhere hand leite und durch Blut und Tränenströme ihren Ratschluß zu Ende führe." Heinrich Graetz, *Geschichte der Juden* 9, 306. On the same page, writing about the origins of modern Jewish historical thinking, Graetz refers to a "few thoughtful Jews" (*einige gedankenreiche Juden*) who, at the time, were able to see or discern in the "wild, apparently capricious and disorderly course of general and Jewish history, the work of Providence" ("*in der wilden, scheinbar launenhaften und unregelmäßigen Strömung der allgemeinen und jüdischen Geschichte ein Werk der Vorsehung zu erblicken*").

73. Graetz, "Historic Parallels in Jewish History," 8.

74. Ibid., 9.

75. Ibid., 11.

76. For a particularly perceptive discussion of the non-Jewish representation of this see Jonathan Freedman, *The Temple of Culture*, 123–4, and passim.

77. Mitchell Hart, *Social Science and the Politics of Modern Jewish Identity.*

78. Paul Popenoe and Roswell Johnson, *Applied Eugenics*, 133, quoted in Freedman, *The Temple of Culture*, 124.

79. William Schrock "Man According to Nature," 208.

80. G. Stanley Hall, "Yankee and Jew," 88.

81. Charles W. Eliot, "The Potency of the Jewish Race," 142.

82. *JAMA*, "Ritualistic Sanitation of the Jews," 801.

83. Ibid., 802.

84. Ratner, "Die Rassenhygiene," 249.

85. G. Levin, *Higiene bei Yidn Amol un Itend*, 12. Levin's work constitutes a departure from the narratives I am dealing with here. He argued that one might be led to believe that, given the fact that "the Jews possessed a modern social hygiene already in ancient times, when most modern civilized nations did not yet exist, or were living at a primitive level... that the level of hygiene among Jews today would be very high, and that we, as a 'holy and pure nation' could serve as a model with regard to purity for all other nations. However, this is not the case" (30). The most observant Jews, he claimed, do not pay much heed to common

rituals of cleanliness; nor are the so-called enlightened Jews much better (31). "It is no wonder then," he concluded, "that we see all sorts of illnesses affecting us, which hinder immigration, and which produce large-scale losses during times of epidemic" (31). Thus, while Levin's work fits into the interpretive tradition under analysis here, insofar as he embraces the idea that the Jews possessed a code of social hygiene in ancient times, he departs in his evaluation of contemporary Jewry. They are not healthy, but dirty and diseased. But, it still needs to be pointed out, this was due to their unwillingness to follow their own laws, not to anything deficient in their natures. In other words, it was a matter of will rather than race.

86. Saleeby, *Parenthood and Race Culture*, 317. On Saleeby and the Jews see also Christine Rosen, *Preaching Eugenics*, 37.
87. David Macht, "Embryology and Obstetrics in Ancient Hebrew Literature," 8.
88. Beth Wenger, "Mitzvah and Medicine: Gender, Assimilation, and the Scientific Defense of 'Family Purity,'" 179.
89. Joseph Jacobs, *Studies in Jewish Statistics: Social, Vital, and Anthropometric*, 56–7. Jacobs also noted that the German (and non-Jewish) statistician Ernst Nagel attributed the preponderance of males born to Jewish women to, first, the greater care Jewish wives took of their own health, and, second, fewer illegitimate births.
90. Cited in Laura Doyle, *Bordering on the Body: The Racial Matrix of Modern Fiction and Culture*, 19.
91. Danzis, "The Jew in Medicine from Biblical to Modern Times," 4.
92. Fishberg, "Rassenzüchtung der Juden," 75.
93. Ibid., 77. Fishberg's assertion was echoed in an essay, published in the same volume, by the Berlin health official and B'nei Brith officer Louis Maretzki. See Maretzki, "Die Gesundheitsverhältnisse der Juden," 146.
94. Fishberg, "Rassenzüchtung der Juden," 77.
95. Rice, *Racial Hygiene*, 349–50.
96. Reichler, *Jewish Eugenics*, 11.
97. Ibid., 11–12.
98. Alfred Nossig, *Materialien zur Statistik des jüdischen Stammes*, 55–6.
99. Ibid., 56.
100. In this, they echoed some of the more popular eugenic authorities of the period. For example, the geneticist W. E. Castle, in his popular textbook *Genetics and Eugenics*, cited late marriages as one of the two main reasons for a "dysgenic" trend in society. See Doyle, *Bordering on the Body*, 18.
101. Reichler, *Jewish Eugenics*, 11, 14.
102. Feldman," Ancient Jewish Eugenics," 31.
103. Jacobs, *Studies in Jewish Statistics*, 52.
104. Hall's paper, delivered at a health congress in Leeds, England, was summarized in *JAMA*. It is worth noting that the editors, in titling its summary, changed Hall's "Aryan" to Gentile and "Semitic" to Jewish: William Hall, "The Influence of Feeding on the Development of Jewish and Gentile Children," 54. For another example of this sort of celebration of the Jewish family, without the explicit language of eugenics, see Maretzki, "Die Gesundheitsverhältnisse der Juden," 129.

5. TB or Not TB, That Was a Jewish Question

1. Medicus, "The Tuberculosis Problem."
2. Winslow Anderson, "Tuberculosis and Its Prevention," 300.
3. Ibid., 302.
4. Ibid., 302–3.
5. D. H. Bergey, "Bovine Tuberculosis as a Factor in the Production of Human Tuberculosis, through the Use of Meat and Milk," 102.
6. For a contemporary summary of the prodigious efforts to produce a vaccine see Edward R. Baldwin, "Immunity in Tuberculosis: With Special Reference to Racial and Clinical Manifestations," esp. 829–32.
7. Noah Ephraim Aronstam, *Jewish Dietary Laws from a Scientific Standpoint*, 22.
8. Ibid., 22–4, emphasis in the original.
9. In addition to the works cited in this chapter, see for example Dr. G. A. Heron, *Evidences of the Communicability of Consumption*. In this work, Heron, a fellow at the Royal College of Physicians in London, discussed the immunity of Jews from TB and dwelt on the careful inspection of meat that "carefully conforming Jews" require. He argued that about 4 percent of meat in Great Britain was infected with the tubercle germ, and that if the rigid inspections and rules regarding meat practiced by Jews were introduced into the general society, many more lives would be saved. A brief discussion of Heron's work appeared in the *Journal of the American Medical Association*, *Medical News*, and the German periodical *Hygienische Rundschau*. See *JAMA*, "Immunity of Jews from Tuberculosis"; *Medical News*, "Review of G. A. Heron, *Evidences of the Communicability of Consumption*"; *Hygienische Rundschau*, "Review of G. A. Heron, *Evidences of the Communicability of Consumption*."
10. William Z. Ripley, *The Races of Europe*, 384. Cited in Sander Gilman, *Franz Kafka, The Jewish Patient*, 53. For a similar invocation of the Jews within the British context, see Michael Worboys, "Tuberculosis and Race in Britain and Its Empire, 1900–1950."
11. Eduard Glatter, *Über die Lebens-Chancen der Israeliten gegenüber der christlichen Confessionen*. Cited in Hugo Hoppe, *Krankheiten und Sterblichkeit bei Juden und Nichtjuden*, 1.
12. Hans Ullmann, "Zur Frage der Vitalität und Morbidität der jüdischen Bevölkerung"; H. Strauss, "Das Tuberkuloseproblem bei den Juden."
13. Hoppe, *Krankheiten und Sterblichkeit*, 19–21. Five years later, writing about the Jews and TB in London, Hoppe summarized a *British Medical Journal* article that demonstrated, on the basis of statistics gathered between 1891 and 1900, that Jews evinced a lower percentage of deaths from TB. This held true for the East End as well as for better-off parts of the city. Jews, according to the British article, have shown similar resistance to other infectious diseases, including plague, malaria, and cholera. The author of the article attributed this to a racial immunity. Hoppe refuted this, insisting that the explanation lay with different living conditions and relations: stronger family sense among poor Jews, greater concern with education, greater care with diet and clothing, religious dietary laws, particularly those dealing with meat, and moderation with alcohol. See Hoppe, "Die Tuberkulose unter den Juden in London."

14. Leo Sofer, "Zur Biologie und Pathologie der jüdischen Rasse," 85–92.
15. Ludwig Silvagni, "La patologia comparata negli Ebrei." The article is summarized in B. L., "Zur Pathologie der jüdische Rasse."
16. Samuel Weissenberg, "Zur Sozialbiologie und Sozialhygiene der Juden," 410–11.
17. Jean Flamant, *Contribution à l'étude de la Pathologie des Israélites*, 15–19. John Efron has examined this notion of Jewish immunity to a host of diseases, including tuberculosis, in his *Medicine and the German Jews: A History*, ch. 4.
18. C. R. Drysdale, "Letter to the Editor."
19. Tuberculosis, it should be noted, was not the only disease that generated debate over Jewish immigration, Jewish identity (i.e., are the Jews a race or a religion?), and the possibility and desirability of Jewish assimilation. And politics, in turn, directly affected the way medical researchers and others conceived of certain diseases. Recent work in the history of medicine has shown how vital the politics of race and immigration were, for instance, to the construction of Tay-Sachs as a "Jewish (Ashkenazik) disease" in the early 1880s, and the response to the typhus and cholera epidemics of 1892 in New York. See S. Z. Reuter, "The Genuine Jewish Type: Racial Ideology and Anti-Immigrationism in Early Medical Writing about Tay-Sachs Disease"; Howard Markel, *Quarantine! East European Jewish Immigrants and the New York City Epidemics of 1892*.
20. On Jack the Ripper as a Jew, see Sander Gilman, *The Jew's Body*, ch. 4; Sara Blair, "Henry James, Jack the Ripper, and the Cosmopolitan Jew: Staging Authorship in The Tragic Muse."
21. See Bernard Harris, "Pro-Alienism, Anti-Alienism and the Medical Profession in Late-Victorian and Edwardian Britain."
22. Henry Behrend, "The Communicability to Man of Diseases from Animals Used as Food"; Henry Behrend, "Diseases Caught from Butcher's Meat."
23. For Behrend's biography see Lipkin Goodman, "Henry Behrend."
24. Behrend, "The Communicability to Man of Diseases from Animals Used as Food," (1880), 12.
25. Thomas Dormandy, *The White Death: A History of Tuberculosis*, 133.
26. On the history of the debate in general see Barbara Gutmann Rosenkrantz, "The Trouble with Bovine Tuberculosis."
27. Ibid., 156.
28. Hermann Gollancz, *The Dietary Laws*, 5.
29. Dormandy, *The White Death*, 331.
30. The Royal Commission followed up its initial report with four more, in 1907, 1910, 1913, and 1914. Unlike in the United States and many other countries, in Great Britain the battle to reform the laws and practices concerning cattle and milk met strong resistance, mainly from the agricultural sectors. But a number of prominent medical authorities also still maintained that no concrete proof existed that humans, especially children, contracted tuberculosis by drinking the milk of diseased animals. See Dormandy, *The White Death*, ch. 29.
31. S. Steinthal, *Die Hygiene in Bibel und Talmud*, 27–8.
32. See Uli Linke, *Blood and Nation: The European Aesthetics of Race*.

33. Abbé Henri Baptiste Grégoire, "An Essay on the Physical, Moral and Political Reformation of the Jews" (1789), 52.

34. Solomon Solis-Cohen, "Health Laws of the Jews," 131.

35. Ibid., 130.

36. Behrend, "The Communicability to Man of Diseases from Animals Used as Food," (1880), 12. Alfred Nossig cited Behrend's 1880–81 *Jewish Chronicle* articles in reinforcing the opinion of Dr. Gibbon, who demonstrated that certain illnesses (*gewisse Krankeheiten*) are almost unknown among Jews. Nossig, *Materialien zur Statistik des jüdischen Stammes*, 3–4.

37. Behrend, "The Communicability to Man of Diseases from Animals Used as Food," (1881), 15.

38. Ibid., (1881), 15.

39. Behrend, "Diseases Caught from Butcher's Meat."

40. Ibid., 412.

41. Behrend quoted from the *International Review* (October 1888): "The civilized world is rather apathetic about consumption. It has gotten rid of the plague and nearly rid of typhus epidemics; leprosy has been driven out of England, and smallpox has been rendered manageable; but one death in seven from all causes is still due to tubercle of the lung, and a part of the remainder is due to other tuberculous diseases. If we feared these as they merit, we should in turn suffer less from their ravages. But we have strangely grown used to them, and view them with a sort of fatalistic indifference", ibid., 416.

42. Ibid., 416–17.

43. Behrend also invoked the esteemed French journal *Revue Scientifique*, which had recently noted that Jews "are comparatively exempt from tuberculous maladies; and it ascribes these biological privileges, in a great degree, to the faithful observance of the hygienic rules prescribed by their religious observances", ibid., 421.

44. Ibid., 417.

45. Ibid., 417.

46. Ibid., 418–19.

47. Marcus N. Adler, "The Health Laws of the Bible, and Their Influence upon the Life-Condition of the Jews," 139. See as well Flamant, *Contribution à l'étude de la Pathologie des Israélites*, 15–18.

48. Marcus N. Adler, "The Health Laws of the Bible," 139.

49. Maurice Fishberg, "The Relative Infrequency of Tuberculosis Among Jews"; Maurice Fishberg, "The Jews as Immigrants – From a Medical Standpoint"; Maurice Fishberg, *Health Problems of the Jewish Poor* (1903); Maurice Fishberg, "Tuberculosis Among the Jews." Alan Kraut, in his work *Silent Travelers: Germs, Genes, and the 'Immigrant Menace'*, has analyzed Fishberg's writings on tuberculosis in some detail. My summary here of Fishberg's analysis will therefore be familiar to anyone who has read Kraut's work. But my iteration of Fishberg's ideas occurs in a far different narrative context than Kraut's. Kraut, as the title of his work suggests, is mainly interested in Fishberg within the context of the American racialism and nativism of the early twentieth century, and the identification of the Jews with disease. My interest is in placing Fishberg

within the longer and broader context of the discourse on Jews, Judaism and health. Kraut mentions Fishberg's argument about TB and Jewish dietary laws, but does not offer any extensive analysis of this, nor does he place it within the intellectual tradition I am attempting to trace here.

50. Fishberg, "The Relative Infrequency of Tuberculosis Among Jews," 697–8.

51. Lombroso argued that it was due to the fact that Jews worked mainly indoors, and so avoided severe weather. Drs. Tostivint and Remlinger, looking at the ethnic and religious groups of Tunis, rejected the racial factor, since the Arabs there were also Semitic, and they suffered at much higher rates than their Jewish compatriots. Nor could they explain disparity with other recognized factors such as poverty, dwelling, clothing, and levels of sanitation. All these the Jews and Arabs shared. Only one difference had been noted: "The Jews abhor the dusting-brush and instead of using it they wipe all surfaces, in some instances several times daily, with damp cloths. By this means very much less dust is raised than by brushing, the risk of inhaling air laden with tubercle bacilli is lessened." Quoted in Fishberg, "The Relative Infrequency of Tuberculosis Among Jews," 608.

52. Ibid., 608. Fishberg noted that Robert Koch, at the recent Tuberculosis Congress, had repudiated the idea that TB could be traced back to cattle, but the majority of experts insisted that there was such a causal connection. The Congress had passed a resolution "in favor of a careful meat inspection for the prevention of tuberculosis."

53. *JAMA*, "Jewish Immunity to Cancer Denied." Note the fluidity of categories when it came to identifying and analyzing the Jews. In one brief piece, the Jews are labeled a race, and then compared to Christians, so that religious identity is blurred with the racial. This was an ambiguity and confusion that accompanied much of the medical and scientific discourse about the Jews during the half-century or so under discussion here.

54. Jean Flamant, for instance, begins his chapter on Jews and cancer by noting that opinions diverge tremendously on the question and that it is quite difficult to come to any definitive conclusions. Flamant, *Contribution à l'étude de la Pathologie des Israélites*, ch. 2.

55. Leonard Glick, *Marked in Your Flesh: Circumcision from Ancient Judea to Modern America*, 194.

56. Maurice Sorsby, a British Jewish physician, made the same claim in his 1931 volume *Cancer and Race: A Study of the Incidence of Cancer Among Jews*. He, too, saw a low incidence of cervical cancer among Jewish women, and ascribed this to "the Mosaic code with its insistence on sexual hygiene." Cited in Glick, *Marked in Your Flesh*, 315, n60.

57. N. Haltrecht, "Das Tuberkuloseproblem bei den Juden: Eine rassen- und sozial-pathologische Studie," 29.

58. Louis Maretzki, "Die Gesundheitsverhältnisse der Juden."

59. Shimshon Kreinermann, *Über das Verhalten der Lungentuberkulose bei der Juden.*

60. Maretzki, "Die Gesundheitsverhältnisse der Juden," 137–40.

61. Ibid., 141.

62. Theodore B. Sachs, "Tuberculosis in the Jewish District of Chicago."

63. Among the many general studies of tuberculosis, see Sheila Rothman, *Living in the Shadow of Death: Tuberculosis and the Social Experience of Illness in American History*, particularly 181f.

64. Sachs, "Tuberculosis," 395.

65. *JAMA*, "Natural Race Immunity," 539.

66. Maurice Fishberg, "Tuberculosis Among the Jews." Daniel Bender has argued that Fishberg reversed himself on tuberculosis and the Jews in 1908. According to Bender, Fishberg did not understand the contraction of the disease as a matter of bacterial infection; he believed that there was a direct causal relation between the shape of the Jew's body, particularly the chest, and susceptibility to the illness. In Bender's words: "Poor lungs and chests and deformed skeletons invited consumption"; conditions in the factories and sweatshops did the rest. Daniel Bender, "'A Hero...for the Weak': Work, Consumption, and the Enfeebled Jewish Worker, 1881–1924," 6–7, for quote and discussion of Fishberg.

67. Fishberg, "Tuberculosis Among the Jews," 420.

68. Ibid., 420. Reibmayr's works were *Inzucht und Vermischung beim Menschen*, and *Die Ehe Tuberculöser und ihr Folgen*.

69. Fishberg, "Tuberculosis Among the Jews," 421–2. By no means did this lead Fishberg to condone intermarriage. On the contrary, he believed it would, if unchecked, lead to the "extinction" of the Jews as a people. However, he was quick to point out that the "introduction of 'Jewish blood' into the veins of other white peoples" posed no danger to the quality of the white race. See his article "Intermarriage Between Jews and Christians," quoting from 132.

70. Fishberg, "Tuberculosis Among the Jews," 424.

71. Arthur Ruppin, *Die Soziologie der Juden*, 265–8.

72. Haltrecht, "Das Tuberkuloseproblem bei den Juden," 32.

73. Baldwin, "Immunity in Tuberculosis," 829, 838.

74. *Washington Post*, "Mosaic Laws Sanitary." The *Post* article is a summary of an article that ran in *Harper's Weekly*.

75. *New York Times*, "Why Tuberculosis Doesn't Attack Jews"; *Washington Post*, "Immune by City Life." A similar article also appeared in the popular journal *Health* 60 (1910), 78.

76. "Old-Time Remedy Has Been Found Efficient in Treatment of Tuberculosis." On the notion of garlic as a medicinal and as a cure for TB, see James Harvey Young, *Medical Messiahs: A Social History of Health Quackery in Twentieth-Century America*, 352 and passim.

77. A century and a quarter earlier, both garlic and onions had been invoked by the Abbé Grégoire in his essay on the regeneration of the Jews. Writing on the long-standing notions that the Jews suffered from particular diseases and that they gave off a peculiar smell all their own – notions that he dismissed as ridiculous – Grégoire noted one of the common explanations for this: "Others ascribe these effects to the frequent use of herbs, such as onions and garlic, the smell of which is penetrating; and some to their eating the flesh of he-goats; while others pretend, that the flesh of geese, which they are remarkably fond of, renders them melancholy and livid, as this food abounds with viscous and gross juices." Thus, traditional Jewish culinary practices produce not health, but disease and fetidness. Grégoire also called attention to the inefficacy or

counter-productivity of other Jewish rituals. The ritual bath, which might be expected to produce cleanliness among the Jews, does not have that effect. More relevant to our discussion here, as discussed earlier in this chapter, Grégoire noted the ill-effects of the removal of blood by the koshering process. Abbé Grégoire, "An Essay on the Physical, Moral and Political Reformation of the Jews," 52.

78. Interestingly, in a 1920 popular medical text in Yiddish, Benjamin Dubovsky asked rhetorically "Is eating onions a remedy against tuberculosis?" The belief that onions can prevent or cure tuberculosis, he said, was a belief particularly common "in our southern states." Experiments have been done, he wrote, but there was no proof that this was the case. Dubovsky, *Gezunt un Leben*, 126–7.

79. Elsewhere, in an article on North African Jews, Fishberg had explained the relative immunity of these Jews to tuberculosis with reference to another cultural custom. He could discern no real social or economic differences between the Jews of North Africa and their Muslim neighbors, and yet the Muslims suffered at much higher rates from tuberculosis than did the Jews. The only difference seemed to be that Jews made a habit of cleaning their floors and furniture with a damp cloth, while Muslims dry dusted. Dry dusting allowed bacilli to scatter, while damp dusting prevented their spread. Eight years before, the *Lancet* ("The Rarity of Tubercle Among the Israelites of Tunis") had reported on a study published in the *Revue d'Hygiene et de Police Sanitare* on the comparative rates of death from the disease among the different groups in Tunis. The study had come to the same conclusion about the disparity between Muslim and Jewish susceptibility to tuberculosis. "Ethnical" differences, according to the two French authors, could not have been in play because both Jews and Arabs belong to "the Semitic race" (1826). The authors also dismissed nourishment, clothing, or economic conditions in general as possible reasons, since Jews were as poor as Arabs in Tunis. "There is, however, one custom peculiar to the Israelites to which the small incidence of tuberculosis is, in the view of the writers, attributable. The Israelites abhor the dusting-brush, and in its stead they wipe all surfaces, in some instances several times daily, with damp cloths. By this means the dust raised by dry dusting is largely reduced, and hence also is lessened the risk of inhaling air-borne tubercle bacilli" (1827).

80. Emil Bogen, "Tuberculosis Among the Jews," 124.

81. For an early twentieth-century example of this argument, with references to other authorities arguing this position, see Maretzki, "Die Gesundheitsverhältnisse der Juden," 128.

82. Bogen, "Tuberculosis Among the Jews," 127.

83. Joseph Rakower, "Tuberculosis Among Jews," 85.

84. Rakower, "Tuberculosis Among Jews," 91.

85. Jeanne Abrams, "Chasing the Cure in Colorado: The Jewish Consumptives' Relief Society"; Marjorie Hornbein, "Dr. Charles Spivak of Denver: Physician, Social Worker, Yiddish Author." For a broader survey, see Jeanne Abrams, *Blazing the Tuberculosis Trail: The Religio-ethnic Role of Four Sanatoria in Early Denver.*

86. See Haltrecht, "Das Tuberkuloseproblem bei den Juden," who takes the Jewish community to task and offers up numerous suggestions on how to start up an effective anti-tuberculosis campaign.
87. Bender, "A Hero . . . for the Weak," 3.
88. Nancy Tomes, *The Gospel of Germs: Men, Women, and the Microbe in American Life*, 183–4.
89. Rothman, *Living in the Shadow of Death*, 182. On popular Yiddish guide books to health and civility at this time, see Eli Lederhendler, "Guides for the Perplexed: Sex, Manners, and Mores for the Yiddish Reader in America."
90. I have found at least one exception to my argument here, an argument that is admittedly tentative. In his Hebrew language study *Talmud and Medical Knowledge (Ha-Talmud ve-Chochmat Ha-Refuah)*, Yehuda Katznelson explicitly tells his readers that a proper discussion of medical matters presupposes a knowledge of the body's organs and functions, and, therefore, he begis his study with detailed introductory remarks on the science of anatomy. These lessons in anatomy "are not intended for physicians, but for those individuals who have studied nothing else but the Talmud" (9), and therefore he would write about technical matters in as clear and simple a way as possible. His book, written not in Yiddish but in Hebrew, was intended for the non-specialist, and intended to teach Jews about medical matters. But it was a highly technical rather than a popular work.
91. A. Sztylman, *Layb un Leben*, 98.
92. M. Jevnin, *Reinlichkeit un Gezunt*, 1–2. A similar assertion about the dirtiness of contemporary Jews appears in Gershon Levin, *Higiene bei Yidn Amol un Itend*. In the forward to the book, Dr. Z. Bichovski, identified as the vice-president of the *Gesellschaft tsu shitzen di Gesundhayt fun di Yidn in Polin* (the Society for the Protection of the Health of the Jews in Poland), writes that "Jewish life is full of paradoxes," and one of the greatest is in the realm of hygiene. The Jewish holy books contain hundreds of paragraphs dealing with purity, washing, bathing, etc. "Whole books have been written about the wisdom of the hygienic measures to be found in the Torah and Talmud, whose profundity and significance are only now being recognized by science" (i). You would think, he continues, that given all our rules and beliefs about purity and cleanliness, that we, the Jews, would be the masters of cleanliness; "but it is an embarrassment to have to admit that we as a people are in fact filthy [*brudig*], maybe the dirtiest people among all the cultured peoples" (ii). Levin echoed these sentiments in his text, and repeated them in his later work, *Di Entviklung fun sozialer Higiene un Medizin bei Yidin in 20th Yohrhundert*.
93. Jevnin, *Reinlichkeit un Gezunt*, 2–4.
94. Ibid., 13.
95. The *Arbeter Ring* referred to tuberculosis as the "proletarian sickness" (*proletarische krankheit*). See Bender, "A Hero . . . for the Weak," 14.
96. A. Kaspe, "Medizin fun sotzialen Standpunkt." For other examples, see M. Barber, "Bacteriologia"; M. Girshdonski, "Tuberkulosis."
97. Kaspe, "Medizin fun sotzialen Standpunkt," 406; Y. A. Merrison, *Higiene: Di Lehre vi tzu verhitten dos Gezunt*; N. M. Ginzburg, *Tuberkoliz un vi kempf man kegen im*.

98. Dubovsky, *Gezunt un Leben* 227.
99. L. V. Zwisohn, *Vi sich tzu verhiten fun Tuberkulosis unt vi tzu haylin oystzehrung*, 4–6.
100. There are numerous examples from the pages of the *YIVO Bleter*. The journal included articles and book reviews dealing with Jews and health, and also summaries and discussions of articles on the subject that had appeared in mainstream medical journals. See, for instance, the series of reviews of articles on Jews and tuberculosis, diabetes, Jewish hospitals, among other topics, contained under the heading "Problemen fun Medizin, Higiene, Anthropologie" ("Problems in medicine, hygiene, and anthropology"), *YIVO Bleter* 18 (1941), 242–8; Max Weinberg, "Diabet bei Yidn" ("Diabetes among the Jews"), *YIVO Bleter* 19 (1942), 375–80; Max Weinberg, "Di Starbigkeit fun Tuberkuloz" ("Mortality from Tuberculosis"), review of Eugene Gagnon, "The Low Mortality Rate from Tuberculosis in the Jewish Race," *Canadian Public Health Journal* 31 (1930), 13–15, in *YIVO Bleter* 21 (1943), 248–9. For examples of monographs, see *Higiene bei Yidn Amol un Itend*, and Levin, *Di Entviklung fun Sozialer Higiene un Medizin bei Yidin in 20th Yohrhundert*.
101. It is worth noting, though, that certainly not all Jewish elites accepted this, not even all those who actively participated in debates framed anthropologically and medically. Joseph Jacobs, for instance, rejected the notion that Jewish religious laws were efficacious in preventing disease, including tuberculosis. He also rejected the argument that Jews enjoyed an immunity from TB on racial grounds; nor were Jews "liable as a race" to diseases such as diabetes or hemorrhoids. See Jacobs, "On the Racial Characteristics of Modern Jews," in *Studies in Jewish Statistics: Social, Vital, and Anthropometric*, viii, footnote 1.

6. "Then What Advantage Does the Jew Have?"

1. Cited in Yaakov Shavit, *Athens in Jerusalem: Classical Antiquity and Hellenism in the Making of the Modern Secular Jew*, 23.
2. On this see Suzanne Marchand, *Down from Olympus: Archaeology and Philhellenism in Germany 1750–1970*; Frank M. Turner, *The Greek Heritage in Victorian Britain*; Frank M. Turner, "Why the Greeks are not the Romans in Victorian Britain"; Carl Diehl, *Americans and German Scholarship, 1770–1870*.
3. In his recent work *The Jewish Century*, Yuri Slezkine has argued that this idea of the Jews as models became universal, the hallmark of modernity. My ambition here is far more modest, limited only to showing that some Christians advanced this notion in the realm of health. Slezkine, moreover, argues that at the root of this modeling process is the image of the Jew as reified "mind" or intellect. My argument here is that, at least in the realm of hygiene and health, it is the Jew as "body" that is attractive and held up as a model for Christians.
4. Petrus Cunaeus, *De republica Hebraeorum* (Leiden, 1617), cited in Charles Berlin and Aaron Katchen (eds), *Christian Hebraism: The Study of Jewish Culture by Christian Scholars in Medieval and Early Modern Times*, 24. See also the discussion in Jonathan Karp, "The Mosaic Republic in Augustan Politics: John Toland's 'Reasons for Naturalizing the Jews,'" 478f.

5. Max Grunwald, "Zur Einführung," in Grunwald (ed.), *Die Hygiene der Juden*, 2. Grunwald's reference was to Alexander Rattray, *Divine Hygiene: Sanitary Science and Sanitarians of the Sacred Scriptures and Mosaic Code.*

6. Charles Richson, *The Observance of the Sanitary Laws, Divinely Appointed, in the Old Testament Scriptures, Sufficient to Ward off Preventable Diseases from Christians as Well as Israelites*, 9.

7. Ibid., 11–13.

8. Ibid., 18.

9. Ibid., 19–23. Richson and Sutherland were hardly the first Englishmen to see the ancient Hebrews as a model for English public life. Already in the seventeenth century, as Adam Sutcliffe has written, "Puritans, striving to make the English into a 'godly people,'" understood "the governmental and legal structures of the ancient Hebrews...as intensely relevant to their contemporary struggle. Hebraic identification in this period was extremely widespread, and in the prelude to the civil war grew increasingly polyvalent." Adam Sutcliffe, *Judaism and Enlightenment*, 45–6. On the "moral kinship" that British and American Christians felt for the ancient Hebrews, see Tudor Parfitt, "The Use of the Jew in Colonial Discourse," 57.

10. Richson, *The Observance of the Sanitary Laws*, 26.

11. Ibid., 27, 31.

12. Ibid., 34. Richson's figures about the Jews' low rate of mortality from cholera were taken from the *Report of the General Board of Health on Asiatic Cholera*, Appendix B, p. 82.

13. Richson, *The Observance of the Sanitary Laws*, 28–9.

14. G. S. Franklin, "Purification and Sanitation by Fire."

15. Ibid., 618–19.

16. Edward T. Williams, "Moses as a Sanitarian," 6. The article originated as a talk before the Norfolk Medical Society on November 29, 1881.

17. Ibid., 7.

18. Ibid., 8.

19. Ibid., 8.

20. Articles in the *Lancet*, March 25, 1876, p. 465, and April 1, 1876, p. 518, cited in Robert Darby, "'Where Doctors Differ': The Debate on Circumcision as a Protection Against Syphilis, 1855–1914," 71. On circumcision in English thought, see also Madge Dresser, "The Painful Rite: Jewish Circumcision in English Thought, 1753–1945."

21. On Hutchinson and circumcision, see Leonard Glick, *Marked in Your Flesh: Circumcision from Ancient Judea to Modern America*; David Gollaher, *Circumcision: A History of the World's Most Controversial Surgery.*

22. Darby, "'Where Doctors Differ,'" 58.

23. Quoted in Darby, "'Where Doctors Differ,'" 58.

24. S. M. I. Henry, *Confidential Talks on Home and Child Life*, 70–1, cited in Darby, "'Where Doctors Differ,'" 62.

25. Quoted in Darby, "'Where Doctors Differ,'" 62–3.

26. The most extensive analysis along these lines is that of Sander Gilman, *The Jew's Body*; Sander Gilman, *Freud, Race and Gender*. For a perceptive reading

of Gilman's analysis, see Naomi Seidman, "Carnal Knowledge: Sex and the Body in Jewish Studies."

27. *New York Times*, "How Races Differ in Disease Immunity." The article was a summary of Lindsay's paper titled "Immunity from Disease Considered in Relation to Eugenics."

28. I have been unable, since I do not read Greek, to discover anything more about the fate of this proposal. It is clear that it was widely disseminated and discussed, but I have no idea whether it ever went further than this. *The New York Times* did not follow up on the story, and I have not been able to find any reference to this proposal in the secondary literature.

29. *Washington Post*, "People of Britain Urged to Follow Jews by Physician."

30. E. Hart, "The Mosaic Code of Sanitation."

31. Darby, "'Where Doctors Differ,'" 72.

32. Williams, "Moses," 6–8.

33. Ibid., 7.

34. Anatole Leroy-Beaulieu, *Israel Among the Nations*, 154. The passage was quoted, approvingly, by Maurice Fishberg, in "The Comparative Pathology of the Jews," 580. This sort of argument could still be found in some quarters into at least the 1960s. In a brief report in *Eugenics Quarterly* on "Jews, Genetics, and Disease," R. H. Post of the University of Michigan made the point that urban populations are exposed to a greater degree than those in rural areas to infectious and contagious diseases, particularly epidemics. He then made an argument reminiscent of those we encountered in Chapter 4 on eugenics: "Heterozygous carriers might have a selective advantage under the stress of these diseases, against which the genes might confer protection. Jewish populations have been subjected more intensively than Gentile populations to contagious diseases during the past two millennia" (164). Post concluded by suggesting that current trends indicate that Gentiles are now moving toward the "traditional Jewish environment – with rapidly growing towns and cities, rapidly increasing protection of slightly handicapped or afflicted persons through modern public health and individual health facilities. . . . " Thus, it seems reasonable to suggest that the particular genetic diseases that traditionally afflict the Jews – "indeed, perhaps all genetic diseases" – will in the future afflict Gentiles to the same degree (164).

35. Glick, *Marked in Your Flesh*, 172–6.

36. These phenomena, however, are no doubt cyclical. Thus, there appears to be a drop in the numbers of circumcisions recently among non-Jews in Britain and to a lesser extent in the United States, as physicians and lay people challenge the necessity of the procedure on both health and moral grounds (i.e., as psychologically detrimental and the only elective surgery that is done without the permission of the patient). On the other hand, the kosher food business in America is booming, in large measure it seems because of the shifting buying habits of non-Jews who believe that kosher food is purer and healthier. For this, see the discussion and notes in Chapter 7.

37. Alan Guttmacher, "Should the Baby Be Circumcised?" Quoted in Glick, *Marked in Your Flesh*, 179.

7. Conclusion

1. See, for example, Fred Rosner, "Judaism, Genetic Screening and Genetic Therapy," especially 407–9. The argument about Moses and preventive medicine could still be found in the medical literature into the late 1960s at least. In a 1968 article in *Medical Times*, the Louisiana physician Gerald N. Weiss insisted that Moses was "the first public health officer" and that he had gathered around him a large number of "health wardens" to administer his hygienic regulations. See Gerald N. Weiss, "The Jews [*sic*] Contribution to Medicine," quoted in Leonard Glick, *Marked in Your Flesh: Circumcision from Ancient Judea to Modern America*, 201. Glick points out that Weiss continued to publish articles into the late 1990s that, while focused on the health benefits of circumcision, included similar celebratory statements about the Jewish contribution to health and medicine in general. For another example, see Henry Enoch Kagan, "God and the Psychiatrist in Psychotherapy," especially 80–2.

2. Over the past few years a number of reports have appeared about the growth in America of the kosher food industry, due in large measure to non-Jews' belief in the health benefits of ritually prepared food. See June Sandra Neal, "Kosher's Charisma: Non-Jews Are Converting to Its Standards, but Dietary Laws Don't Make It all Health Food"; Joe Yonan, "You Don't Have To Be Jewish"; *Business Wire*, "Kosher Food Attracts Non-Jewish Consumers"; Sherri Day, "Forget Rye Bread, You Don't Have To Be Jewish To Eat Kosher."

3. The Internet also offers numerous examples of latter-day versions of the narratives explored in this book. *Historyofcircumcision.net*, for instance, is a scholarly review that deals with the nineteenth-century literature, Jonathan Hutchinson first and foremost. It takes issue with his findings, shows how statistics can be manipulated, and discusses in detail the evidence circulated about Jews, syphilis, and circumcision. The site is maintained by Dr. Robert Darby of Australia, who is both a wonderful resource for literature on the subject and a forceful opponent of the practice of circumcision.

4. James Harvey Young, "Folk into Fake," *Western Folklore* 44 (1985).

5. This includes the large number of works on Jewish law and bioethics that I ignore here. For an overview and analysis see Miryam Wahrman, *Brave New Judaism: When Science and Scripture Collide* (Hanover: University Press of New England, 2002).

6. David M. Feldman, *Health and Medicine in the Jewish Tradition*, 35, my emphasis.

7. In dismissing the idea of Moses as epidemiologist, Feldman cites Yehudah Katznelson (*Ha-Talmud ve-hochmat ha-Refuah*), who referred to the tradition of Moses as possessing knowledge equivalent to modern scientists, but insisted that those who would make such a claim take the biblical verses out of context: Feldman, *Health and Medicine in the Jewish Tradition*, 36.

8. See, for instance, Ronald Isaacs, *Judaism, Medicine, and Healing*, 49f.

9. M. Goldberger, *Treat Yourself Right! Torah Guidelines for Maintaining Your Health and Safety*, 21. The author does not provide any bibliographic reference beyond the title of the journal.

10. See, for instance, Paul Root Wolpe, "If I Am Only My Genes, What Am I? Genetic Essentialism and a Jewish Response"; Paul Root Wolpe, "Bioethics, the Genome, and the Jewish Body."

11. Isaac Bashevis Singer, "The Yiddish Writer and His Audience," 40.

12. For recent examples see Nicholas Wade, "Diseases Common in Ashkenazim May Be Random." Wade reported on the findings of a Stanford researcher, Neil Risch, whose paper on Jews and genetic disease was published in the *American Journal of Human Genetics*. See also Nicholas Wade, "Two Scholarly Articles Diverge on Role of Race in Medicine"; Steven Pinker, "Groups and Genes: The Lessons of the Ashkenazim."

13. Gregory Cohran, Jason Hardy, and Henry Harpending, "Natural History of Ashkenazi Intelligence," 3.

14. Ibid., 7f. See as well the summary and discussion of Pinker, "Groups and Genes." And, on the history of the idea of a Jewish intellectual superiority, see Sander Gilman, *Smart Jews: The Construction of the Image of Jewish Superior Intelligence*.

15. Cohran, Hardy, and Harpending, "Natural History," 12. This theory of Ashkenazi Jews and higher intelligence due to natural selection now appears in a recent popular work on evolution. See Nicholas Wade, *Before the Dawn: Recovering the Lost History of Our Ancestors* (New York: Penguin, 2006). Wade takes the argument directly from the Utah study. See the review of Wade's work, including a severe critique of his "adaptive tales," by H. Allen Orr, "Talking Genes."

16. Pinker, "Groups and Genes," 25.

17. Ibid., 27–8.

Bibliography

Abbreviations

JAMA   *Journal of the American Medical Association*

Primary Sources

Adler, Hermann. "Sanitation and the Mosaic Law," *Lancet* 2 (1893), 1340–1.

Adler, Marcus N. "The Health Laws of the Bible, and Their Influence upon the Life-Condition of the Jews," *Asiatic Quarterly Review* 3, series 2 (1892), 136–46.

Anderson, Winslow. "Tuberculosis and Its Prevention," *JAMA* 23 (1894), 300–5.

Aronstam, Noah Ephraim. *Jewish Dietary Laws from a Scientific Standpoint* (New York: Bloch, 1912).

Askenasi, Jules. *Contribution des Juifs á la Fondation des Écoles de Médecine en France au Moyen-Age* (Paris: Librarie Lipschutz, 1937).

Baldwin, Edward R. "Immunity in Tuberculosis: With Special Reference to Racial and Clinical Manifestations," *American Journal of the Medical Sciences* 149 (1915), 822–39.

Barber, M. "Bacteriologia," *Di Zukunft* 7 (1902), 42–5.

Beach, William Morrow. "The Importance of Sanitation," *JAMA* 2 (1884), 253–6.

Behrend, Henry. "The Communicability to Man of Diseases from Animals Used as Food," *Jewish Chronicle* (Nov. 12, 1880), 12–16; (and Nov. 11, 1881), 15–16.

Behrend, Henry. "Diseases Caught from Butcher's Meat," *The Nineteenth Century* 26 (1889), 409–22.

Bendell, Herman. "The Physician of Sacred History," *Transactions of the Medical Society of the State of New York* (1894), 57–69.

Bergey, D. H. "Bovine Tuberculosis as a Factor in the Production of Human Tuberculosis, through the Use of Meat and Milk," *Medical News* (January 23, 1897).

Bertin-Sans, E. "Hygiene," in *Dictionnaire encyclopédie des sciences médicales* (Paris: 1888).

Bevan, Edwyn, and Charles Singer (eds). *The Legacy of Israel* (Oxford: Clarendon Press, 1927).

Bitting, W. C. "Address: Biblical Medicine," *Transactions of the New York State Medical Association* 8 (1891), 368–86.

B. L. "Zur Pathologie der jüdische Rasse," *Jüdische Rundschau* 7 (1902), 49.

Blumenthal, Mark. "The Sanitary and Dietetic Laws of the Hebrews, as Related to Medicine," *New York Journal of Medicine* (May 1859), series 3, 339–57.

Bogen, Emil. "Tuberculosis Among the Jews," *Medical Leaves* 3 (1940), 123–9.

Breug, Isidore. Dissertation. De medicis illustribus Judaeorum qui inter Arabes vixerunt (Hal. 1843).

Brochard, Marc. *L'Hygiène Publique chez les Juifs, son importance, et sa signification dans l'histoire générale de la civilisation* (Paris: Chez L'Auteur, 1865).

Carcassone, David. *Essai historique sur la médecine des Hebreux anciens et modernes* (Montpellier: Chez Jean Martel âiné, 1818).

Carmoly, Eliakim. *Histoire des médecins juifs, anciens et modernes* (Brussels: Société Encyclographique des Sciences Médicales, 1844).

Castiglione, Arturo. "The Contribution of the Jews to Medicine," in Louis Finkelstein (ed.), *The Jews: Their History, Culture, and Religion*, vol. 2 (Philadelphia: Jewish Publication Society of America, 1949).

Cohen, Israel. *Jewish Life in Modern Times* (London: Methuen, 1914).

Crichton-Browne, James. "Introduction," in W. M. Feldman, *The Jewish Child: Its History, Folklore, Biology and Sociology* (London: Baillière, Tindall, and Cox, 1917).

Danzis, Max. "The Jew in Medicine from Biblical to Modern Times," *Journal of the Medical Society of New Jersey* (1930).

Drysdale, C. R. "Letter to the Editor," *British Medical Journal* (April 6, 1889), 815.

Dubovsky, Benjamin. *Gezunt un Leben* (New York: private printing, 1920).

Eliot, Charles W. "The Potency of the Jewish Race," *Menorah Journal* 1 (1915).

Engländer, Martin. *Die auffälend häufigen Krankheitserscheinungen der jüdischen Rasse* (Vienna: J. L. Pollak, 1902).

Feldman, William M. "Ancient Jewish Eugenics," *Medical Leaves* 2 (1939), 28–37.

Fishberg, Maurice. "The Comparative Pathology of the Jews," *New York Medical Journal* 73 (1901), 537–43.

Fishberg, Maurice. *Health Problems of the Jewish Poor* (New York: P. Cowen, 1903).

Fishberg, Maurice. "Intermarriage Between Jews and Christians," in *Eugenics in Race and State, vol. 2. Papers of the Second International Congress of Eugenics* ([Baltimore: American Museum of Natural History, 1923] New York: Garland, 1985), 125–33.

Fishberg, Maurice. "The Jews as Immigrants – From a Medical Standpoint," *New York Medical Record* 78 (1903), 594–6.

Fishberg, Maurice. *The Jews: A Study in Race and Environment* (New York: Walter Scott Publishing Co., 1911).

Fishberg, Maurice. "Rassenzüchtung der Juden," in *Statistik der Juden: Eine Sammelschrift* (Berlin: Bureau für Statistik der Juden, 1917).

Fishberg, Maurice. "The Relative Infrequency of Tuberculosis Among Jews," *American Medicine* 2 (1901), 695–9.

Fishberg, Maurice. "Tuberculosis Among the Jews," *Medical Record* 74 (1908), 1077–81.

Fishberg, Maurice. "Tuberculosis Among the Jews," *Transactions of the Sixth International Congress on Tuberculosis* 3 (1908), 415–28.

Flamant, Jean. *Contribution à l'étude de la Pathologie des Israélites* (Paris: Librairie Lipschutz, 1934).

Fluegal, Maurice. *Die mosaische Diät und Hygiene: Von physiologischen und ethischen Standpunkte* (Cincinnati: Bloch and Co., 1880).

Franklin, G. S. "Purification and Sanitation by Fire," *JAMA* 7 (1886), 617–19.

Garrison, Fielding H. *An Introduction to the History of Medicine* (Philadelphia: C. P. Saunders, 1922).

Ginzburg, N. M. *Tuberkoliz un vi kempf man kegen im* (Cracow: Meluchosher Natzmindverlag, 1932).

Girshdonski, M. "Tuberkulosis," *Di Zukunft* 11 (1906), 43–8.

Glatter Eduard. *Über die Lebens-Chancen der Israeliten gegenüber der christlichen Confessionen* (Wetzlar: Rathgeber und Cobet, 1856).

Gollancz, Hermann. *The Dietary Laws* (London: Jewish Chronicle Office, 1890).

Gollancz, Hermann. "Preface," in Matthias Schleiden, *The Importance of the Jews for the Preservation and Revival of Learning during the Middle Ages*, trans. Maurice Kleimenhagen (London: Siegle Hill, 1911).

Golsar, Hans (ed.). *Hygiene und Judentum: Eine Sammelschrift* (Dresden: Verlag Jac. Sternlicht, 1930).

Gordon, Arieh, *Mifalot ha-Yehudim: Le'kiyum ha-Chochmat ve-ha-Madayim b'Yamay ha-Baynayim ve-Harchbatam* (Vilna: Y. L. Metz, 1881).

Gordon, Benjamin Lee. *Between Two Worlds: The Memoirs of a Physician* (New York: Bookman Associates, 1952).

Gordon, Benjamin Lee. "Medicine Among the Ancient Hebrews," *Annals of Medical History* (n.d.), 219–35.

Graetz, Heinrich. *Geschichte der Juden* 9 (Berlin: Arani, 1996, reprint of Leipzig edition, 1907).

Graetz, Heinrich. "Historic Parallels in Jewish History," in *Papers Read at the Anglo-Jewish Historical Exhibition 1887* (London: Jewish Chronicle Office, 1888).

Grégoire, Abbé Henri Baptiste. "An Essay on the Physical, Moral and Political Reformation of the Jews" (1789), translated in Paul Mendes-Flohr and Jehuda Reinharz (eds), *The Jew in the Modern World*, 2nd edn (Oxford: Oxford University Press, 1995).

Grunwald, Max (ed.). *Die Hygiene der Juden* (Dresden: Verlag der Historischen Abteilung der Internationalen Hygiene-Ausstellung, 1911).

Guéneau de Mussy, Noël. "The Hygienic Laws of Moses," *New York Medical Abstract* 5 (n.d.), 81–5, trans. unknown.

Haeser, Heinrich. *Lehrbuch der Geschichte der Medicin und der epidemischen Krankheiten* (Jena: Dufft, 1875).

Hall, G. Stanley. "Yankee and Jew," *Menorah Journal* 1 (1915).

Hall, William. "The Influence of Feeding on the Development of Jewish and Gentile Children," *JAMA* 53 (1909), 880.

Haltrecht, N. "Das Tuberkuloseproblem bei den Juden: Eine rassen- und sozial-pathologische Studie," *Zeitschrift für Demographie und Statistik der Juden* 2, new series (1925), 28–33.

Harden, John M. B. "Notes on the Medicine of Moses," *Southern Medical and Surgical Journal* 3, new series (1847), 257–69.

Hart, E. "The Mosaic Code of Sanitation," *Sanitary Record* 6 (1877), 199.

Henry, S. M. I. *Confidential Talks on Home and Child Life* (Edinburgh, n.p.: 1898).

Heron, G. A. *Evidences of the Communicability of Consumption* (London: 1890).

Hirsch, August. *Geschichte der medizinsche Wissenschaft in Deutschland* (Munich: R. Oldenbourg, 1893).

Hoppe, Hugo. *Krankheiten und Sterblichkeit bei Juden und Nichtjuden* (Berlin: Calvary, 1903).

Hoppe, Hugo. "Die Tuberkulose unter den Juden in London," *Zeitschrift für Demographie und Statistik der Juden* 4 (1908), 122–4.

Hosmer, James K. *The Jews: Ancient, Medieval, Modern* (London, T. Fisher Unwin, 1890).

Hygienische Rundschau. "Review of G. A. Heron, *Evidences of the Communicability of Consumption*," *Hygienische Rundschau* 1 (1891), 256.

Imber, Nuphtuli Herz. "The Medical Science of the Talmud," *Denver Medical Times* 19 (1900), 513–14.

Irwell, Lawrence. "Talmudic and Jewish Medicine," *Medicine* (Detroit), 6 (1900), 471–7.

Jacobs, Joseph. *Jewish Contributions to Civilization: An Estimate* (Philadelphia: Jewish Publication Society of America, 1919).

Jacobs, Joseph. *Studies in Jewish Statistics: Social, Vital, and Anthropometric* (London: D. Nutt, 1891).

JAMA. "Immunity of Jews from Tuberculosis," *JAMA* 16 (1891), 22.

JAMA. "Jewish Immunity to Cancer Denied," *JAMA* 17 (1891), 34.

JAMA. "Natural Race Immunity," *JAMA* 45 (1905), 539–40.

JAMA. "Ritualistic Sanitation of the Jews," *JAMA* 48 (1907), 801–2.

Jevnin, M. *Reinlichkeit un Gezunt* (Vilna: B. Jaffe, 1901).

Jewish Chronicle. "Eugenics and the Jew: Interview for *The Jewish Chronicle* with Sir Francis Galton," *Jewish Chronicle* (July 29, 1910), 16.

Jewish Chronicle. "Jews and Eugenics," *Jewish Chronicle* (July 29, 1910), 6.

Julius Preuss' Biblical and Talmudic Medicine, trans. Fred Rosner (New York: Sanhedrin Press, 1978).

Kagan, Solomon. "Professor Max Neuburger: A Biography and Bibliography," *Bulletin of the History of Medicine* 14 (1943), 423–48.

Kagan, Solomon. "Talmudic Medicine," *Medical Leaves* 3 (1940), 164–73.

Kaspe, A. "Medizin fun sotzialen Standpunkt," *Zukunft* (June 1917), 358–60; (July 1917), 405–8; (August 1917), 464–8.

Katznelson, Yehuda. *Ha-Talmud ve-Chochmat ha-Refuah* (Berlin: Hayim, 1928).

Kleimenhagen, Maurice. "Introduction," in Matthias Schleiden, *The Importance of the Jews for the Preservation and Revival of Learning during the Middle Ages*, trans. Maurice Kleimenhagen (London: Siegle Hill, 1911).

Kreinermann, Shimshon. *Über das Verhalten der Lungentuberkulose bei der Juden* (Basel: Benno Schwabe and Co., 1915).

Lancet. "The Rarity of Tubercle Among the Israelites of Tunis," *Lancet* (Dec. 22, 1900), 1826–7.

Lanterne. "Correspondence," *Medical News* (August 31, 1889), 248.

Leroy-Beaulieu, Anatole. *Israel Among the Nations* (New York: G. P. Putnam's Sons, 1895).

Levin, Gershon. *Di Entviklung fun sozialer Higiene un Medizin bei Yidn in 20th Yohrhundert* (Warsaw: TOZ, 1939).

Levin, Gershon. *Higiene bei Yidn Amol un Itend* (Warsaw: TOZ, 1922).

Levy, Max. "Jewish People and the Laws of Evolution," *Maccabaean* 7 (1905).

Levyn, Lester. "Biostatistics of the Jewish Race: Pertaining Especially to Immunity and Susceptibility," *New York Medical Journal* (May 10, 1913, reprint New York, 1913), 982–4.

Lombroso, Cesare. *Der Antisemitismus und die Juden im Lichte der modernen Wissenschaft*, trans. H. Kurella (Leipzig: G. H. Wigand, 1894).

Long, Esmond R. "The Decline of Tuberculosis with Special Reference to Its Generalized Form," *Bulletin of the History of Medicine* 8 (1940), 819–43.

Macht, David. "Embryology and Obstetrics in Ancient Hebrew Literature," *Johns Hopkins Hospital Bulletin* 22 (1911).

Magil, Julius. "Medicine and Physicians Among the Jews – From Bible, Talmud, and Ancient History," *Fort Wayne Medical Journal-Magazine* 18 (1898), 33–43.

Mann, Günter. "Rassenhygiene – Sozialdarwinismus," in Günter Mann (ed.), *Biologismus im 19. Jahrhundert* (Stuttgart: Enke, 1973), 73–93.

Maretzki, Louis. "Die Gesundheitsverhältnisse der Juden," in *Statistik der Juden: Eine Sammelschrift* (Berlin: Jüdischer Verlag, 1917), 123–51.

Medical News. "Review of G. A. Heron, *Evidences of the Communicability of Consumption*," *Medical News* 59 (1891), 724.

Medical News. "Summary of the Proceedings of the International Congress of Dermatology and Syphilography, Held in Paris in 1889," *Medical News* (Aug. 31, 1889), 248.

Medicus. "The Tuberculosis Problem," *New York Times* (March 18, 1900), 23.

Merrison, Y. A. *Higiene: Di Lehre vi tzu verhitten dos Gezunt* (New York: Educational Company of the Arbiter Ring, 1916).

"Mitteilungen," *Zeitschrift für Demographie und Statistik der Juden* 4 (1908), 112.

Morrison, Hyman. "A Biologic Interpretation of Jewish Survival," *Medical Leaves* 3 (1940), 97–103.

Munz, Isak. *Die jüdischen Aerzte im Mittelalter* (Frankfurt a.M.: J. Kauffmann, 1922).

Neuburger, Max. "Jewish Physicians at the Beginning of Modern Times," *Medical Leaves* 2 (1939), 145–7.

New York Times. "How Races Differ in Disease Immunity," *New York Times* (Aug. 26, 1912), 6.

New York Times. "Why Tuberculosis Doesn't Attack Jews," *New York Times* (Nov. 16, 1908), 6.

Nossig, Alfred. "Die Auserwähltheit der Juden im Lichte der Biologie," *Zeitschrift für Demographie und Statistik der Juden* 1 (1905).

Nossig, Alfred. "Die jüdische Sozialhygiene als Erzieherin zur seelischen Vervollkommung," in Hans Golsar (ed.), *Hygiene und Judentum: Eine Sammelschrift* (Dresden: Verlag Jac. Sternlicht, 1930), 42–3.

Nossig, Alfred. *Materialien zur Statistik des jüdischen Stammes* (Wien: C. Conegen, 1887).

Nossig, Alfred. *Die Sozialhygiene der Juden und des altorientalischen Volkerkreises* (Stuttgart: Deutsche Verlags-Anstalt, 1894).

Nossig, Alfred. "Das social-wirtschaftliche Revisionssystem nach der altjüdischen Verfassung," *Die Welt* 5, 14 (1901), 14–16.

Pastoret, Claude Emmanuel de. *Moyse, considéré comme législateur et comme moraliste* (Paris: Buisson, 1788).

Philo of Alexandria, *Life of Moses* Book I, (trans. F. H. Colson, Cambridge, Mass.: Harvard University Press, Loeb edition 1949).

Popenoe, Paul, and Roswell Johnson. *Applied Eugenics* (New York: Macmillan, 1918).

Post, R. H. "Jews, Genetics, and Disease," *Eugenics Quarterly* 12 (1960), 162–4.

Rakower, Joseph. "Tuberculosis Among Jews," *American Review of Tuberculosis* 67 (1953), 85–93.

Ratner. "Die Gedächtnishygiene in den jüdischen Bräuchen sowie in der altjüdischen Literatur," *Hygienische Rundschau* 20 (1910), 1321–6.

Ratner. "Die Geschlechtliche Hygiene in der altjüdischen Literatur," *Hygienische Rundschau* 22 (1912), 69–76.

Ratner. "Die perverse Geschlechtsempfindung in der jüdischen Lehre. Sexual-hygienische Skizze," *Hygienische Rundschau* 20 (1910), 993–5.

Ratner. "Die Psychotherapie und Volksmedizin bei den Juden," *Hygienische Rundschau* 19, 24 (1909), 1385–8.

Ratner. "Die Rassenhygiene, Familienforschung, Eugenik und einiges über die Vererbung geistiger Eigenschaften im altjüdischen Schriftum," *Hygienische Rundschau* 28 (1918), 249–52.

Ratner. "Sociale und hygienische Fürsorge im altjüdischen Staate," *Hygienische Rundschau* 20 (1910), 1153–9.

Rattray, Alexander. *Divine Hygiene: Sanitary Science and Sanitarians of the Sacred Scriptures and Mosaic Code* (London: Nisbet, 1903).

Reeves, James E. "The Eminent Domain of Sanitary Science, and the Usefulness of State Boards of Health in Guarding the Public Welfare," *JAMA* 1 (1883), 612–17.

Reibmayr, Albert. *Die Ehe Tuberculöser und ihr Folgen* (Leipzig: Deutike, 1894).

Reibmayr, Albert. *Inzucht und Vermischung beim Menschen* (Leipzig: Deutike, 1897).

Reichler, Max. *Jewish Eugenics and other Essays* (New York: Bloch Publishing Co., 1916).

Renan, Ernest. *Etudes d'histoire religieuse* (Paris: M. Lévy frères, 1862).

Report of the London General Board of Health on Asiatic Cholera (Montreal: J. Starke and Co., 1849).

Rice, Thurman B. *Racial Hygiene: A Practical Discussion of Eugenics and Race Culture* (New York: Macmillan, 1929).

Richson, Charles. *The Observance of the Sanitary Laws, Divinely Appointed, in the Old Testament Scriptures, Sufficient to Ward off Preventable Diseases from Christians as Well as Israelites* (London: Charles Knight, 1854).

Ripley, William Z. *The Races of Europe* (New York: D. Appleton, 1899).

Rosin, Heinrich. *Die Juden in der Medizin* (Berlin: Philo, 1926).

Rosner, Fred. "Judaism, Genetic Screening and Genetic Therapy," *Mount Sinai Journal of Medicine* 65 (1998), 406–13.

Ruppin, Arthur. *Die Juden der Gegenwart* (Köln: Jüdischer Verlag, 1911).

Ruppin, Arthur. "Die sozialen Verhältnisse der Juden in Preussen und Deutschland," *Jahrbücher für Nationalökonomie und Statistik* 23 (1902), 374–86, 760–85.

Ruppin, Arthur. *Die Soziologie der Juden* (Berlin: Jüdischer Verlag, 1930–1931).

Sachs, Theodore B. "Tuberculosis in the Jewish District of Chicago," *JAMA* 43 (1904), 390–5.

Saleeby, Caleb. *Parenthood and Race Culture: An Outline of Eugenics*, 5th edn, (London: Cassell and Co., 1915 [1909]).

Schleiden, Matthias. *The Importance of the Jews for the Preservation and Revival of Learning during the Middle Ages*, trans. Maurice Kleimenhagen (London: Siegle Hill, 1911).

Schrock, William. "Man According to Nature," *JAMA* 1 (1883), 207–10.

Sigerist, Henry E. "The Philosophy of Hygiene," *Bulletin of the Institute of the History of Medicine* 1 (1933), 323–31.

Silvagni, Ludwig. "La patologia comparata negli Ebrei," *Rivista critica di Clinica Medica* (August, 1901).

Simon, Isidore. "La Gynécologie, L'Obstétrique, L'Embryologie et la Puériculture dans la Bible et le Talmud," in Gad Freudenthal and Samuel Kottek (eds), *Melanges d'histoire de Médecine Hébraïque* (Leiden: Brill, 2003), 3–39. First published in *Revue d'Histoire de la Médecine Hébraïque* 4 (1949), 35–64.

Snowman, J. *Jewish Law and Sanitary Science* (London, n.d.), Pamphlet, reprinted from *Medical Magazine* 6 (1896).

Sofer, Leo. "Zur Biologie und Pathologie der jüdischen Rasse," *Die Zeitschrift für Demographie und Statistik der Juden* 2 (1906), 85–92.

Solis-Cohen, Solomon. "Health Laws of the Jews," *Saturday Evening Post*, February 16, 1907. Reprinted in his *Judaism and Science* (Philadelphia: private printing, 1940).

Sorsby, Maurice. *Cancer and Race: A Study of the Incidence of Cancer Among Jews* (London: J. Bale, Sons and Danielsson, 1931).

Stebbins, N. D. "Evidences of a General System of Medical Practice Being Taught by Scripture, and a Comparison of this System with Rational Medicine and Exclusive Homeopathy," *Peninsular Journal of Medicine and the Collateral Sciences* 5(1857), 3–21, 57–75, 113–32, 169–92.

Steinschneider, Moritz. *Die hebräischen Übersetzungen des Mittelalters und die Juden als Dolmetscher* (Berlin: Bibliographisches Bureau, 1893).

Steinschneider, Moritz. "Schriften über Medicin in Bibel und Talmud und über jüdische Aerzte." *Wiener klinische Rundschau* 25 (1896), 433–5; and 26 (1896), 452–3.

Steinthal, S. *Die Hygiene in Bibel und Talmud* (Berlin: H. Steinitz, 1907).

Stewart, David A. "Diseases and History," *Annals of Medical History* (New York) (July 1935).

Stoddard, Lothrop. *Reforging America* (New York: C. Scribner's Sons, 1927).

Strack, Hermann. *The Jew and Human Sacrifice: Human Blood and Jewish Ritual*, trans. Henry Blanchamp (New York, 1911).

Strauss, H. "Das Tuberkuloseproblem bei den Juden," *Zeitschrift für Demographie und Statistik der Juden* 3, new series (1926), 41–5.

Sztylman, A. *Layb un Leben* (Warsaw: Kooperativer Ferlag, 1932).

Tennovim, Yosef. "Review of *Torat ha-Hygienia* by Dr. A. Goldenstein," *Ha-Rophe ha-Ivri* 1 (1927), 58–60.

Theilhaber, Felix. *Der Untergang der deutschen Juden* (Berlin: Jüdischer Verlag, [1913] 1921).

Thorek, Max. "The Jew in Medicine," *Chicago Jewish Forum* 1 (1942–43), 51–4.

Ullmann, Hans. "Zur Frage der Vitalität und Morbidität der jüdischen Bevölkerung," *Archiv für Rassen- und Gesellschafts-Biologie einschließlich Rassen- und Geschlechtshygiene* 18 (1926).

Von Klein, C. H. *Jewish Hygiene and Diet, the Talmud and Various Other Jewish Writings Heretofore Untranslated* (Washington, D. C., n.p., 1884).

Walker, J. K. "On the State of the Medical Art Among the Jews, as Recorded in the Bible," *Midland Medical and Surgical Reporter* 9 (1830), 163–73.

Wallerstein, L. "Behind the Pioneer Role of Jews in Medicine: The Traditional 'Jewish Doctor' Explained," *Commentary* 19 (1955), 244–50.

Washington Post. "Immune by City Life," *Washington Post* (Nov. 17, 1908), 2.

Washington Post. "Mosaic Laws Sanitary," *Washington Post* (June 8, 1913), ES4.

Washington Post. "Old-Time Remedy Has Been Found Efficient in Treatment of Tuberculosis," *Washington Post* (June 11, 1916), M2.

Washington Post. "People of Britain Urged to Follow Jews by Physician," *Washington Post* (June 12, 1910), 10.

Weiss, Charles. "Medicine in the Bible," *Scientific Monthly* 50 (1940), 266–71.

Weiss, Gerald N. "The Jews Contribution to Medicine," *Medical Times* 96 (1968), 797–802.

Weissenberg, Samuel. "Zur Sozialbiologie und Sozialhygiene der Juden," *Archiv für Rassen- und Gesellschaftsbiologie* 19 (1927), 402–18.

Wiener, Adolf. *Die jüdische Speisegesetze nach ihren verschiedenen Gesichtspunkten zum ersten Male wissenschaftlich methodisch beleuchtet* (Breslau: S. Schottlaender 1895).

Williams, Edward T. "Moses as a Sanitarian," *Boston Medical and Surgical Journal* (Jan. 1882), 6–8.

Wirth, Louis. *The Ghetto* (Chicago: University of Chicago Press, 1928).

Wood, Percival. *Moses: The Founder of Preventive Medicine* (London: Society for Promoting Christian Knowledge, 1920).

Zangwill, Israel. "The Jewish Race," in G. Spiller (ed.), *Inter-Racial Problems* (London: P. S. King, 1911), 268–79.

Zwisohn, L. V. *Vi sich tzu verhiten fun Tuberkulosis unt vi tzu haylin oystzehrung* (New York: o. fg., 1904).

Secondary Sources

Abrams, Jeanne. *Blazing the Tuberculosis Trail: The Religio-ethnic Role of Four Sanatoria in Early Denver* (Denver: Colorado Historical Society, 1990).

Abrams, Jeanne. "Chasing the Cure in Colorado: The Jewish Consumptives' Relief Society," in Moses Rischin and John Livingston (eds), *Jews of the American West* (Detroit: Wayne State University Press, 1991), 95–115.

Adams, Mark (ed.). *The Wellborn Science: Eugenics in Germany, France, Brazil, and Russia* (New York: Oxford University Press, 1990).

Almog, Shmuel. "Alfred Nossig: A Reappraisal," *Studies in Zionism* 7 (1983), 1–29.

Anidjar, Gil. *The Jew, the Arab: A History of the Enemy* (Stanford: Stanford University Press, 2003).

Anidjar, Gil. *Semites: Race, Religion, Literature* (Stanford: Stanford University Press, forthcoming).

Aschheim, Steven. *Brothers and Strangers: The East European Jews in German and German-Jewish Consciousness, 1800–1923* (Madison: University of Wisconsin Press, 1982).

Aschheim, Steven. "The East European Jew and German Jewish Identity," *Studies in Contemporary Jewry* 1 (1984), 3–25.

Assman, Aleida. "Translation as Transformation," in Carola Hilfrich-Kunjappu and Stéphane Mosès (eds), *Zwischen den Kulturen: Theorie und Praxis des interkulturellen Dialogs* (Tübingen: M. Niemeyer, 1997), 21–33.

Assman, Jan. *Moses the Egyptian: The Memory of Egypt in Western Monotheism* (Cambridge, Mass.: Harvard University Press, 1997).

Band, Arnold J. "The Moses Complex in Modern Jewish Literature," *Judaism* 51 (2002), 302–14.

Barclay, John M. G. "Manipulating Moses: Exodus 2.10–15 in Egyptian Judaism and the New Testament," in Robert P. Carroll (ed.), *Text as Pretext: Essays in Honor of Robert Davidson*, (Sheffield: JSOT Press, 1992), 28–46.

Bein, Alex. "Der jüdische Parasit: Bemerkungen zur Semantik der Judenfrage," *Vierteljahrshefte für Zeitgeschichte*, 13 (1965), 121–49.

Bender, Daniel. "'A Hero . . . for the Weak': Work, Consumption, and the Enfeebled Jewish Worker, 1881–1924," *International Labor and Working-Class History* 56 (1999), 1–22.

Bender, Daniel. *Sweated Work, Weak Bodies: Anti-Sweatshop Campaigns and Languages of Labor* (New Brunswick, N.J.: Rutgers University Press, 2004).

Berlin, Charles, and Aaron Katchen (eds). *Christian Hebraism: The Study of Jewish Culture by Christian Scholars in Medieval and Early Modern Times* (Cambridge, Mass.: Harvard University Press, 1988).

Bernal, Martin. *Black Athena: The Afroasiatic Roots of Classical Civilization*, vol. 1 (New Brunswick, N. J.: Rutgers University Press, 1987).

Biale, David. *Gershom Scholem: Kabbalah and Counter-History* (Cambridge, Mass.: Harvard University Press, 1979).

Biale, David (ed.). *Cultures of the Jews* (New York: Schocken, 2002).

Blair, Sara. "Henry James, Jack the Ripper, and the Cosmopolitan Jew: Staging Authorship in The Tragic Muse," *ELH* 63 (1996), 489–512.

Boraleva, Lea Campos. "Classical Foundational Myths of European Republicanism: The Jewish Commonwealth," in Martin van Gelderen and Quentin Skinner (eds), *Republicanism: A Shared European Heritage* (Cambridge: Cambridge University Press, 2002), 247–62.

Boyarin, Daniel. *Carnal Israel: Reading Sex in Talmudic Culture* (Berkeley: University of California Press, 1993).

Boyarin, Daniel. "Tricksters, Martyrs, and Collaborators: Diaspora and the Gendered Politics of Resistance," in Jonathan Boyarin and Daniel Boyarin, *Powers of Diaspora: Two Essays on the Relevance of Jewish Culture* (Minneapolis: University of Minnesota Press, 2002).

Boyarin, Daniel. *Unheroic Conduct: The Rise of Heterosexuality and the Invention of the Jewish Man* (Berkeley: University of California Press, 1997).

Brooke, John Hedley. *Science and Religion: Some Historical Perspectives* (Cambridge: Cambridge University Press, 1991).

Business Wire. "Kosher Food Attracts Non-Jewish Consumers," *Business Wire* (September 27, 2005).

Bynum, Caroline. "Why All the Fuss About the Body? A Medievalist's Perspective," in Victoria E. Bonnell and Lynn Hunt (eds), *Beyond the Cultural Turn: New Directions in the Study of Society and Culture* (Berkeley: University of California Press, 1999).

Cala, Alina. "The Discourse of 'Ghettoization' – Non-Jews on Jews in 19th and 20th Century Poland," *Jahrbuch des Simon-Dubnow-Instituts* 4 (2005), 445–58.

Camporesi, Piero. *The Juice of Life: The Symbolic and Magic Significance of Blood*, trans. Robert R. Barr (New York: Continuum, 1995).

Canguilhem, Georges. "P. J. G. Cabanis," *Dictionary of Scientific Biography* 3 (1971), 1–3.

Charpa, Ulrich. "Matthias Jakob Schleiden (1804–1881): The History of Jewish Interest in Science and the Methodology of Microscopic Biology," *Aleph* 3 (2003), 213–45.

Cherry, Shai. "Creation, Evolution and Jewish Thought," Ph.D. thesis, Brandeis University (2001).

Cherry, Shai. "Three Twentieth-Century Jewish Responses to Evolutionary Theory," *Aleph* 3 (2003), 247–90.

Claeys, Gregory. "The 'Survival of the Fittest' and the Origins of Social Darwinism," *Journal of the History of Ideas* 61 (2000), 223–40.

Cohen, Naomi. "The Challenges of Darwinism and Biblical Criticism to American Judaism," *Modern Judaism* 4 (1984), 121–57.

Cohen, Richard I. "Urban Visibility and Biblical Visions: Jewish Culture in Western and Central Europe in the Modern Age," in David Biale (ed.), *Cultures of the Jews*, vol. 3 (New York: Schocken, 2002), 9–74.

Cohran, Gregory, Jason Hardy, and Henry Harpending. "Natural History of Ashkenazi Intelligence," *Journal of Biosocial Science* (first published online, 2005), 1–35.

Cuddihy, John Murray. *The Ordeal of Civility: Freud, Marx, Levi-Strauss, and the Jewish Struggle with Modernity* (New York: Basic Books, 1974).

Darby, Robert. "'Where Doctors Differ': The Debate on Circumcision as a Protection Against Syphilis, 1855–1914," *Journal for the Society for the Social History of Medicine* 16 (2003), 57–78.

Davis, Edward B. "Fundamentalism and Folk Science Between the Wars," *Religion and American Culture* 5 (1995), 217–48.

Day, Sherri. "Forget Rye Bread, You Don't Have to Be Jewish To Eat Kosher," *New York Times* (June 28, 2003).

Dibelius, Martin. *Studies in the Acts of the Apostles*, ed. Heinrich Greeven, trans. Mary Ling (New York: Scribner's, 1956).

Diehl, Carl. *Americans and German Scholarship, 1770–1870* (New Haven: Yale University Press, 1978).

Diner, Hasia. *A Time for Gathering: The Second Migration 1820–1880* (Baltimore: Johns Hopkins University Press, 1992).

Dormandy, Thomas. *The White Death: A History of Tuberculosis* (London: Hambledon Press, 2001).

Doron, Joachim. "Rassenbewusstein und Naturwissenschaftliches Denken im Deutschen Zionismus während der Wilhelminischen Ära," *Jahrbuch der Institut für deutsche Geschichte Universität Tel Aviv* 9 (1980), 389–427.

Douglas, Mary. *Purity and Danger: An Analysis of Concepts of Pollution and Taboo* (London: Routledge and K. Paul, 1966).

Doyle, Laura. *Bordering on the Body: The Racial Matrix of Modern Fiction and Culture* (Oxford: Oxford University Press, 1994).

Dresser, Madge. "The Painful Rite: Jewish Circumcision in English Thought 1753–1945," *Jewish Quarterly* 44 (1997), 15–17.

Dubin, Lois C. "Pe'er Ha'Adam of Vittorio Hayim Castiglioni: An Italian Chapter in the History of Jewish Response to Darwin," in Yakov Rabkin and Ira Robinson (eds), *The Interaction of Scientific and Jewish Cultures in Modern Times* (Lewiston: E. Mellen Press, 1995), 87–101.

Efron, John. *Defenders of the Race: Jewish Doctors and Race Science in Fin-de-Siècle Europe* (New Haven: Yale University Press, 1994).

Efron, John. *Medicine and the German Jews: A History* (New Haven: Yale University Press, 2001).

Eilberg-Schwartz, Howard. "Introduction: People of the Body," in Howard Eilberg-Schwartz (ed.), *People of the Body: Jews and Judaism from an Embodied Perspective* (Albany, N.Y.: State University of New York Press, 1992).

Endelman, Todd. "Anglo-Jewish Scientists and the Science of Race," *Jewish Social Studies* 11 (2004), 52–92.

Endelman, Todd. *The Jews of Georgian England, 1714–1830: Tradition and Change in a Liberal Society* (Philadelphia: Jewish Publication Society of America, 1979).

Engelstein, Laura. Review of *The Jew's Body*, by Sander Gilman, *Journal of Interdisciplinary History* 23 (1993), 759.

Eze, Emmanuel Chukwadi (ed.). *Race and the Enlightenment: A Reader* (Oxford: Oxford University Press, 1997).

Faith-Weiss, Sheila. "The Race Hygiene Movement in Germany," *Osiris* 3 (1987), 194–5.

Faur, José. "The Hebrew Species Concept and the Origin of Evolution: R. Benamozegh's Response to Darwin," *La Rassegna Mensile de Israel* 63 (1997), 43–60.

Feldman, David. *Englishmen and Jews: Social Relations and Political Culture, 1840–1914* (New Haven: Yale University Press, 1994).

Feldman, David M. *Health and Medicine in the Jewish Tradition* (New York: Crossroad, 1986).

Feuchtwanger, Edgar. "'Jew Feelings' and Realpolitik: Disraeli and the Making of Foreign and Imperial Policy," in Todd Endelman and Tony Kushner (eds), *Disraeli's Jewishness* (London: Vallentine Mitchell, 2002), 180–97.

Fonrobert, Charlotte. "On Carnal Israel and the Consequences: Talmudic Studies since Foucault," *Jewish Quarterly Review* 95, 3 (2005), 462–9.

Fout, John C. "Sexual Politics in Wilhelmine Germany: The Male Gender Crisis, Moral Purity, and Homophobia," *Journal of the History of Sexuality* 2 (1992), 388–421.

Freedman, Jonathan. *The Temple of Culture* (Oxford: Oxford University Press, 2000).

Frevert, Ute. "Professional Medicine and the Working Classes in Imperial Germany," *Journal of Contemporary History* 20 (1985), 637–58.

Friedenwald, Harry. *The Jews and Medicine: Essays* (Baltimore: Johns Hopkins University Press, 1944).

Friedlander, Henry. *The Origins of Nazi Genocide: From Euthanasia to the Final Solution* (Chapel Hill: University of North Carolina Press, 1995).

Funkenstein, Amos. *Perceptions of Jewish History* (Berkeley: University of California Press, 1993).

Gager, John G. *Moses in Graeco-Roman Paganism* (Nashville: Abingdon Press, 1972).

Gager, John G. "Moses the Magician: Hero of an Ancient Counter-Culture?," *Helios* 21 (1994).

Gartner, Lloyd. "Anglo-Jewry and the Jewish International Traffic in Prostitution, 1885–1914," *Association of Jewish Studies Review* 7–8 (1982–83), 129–78.

Gelber, Mark H. *Melancholy Pride: Nation, Race, and Gender in the German Literature of Cultural Zionism* (Tübingen: M. Niemeyer, 2000).

Gelber, N. M. *Toldot Ha-Tenuah Ha-Tzionit Be-Galizia 1875–1918*, vol. 1 (Jerusalem: Reuven Mas, 1958).

Gergen, Kenneth. *The Saturated Self: Dilemmas of Identity in Contemporary Life* (New York: Basic Books, 1991).

Gevitz, Norman (ed.). *Other Healers: Unorthodox Medicine in America* (Baltimore: Johns Hopkins University Press, 1988).

Gilman, Sander. *The Case of Sigmund Freud: Medicine and Identity at the Fin de Siècle* (Baltimore: Johns Hopkins University Press, 1993).

Gilman, Sander. *Franz Kafka, the Jewish Patient* (New York: Routledge, 1995).

Gilman, Sander. *Freud, Race and Gender* (Princeton: Princeton University Press, 1993).

Gilman, Sander. *The Jew's Body* (New York: Routledge, 1991).

Gilman, Sander. *Smart Jews: The Construction of the Image of Jewish Superior Intelligence* (Lincoln: University of Nebraska Press, 1996).

Gilman, Sander, and Nancy Leys Stepan. "Appropriating the Idioms of Science: The Rejection of Scientific Racism," in Sandra Harding (ed.), *The Racial Economy of Science* (Bloomington: Indiana University Press), 173–93. First published in Dominick LaCapra (ed.), *The Bounds of Race: Perspectives on Hegemony and Race* (Ithaca: Cornell University Press, 1991).

Glass, James M. "Against the Indifference Hypothesis: The Holocaust and the Enthusiasts for Murder," *Political Psychology* 18 (1997), 129–45.

Glick, Leonard. *Marked in Your Flesh: Circumcision from Ancient Judea to Modern America* (New York: Oxford University Press, 2005).

Goldberger, M. *Treat Yourself Right! Torah Guide Lines for Maintaining Your Health and Safety* (Southfield, M.I.: Targum 2001).

Goldenbogen, Nora (ed.). *Hygiene und Judentum* (Dresden: Verein für regionale Politik und Geschichte, 1995).

Goldenbogen, Nora (ed.). *Medizinische Wissenschaften und Judentum* (Dresden: Verein für regionale Politik und Geschichte, 1996).

Goldstein, Eric. *The Price of Whiteness: Jews, Race, and American Identity* (Princeton: Princeton University Press, 2006).

Gollaher, David L. *Circumcision: A History of the World's Most Controversial Surgery* (New York: Basic Books, 2000).

Golling, Ralf, and Peter von der Osten-Sacken (eds). *Hermann L. Strack und das Institutum Judaicum in Berlin* (Berlin: Institut Kirche und Judentum, 1996).

Goodman, Lipkin. "Henry Behrend," *The Jewish Encyclopedia*, vol. 2 (New York: Funk and Wagnalls, 1901–1906), 644.

Gross, Johannes T. *Ritualmordbeschuldigungen gegen Juden im deutschen Kaiserreich, 1871–1914* (Berlin: Metropol, 2002).

Guttmacher, Alan. "Should the Baby Be Circumcised?" *Parents' Magazine* 16 (1941), 76–8.

Haller Jr., John S. *American Medicine in Transition, 1840–1910* (Urbana: University of Illinois Press, 1981).

Harding, Sandra (ed.). *The 'Racial' Economy of Science* (Bloomington: Indiana University Press, 1993).

Harris, Bernard. "Pro-Alienism, Anti-Alienism and the Medical Profession in Late-Victorian and Edwardian Britain," in Waltraud Ernst and Bernard Harris (eds), *Race, Science and Medicine, 1700–1960* (London: Routledge, 1999), 189–217.

Hart, Mitchell. "Moses the Microbiologist: Judaism and Social Hygiene in the Work of Alfred Nossig," *Jewish Social Studies: History, Culture, Society* 2 (1995), 72–97.

Hart, Mitchell. *Social Science and the Politics of Modern Jewish Identity* (Stanford: Stanford University Press, 2000).

Hau, Michael. *The Cult of Health and Beauty in Germany: A Social History, 1890–1930* (Chicago: University of Chicago Press, 2003).

Hawkins, Mike. *Social Darwinism in European and American Thought, 1860–1945* (Cambridge: Cambridge University Press, 1997).

Herf, Jeffrey. *The Jewish Enemy: Nazi Propaganda During World War II and the Holocaust* (Cambridge, Mass.: Belknap Press, 2006).

Herzberg, Arthur. *The French Enlightenment and the Jews* (New York: Columbia University Press, 1968).

Heyde, Jürgen. "The 'Ghetto' as a Spatial and Historical Construction – Discourses of Emancipation in France, Germany, and Poland," *Jahrbuch des Simon-Dubnow-Instituts* 4 (2005), 431–43.

Heynick, Frank. *Jews and Medicine: An Epic Saga* (Hoboken, N. J.: Ktav Pub. House, 2002).

Hilhorst, Ton. "'And Moses Was Instructed in all the Wisdom of the Egyptians' (Acts 7:22)," in A. Hilhorst and G. H. van Kooten (eds), *The Wisdom of Egypt: Jewish, Early Christian and Gnostic Essays in Honour of Gerard P. Luttikuizen* (Leiden: Brill, 2005), 153–76.

Hoberman, J. *Bridge of Light: Yiddish Film Between Two Worlds* (New York: Museum of Modern Art, 1991).

Hödl, Klaus. *Die Pathologisierung des jüdischen Körpers: Antisemitismus, Geschlecht, und Medizin im Fin de Siècle* (Vienna: Picus Verlag, 1997).

Holmes, Colin. *Antisemitism in British Society 1876–1939* (London: E. Arnold, 1979).

Hornbein, Marjorie. "Dr. Charles Spivak of Denver: Physician, Social Worker, Yiddish Author," *Western States Jewish Historical Quarterly* 11 (1979), 195–211.

Hoy, Suellen. *Chasing Dirt: The American Pursuit of Cleanliness* (New York: Oxford University Press, 1995).

Huerkamp, Claudia. "The Making of the Modern Medical Profession, 1800–1914: Prussian Doctors in the Nineteenth Century," in Geoffrey Cocks and Konrad H. Jarausch (eds), *German Professions, 1800–1950* (Oxford: Oxford University Press, 1990).

Isaacs, Ronald. *Judaism, Medicine, and Healing* (Northvale, N.J.: Jason Aronson, 1998).

Jacobson, Matthew Frye. *Whiteness of a Different Color: European Immigrants and the Alchemy of Race* (Cambridge, Mass.: Harvard University Press, 1999).

Jordan, William. "Problems of the Meat Market of Béziers 1240–47: A Question of Antisemitism," *Revue des Études Juives* 135 (1976), 38–40.

Jordanova, Ludmilla. *Sexual Visions: Images of Gender in Science and Medicine Between the Eighteenth and Twentieth Centuries* (Madison: University of Wisconsin Press, 1989).

Judd, Robin. "Circumcision and Modern Jewish Life: A German Case Study, 1843–1914," in Elizabeth Wyner Mark (ed.), *The Covenant of Circumcision: New Perspectives on an Ancient Jewish Rite* (Hanover: The University Press of New England, 2003), 142–155.

Judd, Robin. "German Jewish Rituals, Bodies, and Citizenship," Ph.D. thesis, University of Michigan, 2000.

Judd, Robin. "Jewish Political Behavior and the 'Schächtfrage', 1880–1914," in Rainer Liedtke and David Rechter (eds), *Towards Normality? Acculturation and Modern German Jewry* (Tübingen: Mohr Siebeck, 2003), 251–69.

Judd, Robin. "The Politics of Beef: Animal Advocacy and the Kosher Butchering Debates in Germany," *Jewish Social Studies* 10 (2003), 117–50.

Jütte, Robert. "The Historiography of Nonconventional Medicine in Germany: An Overview," *Medical History* 43 (1999), 342–58.

Jütte, Robert. "Die jüdische Medizingeschichtsschreibung im 19. Jahrhundert und die Wissenschaft des Judentums," *Aschkenas: Zeitschrift für Geschichte und Kultur der Juden* 9 (1999), 431–45.

Kagan, Henry Enoch. "God and the Psychiatrist in Psychotherapy," *Journal of Religion and Health* 7 (1968), 79–90.

Kagan, Solomon. *Jewish Contributions to Medicine in America*, 2nd edn (Boston: Boston Medical Publishing Company, 1939).

Kalmar, Ivan Davidson, and Derek J. Penslar (eds). *Orientalism and the Jews* (Hanover: University Press of New England, 2005).

Kalmar, Ivan Davidson, and Derek J. Penslar. "Orientalism and the Jews: An Introduction," in Ivan Davidson Kalmar and Derek J. Penslar (eds), *Orientalism and the Jews* (Hanover: University Press of New England, 2005), xiii–xl.

Karp, Jonathan. "The Mosaic Republic in Augustan Politics: John Toland's 'Reasons for Naturalizing the Jews,'" *Hebraic Political Studies* 1 (2006), 462–92.

Kater, Michael. "Professionalization and Socialization of Physicians in Wilhelmine and Weimar Germany," *Journal of Contemporary History* 20 (1985), 677–701.

Katz, David. "Shylock's Gender: Jewish Male Menstruation in Early Modern England," *Review of English Studies*, new series, 50 (1999), 440–62.

Kevles, Daniel. *In the Name of Eugenics: Genetics and the Uses of Human Heredity* (New York: Knopf, 1985).

Kieval, Hillel. "Representation and Knowledge in Medieval and Modern Accounts of Jewish Ritual Murder," *Jewish Social Studies* 1 (1994), 52–72.

Kilgallen, John J. *Stephen Speech: A Literary and Redactional Study of Acts 7* (Rome: Biblical Institute Press, 1976).

Killy, Walther, and Rudolf Vierhaus (eds). *Dictionary of German Biography* (Munich: K. G. Saur, 2004).

Kraut, Alan. *Goldberger's War: The Life and Work of a Public Health Crusader* (New York: Hill and Wang, 2003).

Kraut, Alan. *Silent Travelers: Germs, Genes, and the 'Immigrant Menace'* (New York: Basic Books, 1994).

Kriwaczek, Paul. *Yiddish Civilization: The Rise and Fall of a Forgotten Nation* (New York: Knopf, 2005).

Kugler, Rob. "Hearing the Story of Moses in Ptolemaic Egypt: Artapanus Accommodates the Tradition," in A. Hilhorst and G. H. van Kooten (eds), *The Wisdom of Egypt: Jewish, Early Christian and Gnostic Essays in Honour of Gerard P. Luttikuizen* (Leiden: Brill, 2005), 67–80.

Kushner, Tony. "Stunning Intolerance: A Century of Opposition to Religious Slaughter," *Jewish Quarterly* 35 (1989), 16–20.

Labisch, Alfons. "Doctors, Workers, and the Scientific Cosmology of the Industrial World: The Social Construction of 'Health' and the 'Homo Hygienicus,'" *Journal of Contemporary History* 20 (1985), 599–615.

LaCapra, Dominick. *Rethinking Intellectual History: Texts, Contexts, Language* (Ithaca: Cornell University Press, 1983).

Larson, Edward J. *Summer for the Gods: The Scopes Trial and America's Continuing Debate over Science and Religion* (Cambridge, Mass.: Harvard University Press, 1997).

Latour, Bruno. *The Pasteurization of France* (Cambridge, Mass.: Harvard University Press, 1988).

Leavitt, Judith Walzer, and Ronald L. Numbers. "Sickness and Health: An Overview," in Leavitt and Numbers (eds), *Sickness and Health in America: Readings in the History of Medicine and Public Health*, 3rd rev. edn (Madison: University of Wisconsin Press, 1997), 3–10.

Lederhendler, Eli. "Guides for the Perplexed: Sex, Manners, and Mores for the Yiddish Reader in America," *Modern Judaism* 11 (1991), 321–41. Reprinted in Eli Lederhendler, *Jewish Responses to Modernity* (New York: New York University Press, 1994).

Lefkowitz, Mary, and Guy Maclean Rogers (eds). *Black Athena Revisited* (Chapel Hill: University of North Carolina Press, 1996).

Levenson, Alan. *Between Philosemitism and Antisemitism: Defenses of Jews and Judaism in Germany, 1871–1932* (Lincoln, Nebraska: University of Nebraska Press, 2004).

Light, Donald, Stephen Liebfried, and Florian Tennstedt. "Social Medicine vs. Professional Dominance: The German Experience," *American Journal of Public Health* 76 (1986), 78–83.

Lindberg, David C., and Ronald L. Numbers. "Beyond War and Peace: A Reappraisal of the Encounter Between Christianity and Science," *Church History* 55, 3 (1986), 338–54.

Lindberg, David C., and Ronald L. Numbers (eds). *God and Nature: Historical Essays on the Encounter Between Christianity and Science* (Berkeley: University of California Press, 1986).

Lindquist, Sven. *"Exterminate All the Brutes": A Modern Odyssey into the Heart of Darkness*, trans. Joan Tate (New York: New Press, 1996).

Linke, Uli. *Blood and Nation: The European Aesthetics of Race* (Philadelphia: University of Pennsylvania Press, 1999).

Luft, David. Review of *The Jew's Body*, by Sander Gilman, *Journal of Modern History* 66 (1994), 573.

Marchand, Suzanne. *Down From Olympus: Archaeology and Philhellenism in Germany 1750–1970* (Princeton: Princeton University Press, 1996).

Marchand, Suzanne. "Philhellinism and the *Furor Orientalis*," *Modern Intellectual History* 1 (2004), 331–58.

Mark, Elizabeth Wyner. "Crossing the Gender Divide: Public Ceremonies, Private Parts, Mixed Feelings," in Elizabeth Wyner Mark, *The Covenant of Circumcision: New Perspectives on an Ancient Jewish Rite* (Hanover: Brandeis University Press, 2003).

Markel, Howard. *Quarantine! East European Jewish Immigrants and the New York City Epidemics of 1892* (Baltimore: Johns Hopkins University Press, 1997).

Marrus, Michael. *The Politics of Assimilation: The French Jewish Community at the Time of the Dreyfus Affair* (New York: Oxford University Press, 1971).

Maurer, Trude. "The East European Jew in the Weimar Press: Stereotype and Attempted Rebuttal," *Studies in Contemporary Jewry* 1 (1984), 176–98.

Maurer, Trude. *Ostjuden in Deutschland 1918–1933* (Hamburg: H. Christians, 1986).

Mayr, Ernst. *One Long Argument: Charles Darwin and the Genesis of Modern Evolutionary Thought* (Cambridge, Mass.: Harvard University Press, 1991).

Mazlish, Bruce. *Civilization and Its Contents* (Stanford: Stanford University Press, 2004).

Meeks, Wayne. "Moses as God and King," in J. Neusner (ed.), *Religions in Antiquity: Essays in Memory of Erwin Ramsdell Goodenough* (Leiden: Brill, 1968), 354–71.

Mendelsohn, Ezra. "From Assimilation to Zionism in Lvov: The Case of Alfred Nossig," *Slavonic and East European Review* 14 (1971), 521–34.

Mendes-Flohr, Paul. "Fin-de-Siècle Orientalism, the Ostjuden and the Aesthetics of Jewish Self-Affirmation," *Studies in Contemporary Jewry* 1 (1984), 96–139.

Meyer, Michael. *The Origins of the Modern Jew* (Detroit: Wayne State University Press, 1967).

Moore, James. "Deconstructing Darwinism: The Politics of Evolution in the 1860s," *Journal of the History of Biology* 24 (1991), 353–408.

Mosse, George. *Toward the Final Solution: A History of European Racism* (New York: H. Fertig, 1978).

Muir, Ernest. "The Control of Leprosy," *American Journal of Tropical Medicine* 17 (1937), 51–8.

Müller-Hill, Benno. *Murderous Science* (Oxford: Oxford University Press, 1988).

Neal, June Sandra. "Kosher's Charisma: Non-Jews Are Converting to Its Standards, but Dietary Laws Don't Make It all Health Food," *Hartford Courant* (February 5, 2006), 6.

Neuman, Kalman. "Political Hebraism and the Early Modern 'Respublica Hebraeorum': On Defining the Field," *Hebraic Political Studies* 1 (2005), 57–70.

Numbers, Ronald L. *Darwinism Comes to America* (Cambridge, Mass.: Harvard University Press, 1998).

Numbers, Ronald L. "The Fall and Rise of the American Medical Profession," in Judith Walzer Leavitt and Ronald L. Numbers (eds), *Sickness and Health in America: Readings in the History of Medicine and Public Health*, 3rd rev. edn (Madison: University of Wisconsin Press, 1997), 225–36.

O'Neill, J. C. *The Theology of Acts in its Historical Setting*, 2nd edn (London: S.P.C.K., 1970).

Orr, H. Allen. "Talking Genes," *New York Review of Books* 53, 14 (2006), 22.

Parfitt, Tudor. "The Use of the Jew in Colonial Discourse," in Ivan Davidson Kalmar and Derek J. Penslar (eds), *Orientalism and the Jews* (Hanover: University Press of New England, 2005), 51–67.

Pasto, James. "Islam's 'Strange Secret Sharer': Orientalism, Judaism, and the Jewish Question," *Society for Study of Comparative Society and History* (1998), 450–2.

Penslar, Derek. *Shylock's Children: Economics and Jewish Identity in Modern Europe* (Berkeley: University of California Press, 2001).

Penslar, Derek. *Zionism and Technocracy* (Bloomington: Indiana University Press, 1991).

Peters, Madison C. *Justice to the Jew: The Story of What He Has Done for the World* (New York: F. T. Neely, [1899] 1910).

Pick, Daniel. *Faces of Degeneration: A European Disorder, c. 1848–1918* (Cambridge: Cambridge University Press, 1993).

Pinker, Steven. "Groups and Genes: The Lessons of the Ashkenazim," *New Republic* (June 16, 2006), 25–8.

Porter, Dorothy. *Health, Civilization, and the State: A History of Public Health from Ancient to Modern Times* (UK: Routledge, 1999).

Porter, Roy. *The Greatest Benefit to Mankind: A Medical History of Humanity* (Hammersmith, UK: HarperCollins, 1997).

Proctor, Robert. *Racial Hygiene: Medicine Under the Nazis* (Cambridge, Mass.: Harvard University Press, 1988).

Reinharz, Jehuda. "East European Jews in the *Weltanschauung* of German Zionists, 1882–1914," *Studies in Contemporary Jewry* 1 (1984), 55–95.

Reuter, Shelley Z. "The Genuine Jewish Type: Racial Ideology and Anti-Immigrationism in Early Medical Writing about Tay-Sachs Disease," *Canadian Journal of Sociology* 31, (2006), 291–323.

Rosen, Christine. *Preaching Eugenics: Religious Leaders and the American Eugenics Movement* (Oxford: Oxford University Press, 2004).

Rosen, George. *A History of Public Health* (New York: MD Publications, 1958).

Rosenkrantz, Barbara Gutmann. "The Trouble with Bovine Tuberculosis," *Bulletin of the History of Medicine* 59 (1985), 155–75.

Rothman, Sheila. *Living in the Shadow of Death: Tuberculosis and the Social Experience of Illness in American History* (New York: Basic Books, 1994).

Ruderman, David. *Jewish Thought and Scientific Discovery in Early Modern Europe* (New Haven: Yale University Press, 1995).

Said, Edward. *Orientalism* (London: Penguin, 1995).

Saks, M. (ed.). *Alternative Medicine in Britain* (Oxford: Clarendon Press, 1992).

Sarna, Jonathan. "The Evolution of the American Synagogue," in Robert Seltzer and Norman Cohen (eds), *The Americanization of the Jews* (New York: New York University Press, 1995), 215–29.

Schlich, Thomas. "The Word of God and the Word of Science: Nutrition Science and the Jewish Dietary Laws in Germany, 1820–1920," in Harmke Kamminga and Andrew Cunningham (eds), *The Science and Culture of Nutrition, 1840–1940* (Amsterdam: Rodopi, 1995), 97–128.

Schorsch, Ismar. *From Text to Context: The Turn to History in Modern Judaism* (Hanover: University Press of New England, 1994).

Schorsch, Ismar. *Jewish Reactions to German Antisemitism, 1870–1914* (New York: Columbia University Press, 1972).

Seidman, Naomi. "Carnal Knowledge: Sex and the Body in Jewish Studies," *Jewish Social Studies* 1 (1994), 115–46.

Shatzmiller, Joseph. *Jews, Medicine, and Medieval Society* (Berkeley: University of California Press, 1994).

Shavit, Yaakov. *Athens in Jerusalem: Classical Antiquity and Hellenism in the Making of the Modern Jew*, trans. by Chaya Naor and Niki Werner (London: Littman Library of Jewish Civilization, 1997).

Singer, Isaac Bashevis. "The Yiddish Writer and His Audience," in Bernard Rosenberg and Ernest Goldstein (eds), *Creators and Disturbers: Reminiscences by Jewish Intellectuals in New York* (New York: Columbia University Press, 1982).

Slezkine, Yuri. *The Jewish Century* (Princeton: Princeton University Press, 2004).

Smith, Helmut Walser. *The Butcher's Tale: Murder and Anti-Semitism in a German Town* (New York: W. W. Norton, 2002).

Sorkin, David. *The Transformation of German Jewry, 1780–1840* (New York: Oxford University Press, 1987).

Stanislawski, Michael. *Zionism and the Fin de Siècle: Cosmopolitanism and Nationalism from Nordau to Jabotinsky* (Berkeley: University of California Press, 2001).

Starobinski, Jean. "The Word *Civilization*," in his *Blessings in Disguise; or, The Morality of Evil*, trans. Arthur Goldhammer (Cambridge, Mass.: Harvard University Press, 1993), 1–35.

Starr, Paul. *The Social Transformation of American Medicine* (New York: Basic Books, 1982).

Steffen, Katrin. "Connotations of Exclusion – 'Ostjuden,' 'Ghettos,' and Other Markings," *Jahrbuch des Simon-Dubnow-Instituts* 4 (2005), 459–79.

Stone, Dan. "Of Peas, Potatoes, and Jews: Redcliffe N. Salaman and the British Debate over Jewish Racial Origins," *Jahrbuch des Simon-Dubnow-Instituts* 3 (2004), 221–40.

Sutcliffe, Adam. *Judaism and Enlightenment* (Cambridge: Cambridge University Press, 2003).

Swetlitz, Marc. "American Jewish Responses to Darwin and Evolutionary Theory, 1860–1890," in Ronald L. Numbers and John Stenhouse (eds), *Disseminating Darwin: The Role of Place, Race, Religion, and Gender* (Cambridge: Cambridge University Press, 1999), 209–45.

Swetlitz, Marc. "Responses of American Reform Rabbis to Evolutionary Theory, 1864–1888," in Yakov Rabkin and Ira Robinson (eds), *The Interaction of Scientific and Jewish Cultures in Modern Times* (Lewiston, N.Y.: E. Mellen Press, 1995), 103–25.

Thissen, Rudolf. "Die Sozialhygiene als selbstständige Wissenschaft und ihre Terminologie," in Erna Lesky (ed.), *Sozialmedizin: Entwicklung und Selbstverständnis* (Darmstadt: Wissenschaftliche Buchgesellschaft, 1977), 445–6.

Tomes, Nancy. *The Gospel of Germs: Men, Women, and the Microbe in American Life* (Cambridge, Mass.: Harvard University Press, 1999).

Turner, Frank M. *The Greek Heritage in Victorian Britain* (New Haven: Yale University Press, 1981).

Turner, Frank M. "Why the Greeks and Not the Romans in Victorian Britain," in G. W. Clarke (ed.), *Rediscovering Hellenism: The Hellenic Inheritance and the English Imagination*," (Cambridge: Cambridge University Press, 1989), 61–82.

Volkov, Shulamit. "Juden als wissenschaftliche 'Mandarine' im Kaiserreich und in der Weimarer Republik; neue Überlegungen zu sozialen Ursachen des Erfolgs jüdischer Naturwissenschaftler," *Archiv für Sozialgeschichte* 37 (1997), 1–18.

Wade, Nicholas. *Before the Dawn: Recovering the Lost History of Our Ancestors* (New York: Penguin, 2006).

Wade, Nicholas. "Diseases Common in Ashkenazim May Be Random," *New York Times* (March 4, 2003), F2.

Wade, Nicholas. "Two Scholary Articles Diverge on Role of Race in Medicine," *New York Times* (March 20, 2003), A30.

Wahrman, Miryam. *Brave New Judaism: When Science and Scripture Collide* (Hanover: University Press of New England, 2002).

Waller, John. *The Discovery of the Germ* (Cambridge: Icon Books, 2002).

Weindling, Paul. *Health, Race and German Politics Between National Unification and Nazism, 1870–1945* (Cambridge: Cambridge University Press, 1989).

Weiss, Yfaat. "Central European Ethnonationalism and Zionist Binationalism," *Jewish Social Studies* 11 (2004), 93–117.

Wenger, Beth. "Mitzvah and Medicine: Gender, Assimilation, and the Scientific Defense of 'Family Purity,'" *Jewish Social Studies* 5 (1998/1999), 177–202.

Wertheimer, Jack. *Unwelcome Strangers: East European Jews in Imperial Germany* (New York: Oxford University Press, 1987).

Wiese, Christian. *Challenging Colonial Discourse: Jewish Studies and Protestant Theology in Wilhelmine Germany* (Leiden: Brill, 2005).

Wohl, Anthony S. "'Dizzi-Ben-Dizzi': Disraeli as Alien," *Journal of British Studies* 34 (1995), 375–411.

Wolpe, Paul Root. "Bioethics, the Genome, and the Jewish Body," *Conservative Judaism* 54 (2002), 14–25.

Wolpe, Paul Root. "If I Am Only My Genes, What Am I? Genetic Essentialism and a Jewish Response," *Kennedy Institute of Ethics Journal* 7 (1997), 213–30.

Worboys, Michael. "Tuberculosis and Race in Britain and Its Empire, 1900–1950," in Waltraud Ernst and Bernard Harris (eds), *Race, Science and Medicine, 1700–1960* (London: Routledge, 1999), 144–66.

Xun, Zhou. "The 'Kaifeng Jew' Hoax: Constructing the Chinese Jew," in Ivan Davidson Kalmar and Derek J. Penslar (eds), *Orientalism and the Jews* (Hanover: University Press of New England, 2005), 68–79.

Yonan, Joe. "You Don't Have To Be Jewish," *Boston Globe* (October 4, 2005), F1.

Young, James Harvey. "Folk into Fake," *Western Folklore* 44 (1985), 225.

Young, James Harvey. *Medical Messiahs: A Social History of Health Quackery in Twentieth-Century America* (Princeton: Princeton University Press, 1967).

Index